THE BOUNDARIES OF BLACKNESS

CATHY J. COHEN

THE
BOUNDARIES
OF
BLACKNESS

AIDS AND THE BREAKDOWN
OF BLACK POLITICS

THE
UNIVERSITY OF CHICAGO PRESS
Chicago and London

The University of Chicago Press, Chicago 60637
The University of Chicago Press, Ltd., London
© 1999 by The University of Chicago
All rights reserved. Published 1999
08 07   5 4

ISBN (cloth): 0-226-11288-8
ISBN (paper): 0-226-11289-6

Library of Congress Cataloging-in-Publication Data

Cohen, Cathy J., 1961–
    The boundaries of blackness : AIDS and the breakdown of Black
politics / Cathy J. Cohen.
        p.   cm.
    Includes bibliographical references and index.
    ISBN 0-226-11288-8 (cloth).—ISBN 0-226-11289-6 (pbk.)
    1. AIDS (Disease)—Social aspects—United States.   2. Afro-
Americans—Health and hygiene.   3. Afro-Americans—Diseases.
I. Title.
RA644.A25C575   1999
362.1'969792'008996073—dc21   98-31088
                                                            CIP

To Quinters Jean Dixon Cohen and Charles Frederick Cohen,

and in loving memory of John David Patterson

Contents

PREFACE

This project began as an effort to do something I felt was lacking in many of the seminars that constituted my graduate education: work on issues that were directly tied to the daily survival of individuals and their communities. Such a goal meant that I needed to pursue questions I perceived as directly linked to the experiences and life quality of marginal individuals and groups in this society. Do not get me wrong; I sat through the lectures on roll-call voting in Congress, and over the years acquired an understanding of and even an appreciation for the way such decisions frame the choices available to groups and individuals in this country and elsewhere. However, I also felt a need to turn to work where the link between political science and people's lives was much more direct and meaningful.

Throughout this project, I have never intended to condemn the choices or behavior of any particular group of leaders or organizations, but instead to understand why, when faced with a disease that was threatening significant numbers of African Americans, traditional black leaders seemed to do nothing, or very little. This task led me to investigate fundamental relationships between power, status, and action *within* African-American communities. To understand the response to AIDS in African-American communities entails an exploration of the intragroup, as well as intergroup, relationships that structure opportunities and information and that correspondingly influence the responses of groups and communities to crises. Through this more localized work, we can begin to detail the general impact of power differentials and stratification on the functioning of political actors in dominant and indigenous sites of power. My aims required that I examine not only the obvious acts of dominant actors and institutions which inhibited mobilization, but also the indigenous norms, attitudes, and practices that influenced the participation and mobilization of those concerned about AIDS in African-American communities. Specifically, I wanted to understand how differences in perceived respectability, as defined by both dominant and indigenous norms, were related to power within African-American communities. More broadly, What is the relationship between indigenous standards of membership and dominant ideologies, institutions, and social practices? And finally, By what processes are issues affecting substantial numbers of African Americans deemed "black issues," deserving of attention, resources, and action on the part of other black people?

Insight into any of these questions enhances our understanding of the relationship between participation and power. Yet in spite of the significance of this subject, I still encounter individuals who question the worthiness of this project. They ask, Why a book on, of all things, AIDS mobilization in African-American communities? Clearly, some of the confusion regarding the significance of this project stems from the homophobia, racism, and sexism that condition individuals to look upon research focused on the experiences of oppressed communities as nonscientific. Suspicion about the value of the topic also arises because, as social scientists, we often find it more convenient to explore questions that are distant and less charged with direct implications regarding life, death, and the quality of life. Moreover, in our search for a parsimonious general law, we often avoid questions that seem messy and unresolvable (or at least unresolvable by the time of our tenure review). Nevertheless, it is crucial that we turn our attention to just such issues of institutions, ideology, and agency that are much more subtle, but no less deadly in their impact.

The complaint I found most troubling came from those in and out of black communities who condemned the project as just another book by a black academic trashing black communities. While I do not hold strictly to the rule about not airing our dirty laundry in public, I do not see this book as a "trashing" of black communities. It would be a mistake, in fact, to read this book as an indictment of African-American communities. Far from dismissing the importance of black Americans and of our political leaders and organizations, I offer this project as one more catalyst for generating more thinking about and discussion of the nature of black politics. Increasingly, African-American communities and other marginal groups are confronted with fragmentation and cross-cutting issues. Whether because of the economic progress achieved by some and not others, or the social mobility achieved by, in particular, middle-class black Americans, the dominant myth of a monolithic black community is tearing not only at the seams but throughout its entire fabric. Undoubtedly, many black people continue to operate within a linked-fate political framework, where the struggles of other black people are purported to represent what can happen to any of us. However, a more accurate characterization of the political positioning of most black Americans is that of a qualified linked fate, whereby not every black person in crisis is seen as equally essential to the survival of the community, as an equally representative proxy of our own individual interests, and thus as equally worthy of political support by other African Americans. The AIDS crisis, especially the limited response to this crisis in many African-American communities, provides a classic illustration of the political failings that affect vulnerable populations when an unqualified linked-fate politics is promoted and presumed but is not actually in operation among marginal groups.

In the case of AIDS it would be easier to make a case for the successful working of linked-fate politics if the virus had originally attacked the middle class, the connected, the respected in African-American communities because under that scenario the mobilization of the community would probably have been evident. But this has not been the history of this disease. AIDS began in black communities, apparently, with black gay men, black men who have sex with men, black injection drug users and their sexual partners—groups we are accustomed to ignoring. The actions of national black political organizations, black churches, the black press, and community leaders who silently and "morally" refused to respond to this crisis or delayed their mobilization are barely discernible to an unsuspecting and uncaring public. Unfortunately, neither the public's obliviousness nor the normality of exclusion makes the politics of these institutions, groups, and leaders any less dangerous.

Beyond the statistics and apart from the puzzlement and intrigue of a political scientist, I chose to pursue this topic because something deadly appeared in my communities that demanded my attention. Death is not a new phenomenon in black communities, and, unfortunately, the death of young people is not uncommon in the history and current circumstances of African-American lives. However, to see both young and old die a miserable, painful, and stigmatizing death is hard to ignore. When a family feels forced to lie about the cause of their son's death, when children are left alone because both parents have died of this disease, when friends and family reject those attempting to live and survive with AIDS—these things leave permanent marks in your memory. As all of this happens so frequently that fewer and fewer people can say that they know of no one who has died of AIDS, you see the makings of a monumental tragedy. Finally, if you add to this scenario the fact that some individuals affected by this dual plague of disease and inertia—most often black gay men—decide that they must and will fight against the indifference exhibited toward their lives and now their deaths, then you face some of the most meaningful work of your life.

ACKNOWLEDGMENTS

It has often been written that no book is ever the work of only its author. Never has a statement been more true. I am truly indebted to the family, friends, and colleagues that helped this project come to life and now to completion. For valuable support in allowing me to pursue my rather diverse research agenda I want to thank the Robert Wood Johnson Foundation, particularly the Scholars in Health Policy Research Program. I would also like to thank the Institution for Social and Policy Studies, the Block Fund from the Political Science Department, the Fund for Lesbian and Gay Studies, and the Junior Faculty Fellowship Program, all at Yale University.

Throughout the process of writing this book I received valuable feedback from many individuals and groups. I want to begin by thanking all the participants in the numerous seminars and workshops at universities and conferences around the country who helped clarify the arguments in this book. I also owe a special note of gratitude to the participants in the faculty seminar at The Center for the Study of Race, Inequality and Politics; the scholars' weekly meetings in the Robert Wood Johnson Health Policy Research Program; and the African and African-American Studies Research Workshop, all at Yale. In addition to the group discussions of the book, a number of individuals generously read either individual chapters or the entire manuscript at different stages in its development. There were also those who talked with me for hours about the ideas, experiences, and frustrations documented in this book. So, for their support, I want to thank Katherine Acey, Robert Brown, Hazel Carby, Mario Cooper, Michael Dawson, Licia Fiol-Matta, Josh Gamson, Gil Gerald, Colleen Grogan, Vicky Hattam, Cynthia Horan, Lynne Huffer, David Maurrasse, David Mayhew, Michael Merson, Debra Minkoff, Diane Pinderhughes, Colin Robinson, Mark Schlesinger, Jim Scott, Rogers Smith, Todd Shaw, Jackie Stevens, and Phil Thompson. Finally, I would like to thank John Tryneski, Claudia Rex, and Betsy Solaro at the University of Chicago Press as well as Nick Murray for their helpful editorial suggestions, marketing insights, and undying patience.

A group of exceptional graduate and undergraduate students at Yale were instrumental in amassing the research contained in this book. Thank you Terri Bimes, Sonya Brewer, Jayna Brown, Alethia Jones, Tamara Jones, Alexis Lori McGill, and David Wright. Anthony Foy, Naomi Murakawa, and Dorian Warren provided invaluable help with the final production of the book. Pam LaMonica went beyond the call in transcribing lots of very long interviews. Barbara Dozier and Ella Futrell were incredibly helpful in making sure that all of the research assistants associated with the project were paid on time, while keeping me within my research budget.

Through my work on this book, I have been able to expand not only those I call friends, but just as importantly, those I recognize as committed activists fighting for the radical transformation of people's lives. The individuals are too many to mention but I want to acknowledge all those with whom I have engaged in political work from UCAR to BAM! (Black AIDS Mobilization) to, more recently, the Audre Lorde Project, and all the other organizations in between. I have learned a great deal from the struggles both outside and inside each organization.

The madness of writing this book was made sane in no small part by the incredible group of friends who have been in place since the birth of this project in graduate school at the University of Michigan. To the UCAR crew—plus a few—I thank you for all of your help. To a group of very special black feminists who are family—I thank you. Barbara Ransby, Jocelyn Sargent, Kim Smith, Tracye Matthews, Kim James, Regina Freer, and Tanaquil Jones have each, in their own way, been patient when calls weren't returned, yet firm when I needed to be reminded of the other commitments in my life. You have provided not only a place to come home to, but also a place of principled struggle and challenge. Finally, a special thank-you is reserved for Candy Taaffe, who provided support, patience, laughter, and needed distraction. Her skill as both a bibliographer and a bowler will forever be appreciated.

Anyone who knows me well knows the importance of my family in all its constructions—immediate, extended, political, and chosen. I thank all of them for their support and patience with me through this long process. I owe everything that is good or insightful in this book to the teaching and consciousness instilled in me by my parents,

Charles and Quinters Jean. I owe my willingness to battle for the things that are important to me to my sister Charlene and brother Charles Jr. My concern for the future of black people is undoubtedly rooted in the next generation of Cohens—Terry, Tamara, Charles III, Terica, and Tianna. And for my constant attempts to surround myself with new constructions of family, I thank my brother in-law, aunts, uncles, cousins, and grandparents who epitomize the love, caring, and empowerment that can come from families and communities.

Finally, I want to acknowledge and thank the many individuals who gave of their time to talk to me about AIDS in black communities. Some of these individuals were government officials, some started the first AIDS organizations in black communities, some are living with HIV or AIDS, and others have died since their interviews with me, but all were committed to stopping a plague that continues to devastate the multiple places and communities I call home. I am, therefore, indebted to trailblazers and role models such as Audre Lorde, Essex Hemphill, Pat Parker, Marlon Riggs, Katrina Haslip, Alan Robinson, Donald Woods, Jamie Crankfield, and Craig Harris. All were strong, most were black gay men and lesbians, who in their own way struggled throughout their all too short lives for the liberation of all black people. They each represent a life committed to struggle that we can only hope to emulate.

CHAPTER ONE

The Boundaries of Black Politics

Billy said he had often thought of telling his parents he was HIV positive, but that would mean telling them that he was gay. He even considered breaking the news about his status by taking the more "respectable route" and telling them that he had contracted AIDS by injecting drugs. But he figured they would never believe him, since they had always been a close family and would know if their son was using drugs. The funny thing was, for all their closeness, they didn't seem to know that he was gay, or maybe they just couldn't admit it out loud.

For all his anger about needing their support and not being able to ask for it, he did understand that his being gay was a difficult situation for his parents. To be a black working-class family, to live in a small town where all the black people know you, to be active in the church, to have a son whom you always promoted to the neighbors as being smart, successful, and the ultimate bachelor (single and in his mid-30s), and now to openly deal with the question of whether he was "like that"—he thought this was probably too much to ask. To admit that your son was gay would be to confirm that you did something wrong in bringing him up. It would mean watching him lose the respect of the neighbors as they shook their heads whenever he turned his back. It would mean going to church and openly lying to the minister whenever he asked when Billy was going to get married. In a forgiving sort of way, Billy understood why they had never really pressed him on the lack of girlfriends, the male friends who were constantly around, and his insistence on leaving his small home town and moving to the big city.

In talking with Billy, I often thought that the pain his HIV-positive status caused him, both physically and emotionally, was secondary to his concern about not disappointing his parents. In many ways his positive status had brought all of these issues to a critical point. During the afternoon I spent with Billy, he talked of the hypocrisy he felt in lying to those he loved so dearly. He spoke of the constraints his concern about his parents' finding out that he was gay had imposed on his willingness to confront his status openly. Where could he go for help and information? How could he be active around the politics of this disease without worrying that his picture would end up in some paper, or that someone's son or daughter or cousin from his hometown church might see him?

Throughout our conversation, he repeatedly returned to his feelings of invisibility and powerlessness. The support and approval of the larger black community seemed so important that he was unwilling, and probably unable, to do anything that might jeopardize that support, even if it meant that he was unable to deal aggressively with a disease that threatened his life. He knew in the end he would have to return home and let his mother take care of him. In the meantime, friends—his hand-picked "family" of other black gay men—would fill the caretaking role of his mother. At the same time, he insisted throughout our conversation that he did not want to impose on these friends in his last and most vulnerable moments. In the same way that Billy sought not to burden his friends, he also seemed to shy away from placing any demands upon the black community. Throughout the time I spent with him, I never heard him question why the rejection of "his" black community was so inevitable. I never heard him curse the leadership of the community that refused to mobilize and draw attention to the impact of this disease in the black community. Instead, he seemed to be preoccupied with holding on to what little stability and privacy he had left.

She was an older black woman, the type who over the years has devoted herself not only to raising her own children, but also to caring about her community. As we talked she would often say that she never imagined being in this position after retiring from thirty-one years of teaching. Who was she to be running an AIDS service organization? Yet five years ago people kept saying that the community was being hit hard by AIDS and someone had to do something about it. It seemed only appropriate, with a little convincing of course, that she head up such an effort.

As we talked, it became clear that while she may be one of the most loving individuals you could ever meet—evident in everything from the way she kisses her grandchildren to the way she addresses staff and clients, asking them if they want something to eat—there was still some uneasiness around the subject of AIDS and what she perceived to be the population with whom she was dealing. She repeated over and over again during our conversation, shaking her head all the time, that these poor kids on drugs just had no sense of what they were doing. She seemed determined to talk about drug users as people we should feel sorry for and who need our help. Through her words, one can sense support and caring for those whom many have discarded. Interestingly, statements about empowering this downtrodden segment of black communities never cross her lips. Instead, it seems she perceives her mission to be caring for and serving these individuals. Ideas of empowerment seem almost irrelevant. She did beam proudly, however, as she spoke in detail of the new teen hotline in the center. She hoped that it would enable young people in and out of this community to get the information they need to avoid contracting HIV and AIDS.

Noticeably lacking from our conversation was a discussion of the impact of AIDS on black gay men and lesbians. I looked around the room, where there seemed to be a poster on every space of wall, and I could not find one poster that focused on gay men (I didn't even try to look for anything dealing with lesbians and safe sex). There were posters telling you to wear a condom. There were posters telling you to talk to your sexual partners about AIDS. There were even posters telling you how to bleach your "works" (needle and syringe), a radical stance in almost any environment, especially in a church. But I could see nothing that was aimed at, or spoke directly to, gay men. Don't get me wrong. This woman was well aware that the AIDS epidemic was originally identified with gay white men. This was especially evident as she detailed how the white AIDS organization (specifically the white gay organization) had lots of money, while she, on the other hand, had many more clients and yet struggled to stay afloat financially. It is only my perception, but the resentment I heard in her voice seemed less motivated by homophobia than by a history of always seeing white people as one step ahead. She summed up her battles and victories against the local white AIDS organizations by saying, "I thank God that we have become one of the top AIDS organizations. You see they may be able to step on my toe, but they can't step on my head."

This woman has put in long hours and even longer years to make sure there would be some response to this disease in her community. I asked her about possible funding from the NAACP or the Urban League. She looked at me honestly, with years of battling inside and outside of AIDS written on her face, and asserted that those organizations had done nothing for her clients or her program. Her answer was so matter-of-fact that it was clear she could not be bothered with such trifling behavior. She has larger concerns, namely the survival of her community.

As we finished our conversation, one of her staff members asked why women seem to be the ones doing all the work. The question, I believe, was not meant to negate the efforts of black and white gay men, but instead to represent her reality, her perspective from the basement of the church—that of the black community—where black women, mothers, wives, sisters, lovers, and friends are helping and leading the fight against AIDS. Before she could answer that question, my colleague who accompanied me to this meeting raised the question of black gay men and lesbians, not only because they have been such pioneers in responding to this disease in black communities, but also because they had been made so invisible during this whole conversation. Again with warmth but some nervousness, this older black woman talked about how gays are some of her favorite clients because they don't need anything. "They have insurance; they can go to the hospital; they know what is happening to their body concerning this disease," she said. Being gay or lesbian, while probably raising moral conflicts for this older activist, was presented much more as an issue of class and educational privilege from which most of her other clients have been systematically excluded. Her job is to make sure there are services for all her clients. Therefore, while her work and even her office are based in the black church, she has decided that for right now her individual biases and comfort level will have to take a back seat if the work is going to get finished.

He was late, out ministering to his congregation, he said, so he wanted to make this a relatively short conversation. I reminded him of the subject matter—AIDS in the black community—and he nodded and waved his hands in such a way as to indicate that this would be a short conversation because there just wasn't much to say here. "You have to understand," he started, "it goes against the general tenets of Christianity. How can you expect ministers to accept or acknowledge the behavior that causes AIDS? All we can do is take care of those who are sick—that is our Christian duty."

Throughout our conversation, he kept coming back to what seemed to be a general principle guiding the church's response to this disease:

love the sinner but hate the sin. He recalled that lots of clergy have seen members of their congregations die from this disease. His own church had lost two gay choir directors to AIDS. When I asked how the congregation dealt with the sexuality of their beloved choir directors, he explained that, while everyone knew that they were gay, they were doing the Lord's work, and sometimes you have to overlook specific behavior. He went on to illustrate the point: "Ministers sometimes do things that are wrong because we are of the flesh; however, no minister I know of would ask that their behavior be condoned or recognized as right." Instead, he continued, "we continually struggle to leave that behavior behind us and go in a better way."

For all his words about immorality, the reverend made it clear that in the end he did not believe in turning lesbians and gay men out of the church. He talked of the significant lesbian and gay segment of his own congregation and how he ministered to all his church members equally. He discussed the need for all, including gay men, to settle into monogamous relationships. He seemed resigned to the fact that ultimately it would not be up to him to judge their behavior, and that they would have to come to terms with the Lord's judgment of what is right and wrong. He was also fiercely committed to the idea that the church would have to reevaluate its strategy in responding to those with AIDS in the community if it hoped to improve. Yet he always returned to the position that for most in the church, behaviors that led to AIDS were unacceptable. "You know," he started again, "I have had people leave my church because I talk about AIDS from the pulpit. They come up to me and say, 'Reverend you spend too much time on that disease.' And I try to explain to them that this thing is killing our community and that we must do something."

Throughout most of our conversation, he talked of AIDS as being a disease of gay men and "junkies." Discussions of others infected with the disease only came up when explaining how the church's response had improved. He began another lecture explaining that at one time the church generally did not respond, or when it did, the response was negative. This position was generated in part because leaders of the church, like most people, saw AIDS as a disease of homosexuals, in particular white gay men—"faggots." However, after women, children, and hemophiliacs—those who have no control over this disease—were found to be infected, church leaders began to realize that a more compassionate response was called for.

The question of drug use took even less elaboration. Drug use was bad! It destroyed the community. And, again, you can love the sinner but hate the sin. There seemed to be a bit more recognition of the connection between drug use, AIDS, and a black political agenda. The cause of more drug rehabilitation programs was something he would be willing to fight for, but he stood against the provision of clean needles in the black community. He explained that white people brought drugs into the community, and now they wanted to come and give out free needles. "I guess they figure if AIDS and drugs can't kill us, then they will help the process along by giving kids in the neighborhood needles to shoot up with. And they ask why we think this thing (AIDS) is genocide on the black community," he complained.

We finished our conversation with a discussion of how the black community's response to AIDS might be improved. He seemed to believe that in the end it would be the work of the church and black AIDS service organizations working with the church that would make the difference. He was adamant that groups like ACT UP would never be effective in the black community: "Let me tell you, the tactics of some ACT UP won't work in here. I mean people are already suspicious of the AIDS virus. Lots of people think it's a plot for genocide. So we need to deal with it in our own way. If ACT UP came in here trying to disrupt my service like they did at St. Patrick's, they would get put out, physically. We will deal with this disease, but it will take a while. You have to understand that for many of our poorly educated clergy, homosexuals and drug users are immoral, and that is the end of the story. For those ministers, only by rejecting that behavior and accepting Jesus Christ can these folks be seen as good members of our community."

Although she didn't believe it, she was a great speaker. She captivated the crowd as she explained the path that led her to deal openly with her HIV-positive status. Young and in love, she ended up having a few babies, and to keep her man she began doing drugs with him. To keep the drugs, she began stealing. And then there was prison, where she learned of her status. There was no pre- and post-test counseling, no support networks, no information about the disease, just the notification that she had AIDS (there was no discussion of being HIV positive). I don't remember, but she may have even found out when they moved her to a different ward, the one everyone called the "AIDS chamber."

It was a long time before she admitted to herself or anyone else that, yes, she was positive, and yes, she was going to die. She recalled that it was even longer before she admitted to herself that yes, she was HIV positive, and yes, she was going to live, she hoped, for a long while before she died. The beginning of this new determination to survive came when she began to talk about AIDS with the women on the ward. They quickly schooled her on how to eat better, how to get more information about her "condition," and basically how to use the medical system to her advantage. But the real motivation for her change of heart came from the understanding that she needed to be around for her kids. And the only way to keep her kids was, first, to stay clean and, second, to deal with this disease.

She did stay clean, and she is now out of prison and living with her kids, including a small baby girl. As we talked, she mentioned at least three times with great relief that the baby was negative. Not discounting the love any mother has for her daughter, it seemed additionally important that she not be made to struggle through carrying the stigma of "killing her child"; there was enough pain and stigma in her life already. She talked openly about her past drug use and even pointed out the places where she used to shoot up. "Getting high can feel so great, and it takes all the strength I can muster not to be drawn into that again," she openly acknowledged. On the other hand, she has not forgotten the pain of getting high—not only the physical pain but the times when she would do anything just to get another hit. What social scientists might call the stigma of drug addiction, she described as the tears and final hatred her mother exhibited towards her when she was using. She could not remember how many times she asked family members for money, or how many times she left her kids in the care of relatives, or how many times she had done things she was not proud of just to get some drug. But throughout all of those very difficult experiences, she could not recall a moment when her family was afraid of her. Sure, they were afraid of what she might do to get drugs, but they were never unwilling to touch her; they were never afraid of her body. That came when they learned she had AIDS. She made it clear that her family has been very supportive and that, although it took some time, things were now just like they had been. "They didn't know anything. Hell, I didn't know anything about AIDS," she explained. "They thought it was some disease mostly white gay men got. I mean they knew that junkies could get it, but not their daughter or sister." She emphasized the point that early in the epidemic there weren't a lot of people out there telling black people about this disease.

Things are better now. She goes to a church where she can talk to the minister about anything. Her health also seems to be getting better now that she is no longer using. She has taken active steps to be open about this disease and battle for her life. She still faces problems. She tells me that she is worried about being too public about her status, because her children still need to function in the neighborhood without getting hassled by people. And of course she struggles daily to deal with this disease and "people's shit around it." She points out that when she stopped using, she thought all that stuff where people talk about you and your family was over, but because of her status, it has all intensified. People still talk about her and her family, but now they not only say that she is pitiful—wasting her life—but that she is dangerous and a threat to the life of her children and all those who come into contact with her.

* * *

For many dealing with AIDS (acquired immunodeficiency syndrome) in African-American communities—be it through a positive HIV (human immunodeficiency virus) test, the experiences of a loved one living with the disease, or working to educate, organize, and prevent the spread of HIV and AIDS in the community—the voices above reflect just some of the dilemmas they have encountered. Issues of stigma, fear, rejection, invisibility, classism, sexism, homophobia, and drug phobia all construct just part of the environment in which a response to this disease has developed in black communities. To discuss AIDS in black communities is to discuss a multiplicity of identities, definitions of membership, locations of power, and strategies for the political, social, and economic survival of the community, because all these factors interact with a disease that divides and threatens ever-growing segments of these populations. To investigate the political response to AIDS in African-American communities is to look closely at a much larger phenomenon threatening black and other marginal communities, namely, a changing political environment. The public agenda of African-American communities was once dominated by consensus issues construed as having an equal impact on all those sharing a primary identity based on race. Now, cross-cutting issues structured around and built on the social, political, and economic cleavages that tear at the perceived unity and shared identity of group members are increasingly finding their way into the public spotlight. Cross-cutting issues, while always a part of the historical struggles of marginal groups, are currently generating unprecedented public attention, as African Americans and the multiple issues they confront steadily move into the mainstream of American society.

Using HIV and AIDS as the lens through which I focus my analysis, this book examines the political processes of black communities. Specifically, I contend that where once consensus issues dominated the political agendas of most black organizations, these concerns are now being challenged and sometimes replaced by cross-cutting issues and crises rooted in or built on the often hidden differences, cleavages, or fault lines of marginal communities. Cross-cutting issues are perceived as being contained to identifiable subgroups in black communities, especially those segments of black communities which are the least empowered. Thus these issues further stigmatize group members already constructed as deficient in those characteristics thought to embody the normative standards of the community. The development of such public issues has occurred as African Americans confront a new political context, that of advanced marginalization.[1] In this contradictory political context, more African Americans than ever before have secured access to, and limited power over, dominant institutions and resources. However, despite such advances on the part of some group members, the majority of African Americans still lack the political, economic, and social resources necessary to participate actively in decision-making that significantly influences and structures their lives. Cross-cutting issues underscore these intragroup differences, highlighting the disparate living conditions that define many African-American communities. Moreover, these concerns bring into question how traditional black leaders and organizations will respond to issues that no longer manifest themselves strictly as racial consensus issues, but instead stratify along the lines of class, gender, and sexuality. Will indigenous leaders actively support the struggles of the most vulnerable and marked in their communities, risking the hard-won access, mobility, and respectability of some group members? Or will elites engage in a form of secondary marginalization, further stigmatizing and policing the behaviors of their most disempowered members, while seeking again to prove their legitimacy as full citizens in this society?[2] AIDS, as a cross-cutting issue laced with stigma and rooted in African-American communities, provides some insight into how black leaders, organizations, and community members will respond to the changing political environment that confronts all marginal groups in the twenty-first century.

Homogeneity and Linked Fate

Traditionally scholars, in particular of race and politics, have categorized the political activity of African Americans as representing a level of consensus rarely seen in the political mainstream. Pointing to trends in shared political ideologies, policy preferences, and voting behavior, researchers have assumed a stable and homogenous racial group identity and experience to be at the root of such findings (Barker 1988; Pinderhughes 1987; Schuman, Steeh, and Bobo 1985). Years of economic exploitation, residential segregation, political disempowerment, and cultural appropriation define the experiences of most African Americans, and the marker of race has most consistently been offered, by those inside and outside of black communities, as an explanation or justification for the substantial and systemic inequalities faced by African Americans.

A shared history of oppression, rooted in ideologies and systems of racial hierarchy, has motivated the development among black Americans not only of a common narrative of exclusion, self-reliance, and struggle, but also of a shared consciousness and linked fate (Dawson 1994; Gurin, Hatchett, and Jackson 1989; Bobo 1983). The shared consciousness and linked fate that African Americans use to understand the world and to interact in it might be understood as two psychological processes resulting from living in a racist society, through which African Americans come to see their individual interests or fate as closely, if not directly, tied to the progress and advancement of the entire black or African-American community. Michael Dawson (1994) suggests that the idea of linked fate arises from a shared history and common lived experiences among African Americans as well as from their recognition of significant political, social, and especially economic differences between African Americans and other groups, specifically white Americans. By exaggerating out-group differences and minimizing in-group variation, many African Americans use racial group interests as a proxy for self-interest. The progress of the group, therefore, is understood as an appropriate, accurate, and accessible evaluative measure of one's individual success.

As we might imagine, the political implications of such a calculus are numerous, not the least of which is that shared consciousness, linked fate, and racial group identity have come to serve as crucial, if not essential, resources in efforts at group mobilization. For example, much of the political information which black Americans have had access to or viewed as relevant has been and continues to be structured around racial group interests. Further, the indigenous organizations that have been instrumental in providing alternative or oppositional information as well as leadership for political battles to improve the quality of life for African Americans are institutions which generally emphasize and adhere to a unidimensional racial framework. Consequently, political issues understood or defined in ways that tap into a racial group framework, initiating feelings of linked fate and the perception of advancing the interests of the entire black community, are more likely to be "owned" as community issues meriting group political mobilization.[3] For such issues, framed as somehow important to every member of "the black community," either directly or symbolically, I use the term *consensus issues*. They are often the most visible segments of any black political agenda, and they often receive the bulk of resources and attention from black political leaders and organizations.

Rarely, however, does a concern inherently comprise all the elements necessary to be recognized as a consensus issue. Instead, this designation comes through the framing or manipulation of policy, as political entrepreneurs attempt to satisfy preconceived notions of which issues qualify as meaningful, important, and representative of black communities (Kingdon 1984). In actuality, both inside and outside of black communities, certain segments of the population are privileged with regard to the definition of political agendas. For example, issues affecting men are often presented as representative of the condition of an entire community and thus worthy of a group response. Recently in black communities the troubling and very desperate condition of young black men, who in increasing numbers face homicide, incarceration, and constant unemployment as their only "life" options, has been represented as a marker by which we can evaluate the condition of the whole group. The similarly disturbing and life-threatening condition of young black women, who confront teenage pregnancy, state backlash, and (increasingly) incarceration, however, is not portrayed as an equally effective and encompassing symbol of the circumstances of black communities. This is not to say that the gendered systems of oppression that confront young black women are not also discussed by community leaders and dominant public elites or acted upon by indigenous organizations. Instead, as scholars of women and politics have long noted, the needs, conditions, and actions of women, in this case young black women, may be recognized and deemed important to the private relationships within black communities, but they are not seen as representative of the public struggle for survival, accounts of which most often present black men as the targets of outside/genocidal/community-threatening attacks (White 1990). Further, any insistence by group members that the lived experience of young black women also be recognized as part of the larger community narrative of racial discrimination and struggle is portrayed as denying the more dire position of young black men.

I do not mean to suggest that class, gender, sexual norms, and privilege in black communities mirror their manifestations among dominant groups such as upper-class whites. Even patriarchal privilege is affected and diluted by systems of oppression such as racism. Undoubtedly, the intersection of class, sexuality, and gender in black communities further distinguishes which black men are privileged within the group. However, recognizing the distinct and complicated nature of power in black communities does not deny the ability of patriarchy and sexism, homophobia and heterosexism, as well as classism to define the experiences and concerns of certain group members, primarily middle-class, heterosexual men, as representatives and markers of the progress or threat experienced by the entire community.

Take for example, the transformation in meaning that occurred for many black Americans regarding Clarence Thomas's nomination to the United States Supreme Court. Prior to charges of sexual harassment, Thomas had little name recognition and only tentative support in black communities. However, Thomas's characterization of televised hearings "investigating" the harassment charges against him as a "high-tech lynching" and the efforts of political entrepreneurs (led ironically by some Republican members of the Senate judicial committee) to represent the public spectacle around Thomas as yet another instance of white elites going after a black official mobilized support in black communities. As opposition to Thomas's nomination became redefined in ways that framed it not as a specific attack upon Thomas and his very conservative and reactionary record, but as an attack that encompassed the entire black community (especially black men), support for Thomas—or more realistically, the symbolism of his nomination—grew.

In this case, not even the inscription of the opposition to Thomas on the body of a black woman—Anita Hill—could stop this circling-of-the-wagons phenomenon. Kimberle Crenshaw (1992) writes, in *Race-ing Justice, En-gendering Power,* that

One of the most stunning moments in the history of American cultural drama occurred when Clarence Thomas angrily denounced the hearings as a "high-tech lynching." Thomas's move to drape himself in a history of black male repression was particularly effective in the all-white male Senate, whose members could not muster the moral authority to challenge Thomas's sensationalist characterization. Not only was Thomas suddenly transformed into a victim of racial discrimination, but Anita Hill was further erased as a black woman. . . .

The deification of Thomas and the vilification of Anita Hill were refigured by practices within the black community that have long subordinated gender domination to the struggle against racism. In the process the particular experiences of black men have often come to represent the racial domination of the entire community, as is demonstrated by the symbolic currency of the lynching metaphor and the marginalization of representations of black female domination. (416–17)

As Crenshaw argues, Thomas was successful in invoking a racial consensus or linked-fate framework in which attacks against him were reinterpreted as attacks against the entire black community. Increasingly, however, black Americans and other marginal group members are faced with public issues, constructed or framed in ways that highlight not their relevance to the entire group but their limited or bounded impact on a fragment of the community. Such *cross-cutting issues* are presented as affecting only specific segments of the group. Further, these issues bring into question and cast doubt on the idea that a shared group identity and feelings of linked fate can lead to the unified group resistance or mobilization that has proved so essential to the survival and progress of black and other marginal people. The process of stratification and intersection—in which issues are no longer understood as all-encompassing racial issues or experienced by all community members similarly—is the central focus of this book.

Cross-Cutting Political Issues

The concept of cross-cutting political issues refers to those concerns which *disproportionately and directly* affect only certain segments of a marginal group. These issues stand in contrast to consensus issues, which are understood to constrain or oppress with equal probability (although through different manifestations) all identifiable marginal group members. Cross-cutting issues, in addition to disproportionately impacting one segment of a group, are also often situated among those subpopulations of marginal communities that are the most vulnerable economically, socially, and politically, and whose vulnerable status is linked to narratives that emphasize the "questionable" moral standing of the subpopulation. These issues challenge for prominence in the public imagination the middle-class persona put forth by community leaders attempting to legitimize marginal group members and their concerns to dominant institutions and groups. Issues such as AIDS and drug use in black communities, as well as the extreme, isolated poverty disproportionately experienced by black women—all issues which disproportionately and directly affect poor, less empowered, and "morally wanting" segments of black communities—fall into this category of political issues.

Cross-cutting issues tend not only to mobilize one primary identity, in this case one's racial identity, but also to engage other primary identities, such as those constructed around gender, sexuality, and class. This intersectional structuring of cross-cutting issues leaves their community definition or "ownership" ambiguous, especially when such issues are perceived as mitigating the strength of one's racial identity. So, for example, to talk about the impact of AIDS on black communities, we must discuss the role that race plays in defining this issue to group members. We must also, however, discuss how sexuality, in particular gay male sexual identity and behavior, influences the receptiveness of different segments of black communities toward owning this issue. We have to recognize that a gay sexual identity has been seen in black communities as mitigating one's racial identity and deflating one's community standing. Thus, cross-cutting issues put into full view the question of who is "worthy" of support by the larger black community, specifically by its indigenous political organizations.

Attention to cross-cutting issues and segmentation in black communities has always been a part of the political struggles in black communities. Whether in the writings of Du Bois, the economic and social plans of Washington, or the charity work of middle-class black women involved in the club movement, concerns over class, gender, and respectability have historically influenced which political issues and which segments of black communities were thought to be suitable for public "ownership" (James 1997; Gaines 1996; Higginbotham 1993; Washington 1995; Du Bois 1986). Despite this continuous struggle with difference in black communities, researchers, politicians, and elites, both inside and outside of black communities, have generally constructed the political agendas and lived condition of black Americans as extremely monolithic. Left unexplored were contests over recognition and power among African Americans. However, with the increasing formal incorporation of some African Americans into political, social, and economic institutions of this country and the resulting bifurcated, racialized experiences of, for instance, middle-class and poor African Americans, a unidimensional representation of this group may no longer be possible.[4]

In our current political environment, struggles over the expansion of "the" black political agenda continue at a decidedly quickened and public pace. No longer can consensus issues, structured around a unidimensional racial framework, be put forth as the only concerns that affect and mobilize African Americans. Much more visibly, cross-cutting issues, demanding ownership, wreaking havoc on the lives of many African Americans, and rooted in the multiple identities of group members, are increasingly seen as some of the most fundamental problems facing marginal groups. Cross-cutting issues, those problems originating in the experiences of the most vulnerable in black communities, necessitate that group members previously understood as marginal or a blight on the community be made a central focus of the group's politics. In light of this development, African Americans must weigh concern over the respectability and legitimization of black communities in the eyes of dominant groups against concern over the well-being of those most vulnerable in our communities, as they struggle against very public, stigmatizing issues. It is this tension that informs the indigenous political processes that determine which issues will be embraced by black elites and organizations.

So while academics publish volumes about the intersection of race, class, and gender, a cross-cutting issue such as welfare reform personifies, in the lives of women on welfare, the ways in which identities of gender, class, and race, at the very least, intersect and are manipulated by dominant institutions to construct the special category of delinquent poor women of color—those portrayed as unable or unwilling to make rational reproductive and economic choices (Cohen, Jones, and Tronto 1997; Gilens 1996; Guy-Sheftall 1995; Zinn and Dill 1994). This stigmatized public image not only affects the immediate condition of poor women of color, limiting this subpopulation's access to state assistance, but also creates embarrassment and shame among many middle and working-class black Americans, initiating a process of distancing between those deemed "respectable" black Americans and those deemed "deficient" black Americans. Thus, cross-cutting issues arise out of the multiplicity of identities that marginal group members embody, and they personify the dilemmas that marginal group members face in trying to mold such intersecting identities into a strategy for survival and progress. In concrete ways, cross-cutting issues represent the distinct, racialized experiences of different segments of black communities, the fragmentation that threatens a perceived unified black group identity and interest, and the corresponding reduction in the probability and effectiveness of political mobilization by blacks as a group.

Difference, Membership, and African-American Politics

Researchers familiar with African-American communities have noted that significant class, educational, economic, and political differences have always existed within those communities (Frazier 1957). Whether those differences manifest themselves in the work one pursues or on the street in Harlem on which one lives, difference has been a constant in African-American communities. And as black communities approaching the twenty-first century evolve and confront increasing economic bifurcation, divergent interests, and distinct racial experiences, examples of variation and fragmentation seem to be gaining the attention of scholars. In contrast to the apparent continued congruity in African-American public opinion and voting behavior, less-traditional scholarly work has suggested, increasingly in the last fifteen years, that the cohesiveness of African-American politics is and has always been in question (Dawson 1994; Marable 1991; West 1993). For example, many black feminist scholars have continuously highlighted the intersectional and gendered variations in the racial experiences of African-American men and women (Guy-Sheftall 1995; Omolade 1994; Morrison 1992; Crenshaw 1989; King 1988; hooks 1984; Smith 1983). Further, this field of research has also been instrumental in facilitating, and sometimes participating in, discussions of the ways in which sexuality or "non-normative" sexual identities also create a distinct and often more marginalized racialized existence for both African-American men and women (Cohen 1996a; Harper 1996; Hemphill 1991; Beam 1986; Clarke 1983; Smith 1983). The impact of class in shaping the political attitudes and behavior of both poor African Americans and middle-class African Americans is once again a topic for examination (Gaines 1996; Dawson 1994; Cose 1993; Feagin and Sikes 1994). Further, the roles of age, neighborhood composition, and geographic location, particularly as factors that influence and divide African Americans in their politics, are generating more scholarly attention (Wilson 1987; Cohen and Dawson 1993; Massey and Denton 1993).

Evidence of divisions or variations in African-American politics, however, is not limited to academic analysis; the idea of a unified black community or identity has long been challenged. Black women have loudly and continuously given voice to the distinct, gendered conditions under which they experience racial oppression (Omolade 1994; Giddings 1984; Davis 1981). Poor black people have always recognized and organized around their unique position in the black community (Gordon 1964; Kelley 1990; Piven and Cloward 1979). Further, black lesbian and gay activists and cultural workers have written and organized around their particular understanding and experience with racial, gendered, sexual, and often class oppression (Hemphill 1991; Beam 1986; Smith 1983; Lorde 1982).

Even when we turn our attention to recent public events involving the African-American community, division, not consensus, seems to be the pattern of the politics. Public events such as the Anita Hill–Clarence Thomas hearings, debates over the speeches and role of Nation of Islam leader Minister Louis Farrakhan, the guilt or innocence of O. J. Simpson, and the Million Man March all highlight the multiple points of fragmentation and intersection which structure the politics of African Americans. Interestingly, many of these issues, while fostering real debate and dissension in African-American communities, are portrayed in the mainstream press as nearly consensus issues—all blacks think O. J. Simpson is innocent, or all African Americans support Louis Farrakhan and the Million Man March. However, when we look beyond mainstream press representations of African-American communities and observe the continued change, even bifurcation, in the demographic composition of this group, the cohesion assumed and asserted previously by scholars is much less certain and may now be tearing at the seams in clearly visible ways. For example, Michael Dawson (1994), William Julius Wilson (1987; 1980), and Reynolds Farley (1984) have all written about the increasing economic polarization found in black communities. Gerald Jaynes and Robin Williams (1989) note that this stratification can be found in both individual male earnings and family-income trends:

> Uneven change over time in the average economic position of blacks over the past half century has been accompanied, espe-

cially in the last quarter century, by accentuated differences in status among blacks. One of the most important developments since the 1960s has been that some segments of the black population gained dramatically relative to whites, while others have been left far behind. . . .

Conditions within the black community began to diverge sharply in the 1970s. This divergence can be seen very clearly in the experience of young men. By the early 1980s, black men aged 25–34 with at least some college earned 80–85 percent as much as their white counterparts. . . . At the other end of the group were the one-quarter of black men aged 25–34 who had not finished high school and who could not compete in the stagnant 1970s economy. An increasing number dropped out of the labor force altogether. . . .

Since 1959, inequality among black men has been consistently greater than among white men. The lowest-earning 40 percent of black men earned about 8 percent of the total earnings of black men in 1959, but 5 percent in 1984. The highest-earning 20 percent of black men earned 50 percent of the total in 1959, but 60 percent in 1984.

Polarization of the family income distribution has also taken place. In 1970, 15.7 percent of black families had incomes over $35,000; by 1986, this proportion had grown to 21.2 percent (in 1986 constant dollars). Similarly, the proportion of black families with incomes of more than $50,000 increased from 4.7 percent in 1970 to 8.8 percent in 1986 (22 percent of white families had incomes of more than $50,000 in 1986). During the same years, the proportion of black families with incomes of less than $10,000 also grew, from 26.8 percent to 30.2 percent. (274–75)

In spite of the public fragmentation and stratification evident in the numbers quoted above as well as other changing demographics in black communities, issues thought to be "owned" by the community are still rooted primarily in the experiences of those whom Kimberle Crenshaw (1989) deems the privileged members of the group. The topics talked about and acted upon by black public officials, community leaders, and established black organizations—those considered part of the "black political agenda"—are still largely issues that are deemed legitimate, respectable, and ready for public inspection (Gaines 1996; Hammonds 1997). Thus, while there is a history of contestation around the definition of a broad and expansive black political agenda, one that includes issues affecting all segments of the community, especially those members understood to be defined by multiple marginalizing identities, the political issues that continue most often to be pursued and embraced publicly by community institutions and leaders are those thought to be linked to, or to conform to, middle-class/dominant constructions of moral, normative, patriarchal citizenship.

The struggle that largely characterizes the politics of African-American communities today is contradictory. While multiple identities are not only recognized but increasingly play a significant role in structuring the lived experience of black people, many community organizations and leaders seem determined to espouse a politics rooted in a unidimensional understanding of racial identity, where the status of middle-class, male, or heterosexual provides privilege and attention. It is this evolving tension within African-American politics and the politics of most marginal communities that is at the center of this project. African-American communities' political construction of and response to the AIDS crisis in black communities provide one example of how black people, in particular black leaders, decide whether an issue is to be defined as inherent to the black community—deserving of community attention, resources, and response. What processes of evaluation do community leaders, institutions, and members use to identify which fragmented or cross-cutting issues deserve a place on "the black political agenda"? This question is especially relevant to all those marginal group members who depend on community or indigenous resources and support for their survival, because community political action either addresses their particular needs or motivates dominant institutions and groups to pay at least some attention to their concerns.

Closely connected to these questions of community ownership and group political mobilization are the topics of membership and identity. In our current stratified existence, how does any marginal group determine which members merit the support and mobilization of "the community"? Whose issues are important or broad enough to be included and prioritized for political action? In black communities, who is worthy enough or "black enough" to warrant such community ownership? Is affirmative action, largely thought to affect primarily middle-class black Americans, more of a "black issue" than welfare reform? When we talk about the endangered status of black men, does that discussion include the devastation to black gay men resulting from the AIDS epidemic? Can the politics of any marginal community sustain anything other than a single-dimensional or single-axis approach to politics or liberation?

Thus, if we accept the proposition that identity-based groups are essential to the advancement and progress of oppressed or marginalized communities, then understanding the processes by which seemingly private issues get redefined or framed as community issues and part of the group political agenda is critical. More specifically, as we enter the twenty-first century, where issues will rarely be rooted or located exclusively in one community or rarely experienced equally among all marginal group members (i.e., welfare reform, affirmative action, English-only requirements, immigration restrictions), how does an issue become designated a community issue? Does the increasing variation in lived experiences among African Americans threaten or restructure the potential for group mobilization?

AIDS in Black Communities

As stated above, AIDS is the empirical center of this book. When I started this project in 1989, it was commonly held that between one million and two million people in the United States were already infected with the human immunodeficiency virus, many of whom were expected to be sick with full-blown AIDS by the year 2000 (Fauci 1991). At that time AIDS deaths in the United States exceeded 170,000, and researchers projected that between 1991 and 1993, 165,000 to 215,000 more Americans would die from this disease and its complicating infections.[5] Further, more young Americans were expected to die from AIDS in 1990 and 1991 alone than the 55,000 Americans who died during a decade of the Vietnam War.

Despite such expectations of gloom and death, it seemed that no one, except what appeared to be the predominantly white lesbian and gay community, wanted to talk openly about this growing epidemic.[6] Undoubtedly, the lack of action, from the general public on down to the president, was and is directly tied to the conception of AIDS as a disease of white gay men, black and Latino/a drug users, and other marginal people engaged in "immoral behavior." This image of the disease, propelled by homophobia, racism, and drug phobia, allowed and even promoted indifference toward the deaths of people with AIDS, in particular the large number of gay men diagnosed early with this disease. However, standing in opposition to a seemingly general consensus on the part of the government, the general public, and the media that we need not concern ourselves with the devastation of what was presented as *only* one community, there consistently appeared groups of individuals, most often stigmatized as "perverted dykes and fags," who found old and new ways to make officials and institutions (if not the public) answer to some of their demands. This community developed sophisticated political tactics to respond to the indifference and hostility that government and other institutions displayed regarding people with AIDS (PWAs). Rallies, sit-ins, lobbying, private meetings, civil disobedience, "phone zaps"—few things seemed too far out-of-bounds to make people listen and respond.[7]

And while all this activity on the part of the gay community continued to draw my attention to questions of political mobilization around the AIDS crisis, I knew from personal experiences with friends that white gay men were not the only group being attacked by AIDS. As I researched the statistics, it became glaringly apparent that this was not just a concern for the gay community. Gay and nongay members of black and Latino communities were also increasingly being afflicted by the disease. For instance, in 1990 national surveillance figures indicated that black and Latino/a women, men, and children were disproportionately represented among those with AIDS.[8] Among adult AIDS cases nationally, blacks were found to comprise almost 28 percent of all cases, more than double their 12 percent share of the population. Latino/a adults, correspondingly, represented nearly 16 percent of all adult AIDS cases, nearly double their 9 percent of the population. Among pediatric AIDS cases—those younger than thirteen—black children comprised 52 percent of reported cases, while Latino/a children made up 26 percent of this population in 1990. There was no denying that even in 1990 AIDS had increasingly become a disease of people of color.[9]

In light of the growing number of AIDS cases in black and Latino/a communities, there *appeared* to be a major piece missing from the manifestation of AIDS in these communities, especially as compared to its manifestation in primarily white lesbian and gay communities. Specifically, in "the black community" there appeared to be no major (or minor for that matter) political activism in response to AIDS. There were no rallies and sit-ins. There was no lobbying on Capitol Hill. There were no legislative initiatives by black Congressional members to use government resources to curb the havoc wreaked by this disease in black communities. There were not even established community leaders standing in line to talk about this issue and its devastation on the group. When I looked for mobilization around AIDS in the black community back in 1990, initially I saw nothing.

The unsettling observation of unequal mobilization between the black community and the white gay and lesbian community initially shaped this project. I wanted to understand why two groups facing what appeared on the surface to be the same medical crisis would respond in such different ways. How was it that the gay community could be so forceful in its response and the black community seem to be so silent? Through much of my research and, more importantly, through my political work, I have come to learn that my initial understanding of the black community's response to AIDS, while not completely wrong, was uninformed. After years of graduate school, I did what I was trained to do; I turned to traditional sources of information: books, articles, and data sets. What I found there, when I found anything, undoubtedly skewed my conception of the gay community's response to AIDS as well as the black community's response to this epidemic. Those more traditional sources of information often provided incomplete evaluations of each community's response, trivializing the activities of gay activists and missing entirely those in the black community who lead battles around AIDS. In spite of the inaccuracies, however, the fact remained that each community pursued decidedly different strategies in response to the devastation of AIDS.

Over the years, as I have grown older and the epidemic has increasingly rooted itself in communities of color in the United States, this project has also evolved. What began as a comparison of the political responses to AIDS by a visibly active lesbian and gay community and a seemingly more distant and less confrontational African-American community is now focused much more exclusively on a detailed exploration of the ways in which African-American communities understood and responded politically to this social and health crisis. In part this reformulation has occurred because of statistics that suggest that this epidemic continues to strengthen its hold on black communities in the United States. In 1995, for example, the proportion of those classified with AIDS who were black (40 percent) was for the first time equal to the proportion of those classified with AIDS who were white (40 percent).[10] It is now estimated that blacks comprise 57 percent of all new HIV infections (Stolberg 1998, A1). The disproportionate impact of HIV and AIDS on black communities becomes clear when we consider that whites make up approximately 75 percent of the population, while blacks comprise only 12 percent. Additionally, statistics from the Centers for Disease Control and Prevention (CDC) indicate that as of 1998, blacks comprised the majority of those classified with AIDS among women (56 percent) and children (58 percent).[11] Furthermore, a recent study by Philip S. Rosenberg of the National Cancer Institute underscores the serious threat of AIDS for black Americans. His research indicates that while 1 in 139 white men ages 27–39 were thought to be HIV positive, 1 in 33 black men and 1 in 60 Latino men of the same age group were believed to be infected. Among women, 1 in every 1,667 white women ages 27–39 were thought to be living with HIV, while 1 in 98 black women and 1 in 222 Latina women were thought to be infected. Consequently, The Harvard AIDS Institute (1996) reports that "the latest U.S. data suggest that more African Americans are now infected with HIV than all other racial and ethnic groups combined (4)."

But statistics alone do not fully explain the shift in focus of this project. In part my concentration on the political response to AIDS in African-American communities was also prompted by what I believe is a need or gap in the literature on AIDS. Over the last six or seven years, we have seen a proliferation of books on the AIDS epidemic. The range of subject matter covered stretches from essential health and emotional information for those living with any of the opportunistic infections associated with AIDS to theoretical analyses of the cultural response to this disease and to how gay men who have tested HIV negative are dealing with feelings of guilt and depression. And while the scope of the subject matter continues to expand, nearly all of these studies are centered around the experiences of white individuals and white communities, where whiteness is assumed to serve as the normative or "baseline" experience of those affected by AIDS. I mention this not to discount the increasing number of edited volumes which include at least two or three chapters on people of color and their experiences with AIDS, but instead because I believe this pattern of relative invisibility has sent the wrong message to the general population and especially to black and gay communities. Those who study the impact of media representation commonly hold that we are more likely to pay attention and to associate ourselves with a story or issue if the people being talked about or the images being presented look and sound like ourselves. Thus, while the AIDS epidemic increasingly becomes a disease of people of color, the literature, images, and general representation of the disease stay predominantly white. This misrepresentation suggests that AIDS in communities of blacks and other people of color is something with which the country, the state, and communities of color in particular need not concern themselves. Further, this absence of attention also implies that activities on the part of the government, pharmaceutical companies, community activists, and others involved in the response to AIDS in communities of color do not merit the scrutiny and careful analysis directed at other groups struggling against this disease. My aim here, however, is to affirm that these conditions do warrant the resources and the attention necessary to save lives in communities of color.

Marginalization and Black Communities

Another reason I have chosen to focus on African-American communities' response to AIDS is that I believe there is much to learn about the impact of marginality on the ways that communities deal with political issues, especially those that emphasize and highlight power inequalities within marginal groups. Some people argue that to understand the black community's response to AIDS is to understand any community's response to this disease. They suggest that many people remain ignorant of the facts about HIV and AIDS and thus rely on homophobia, drug phobia, race, class, and gender to construct their understanding of this epidemic. And clearly similar information and learning patterns can be found across communities. It would be silly, for instance, to argue that dominant information sources, such as network news coverage or government agencies like the CDC have not been crucial in shaping how all people in this country, including black Americans, think about HIV and AIDS. But the story of black communities' relationship to this disease does not end with an examination of dominant institutions. I contend that the actions and attitudes of marginal communities are influenced as much by indigenous institutions, leaders, organizations, and information sources as by dominant institutions and systems.

Throughout this book I use the framework of marginalization to examine the response to AIDS in African-American communities. I assume that a group is marginal to the extent that its members have historically been and continue to be denied access to dominant decision-making processes and institutions; stigmatized by their identification; isolated or segregated; and generally excluded from control over the resources that shape the quality of their lives. Much of the material exclusion experienced by marginal groups is based on, or justified by, ideological processes that define these groups as "other." Thus, marginalization occurs, in part, when some observable characteristic or distinguishing behavior shared by a group of individuals is systematically used within the larger society to signal the inferior and subordinate status of the group (Goffman 1963). This stigmatized "mark" often becomes the primary identification by which group members are evaluated and through which they experience the world. Of course, other identities affect the status and position of marginal group members; however, certain constructed identities those we might call primary—come to have a dominant effect on the life chances and life experiences of marginal group members.[12]

In response to their limited access to dominant institutions, marginal group members often come to rely on indigenous sources, information, and organizations to provide resources that are otherwise unavailable to them. These indigenous sources are instrumental in providing marginal group members with alternative or oppositional ways of thinking about issues. Thus, understanding the internal or indigenous structuring of marginal communities, where needed resources and support can be found, is critical to understanding the political actions and attitudes of marginal group members. Recognizing the importance of indigenous resources and institutions, we must also pay close attention to local or internal contexts, issues, and hierarchies that restrict access to indigenous resources for certain marginal group members or segments and thus further marginalize the most vulnerable of the community, increasing the potential harm of crises such as AIDS.

The theory of marginalization I present here and detail further in chapter 2, is structured around at least three major principles that aid in our understanding of the political behavior of marginal groups: first, a focus on the history of power relations and oppression under which groups evolve; second, the centrality of the indigenous structure of marginal communities in understanding their political choices; and third, the recognition that strategies of marginalization are not static but evolve over time, responding in part dialectically to the resistance of marginal group members.

The first principle means that we must incorporate the historical experiences of marginal groups into examinations of their present-day political choices and actions, recognizing that historical experiences of exclusion not only frame the way marginal groups view more dominant institutions and groups but also constrain the way groups view themselves and their ability to mobilize around certain issues. For example, how do we explain a 1990 *New York Times* survey in which nearly one-third of black New Yorkers contacted (29 percent) believed that it was true or might be true that the "virus which causes AIDS was deliberately created in a laboratory in order to infect black people?" Without knowledge of the historical circumstances of black Americans, it would be difficult to understand the mistrust of public health officials exhibited by many African Americans, whose relationship to the medical industry has been informed and defined by a history of blame and manipulation. The most infamous and public example is that of the Tuskegee Syphilis Study where black subjects were denied treatment for syphilis so government health officials could study the progression of this disease (McBride 1991; Jones 1981). Thus, any analysis of the politics of marginal communities must be informed by the history of inequality and oppression under which these groups have developed.

The second principle of this theory reminds us that an understanding of the indigenous structure of marginal communities must be taken into account as we analyze their political activity. Accurate study of the mobilization of marginal groups is nearly impossible without paying strict attention to the ways that indigenous institutions and leaders wield localized power, frame issues, and distribute community resources. Indigenous media sources like the black press, and indigenous organizations and institutions like the NAACP and the black church are all crucial players in internal contests over which issues will be "owned" and which community members will be privileged, having their needs and rights serve as the standard through which justice and equality are measured for the group. Only by paying attention to power relationships within marginal communities can we closely examine variation in the consequences of political choices made by indigenous leaders for different marginal group members.

Finally, the third principle informs us that processes of marginalization are not static, but dialectical, in their relationship with strategies and actions of resistance on the part of marginal group members. For example, one pattern of marginalization may focus on the *categorical exclusion* of all members of a certain class or group from central control over the dominant resources of a society. And while such a strategy might prove effective in directing the policies and interaction of society at one stage in its development, other, more complicated strategies may be needed in a different political environment. Thus, a strategy that allows for the limited mobility of some "deserving" marginal group members—*integrative marginalization*—may be effective in the face of resistance from the excluded group. The pattern of exclusion or marginalization I am most interested in for this analysis—*advanced marginalization*—not only allows for limited mobility on the part of some marginal group members, but also transfers much of the direct management of other, less privileged marginal group members to individuals who share the same group identity.

So, for example, while many African Americans struggle to maintain some decent standard of living under a pattern of advanced marginalization, others have secured unprecedented access to dominant institutions and find themselves solidly integrated at multiple levels into the state apparatus. Those marginal group members who are close to the edges of dominant power, where access and involvement in decision making actually seem possible, confront incentives to promote and prioritize those issues and members thought to "enhance" the public image of the group, while controlling and making invisible those issues and members perceived to threaten the status of the community.[13] It is from such a conflictual position that we increasingly find traditional black elites engaging in their own indigenous form of marginalization—*secondary marginalization*—replicating a rhetoric of blame and punishment and directing it at the most vulnerable and stigmatized in their communities.

Through this framework of marginalization, and with an awareness of the developing bifurcation in the black community, we begin our examination of the community's response to AIDS. I use the theory of marginalization to frame my discussion of AIDS in black communities because it highlights and makes central the indigenous sites of power that help to structure black communities' response to this disease. Moreover, this framework reminds us that we must understand all of the factors that influence the black community's response to AIDS within the context of the historical relationship of distrust and blame that exists between the government and the black community, especially around issues of health and disease. I examine this historical relationship as well as current questions of membership and identity in chapter 2.

Methodology and Data

The research strategy for this book is varied, relying on case study, elite interviewing, content analysis, roll-call vote analysis, and participant observation techniques. Most of the case-specific empirical data comes from conversations and oral interviews with activists, community leaders, elected and appointed officials, and people living with AIDS in New York City between the years 1990 and 1993.[14] Again, I want to emphasize that I do not attempt to provide a complete historical record of activism. Instead I try to provide detail sufficient for a general understanding of activism during the years 1981–1993. Further, while AIDS is a crisis confronting many or most black communities across the country and throughout the world, a significant amount of the evidence and storytelling in this book deals with the manifestation of AIDS in New York City.

In many ways New York City provides the perfect framework for investigating the activities of African Americans in response to AIDS. First, it has an excessively high number of cases, so that no officials from any community can argue that AIDS is not a pressing concern for the entire city as well as specific racial and ethnic groups. In early 1998 the New York City Department of Health reported cumulative adult AIDS cases to be over 100,000.[15] And while many people recognize that AIDS has devastated the gay community, and continues to do so, fewer people realize the increasing wreckage caused by the AIDS epidemic in New York City's black communities. In New York City since 1990 more AIDS cases have come from the black community than any other racial or ethnic group.[16] Currently, nearly 41 percent of those with AIDS in New York City are black, although we must understand this in terms of their representation in New York City, where blacks make up just over 25 percent of the population.[17] Further, since 1991, AIDS has been the leading cause of death among black women ages 15–34 and among black men 25–44 in New York City.[18] Among women, blacks represent over half of all female AIDS cases, comprising 53 percent of this population in New York City. Black children also dominate pediatric AIDS cases, making up 55 percent of all children with AIDS in New York City. Black men, as might be expected, are also overrepresented, comprising 37 percent of all adult male cases of AIDS.[19]

The prominence of this issue for New York City means that the elites who shape community responses are generally accessible. Elites in the black community whom I interviewed include members of the clergy, the black media, individuals in city government, and officials in the city's health-delivery system. I also interviewed community activists who provided insight into the grassroots response to the AIDS epidemic in black communities. In an attempt to compare responses from different groups, I also conducted interviews with members of the gay (primarily white) community, including elites, activists, service providers, as well as people with AIDS. Finally, I also talked with and gathered information from national government officials, including staff at the Centers for Disease Control, members of the mainstream media, and other critical players associated with institutions responding to this crisis. The information gained through these interviews, meetings, conferences, and informal conversations provides the real data for this project.[20]

Again, while the overwhelming focus of this book is on the political response to AIDS in African-American communities, I also use the activities of gay and lesbian communities as a point of departure, engaging in an *informed comparative analysis*. This entails using the history of activism emanating from traditionally recognized gay and lesbian communities—not to make a mirror-image comparison to African-American communities, but to generally inform us of and provide a framework for analyzing the many *possible* political responses to AIDS.[21] The purpose here is to use our understanding of lesbian and gay activism and the similar marginal positions of both blacks and gays in dominant American society to inform and guide the exploration of our central topic—the African-American political response to AIDS. Some understanding of both communities is therefore critically important, not only because it provides a comparative basis for understanding mobilization, but also because through this analysis I may find a way to give voice to concerns that threaten the existence and survival of members of both groups.

Outline of the Book

Chapter 2 extends the discussion of the theoretical framework of marginalization, examining the different patterns of marginalization and exploring in particular the importance of indigenous structures to marginal groups. Once the theory of marginalization has been delineated, I present a brief, general rendering of the black community's response to HIV and AIDS. Using historical texts, personal interviews, and government statistics, chapter 3 details the political context in which AIDS emerged as well as three different stages in the response of African-American communities. In the early stages of this disease, who in African-American communities engaged in acts of education, service, and political struggle? Further, over the years, how has the response to AIDS evolved to include more indigenous institutions? Once we have an understanding of the feelings and actions of African Americans concerning AIDS, we can pose the question, Where did these attitudes and behavior originate?

The remaining chapters detail the different institutions, leaders, and individuals that helped to shape the activity and feelings documented in chapter 3. In chapters 4 and 5, I examine the role of dominant institutions in shaping an understanding of this disease among the general population and specifically among African-American communities. To what degree did the marginalized status of the epidemic's early "victims" affect the willingness of dominant institutions to respond in an effective and forceful manner? Specifically, how did the marginal status of those groups believed to be most at risk for AIDS, gay men and intravenous drug users, influence the early response of dominant institutions? I am interested in how the attention an issue receives from dominant leaders and institutions signals and significantly determines the reaction and response of dominant groups, and to a lesser degree of marginal group leaders, organizations, and members. While some of this information has been presented in books like *And the Band Played On* (Shilts 1988), I try to offer new insights by taking an in-depth look at the framing of this issue on the part of television and print news sources. In chapter 4, I examine the specific role of the Centers for Disease Control in constructing "the facts" and "the victims" of this new disease. In chapter 5, I turn my attention to the role of the mainstream media and its work as a linking institution, shaping and transmitting information on AIDS for the public. Using data from the Vanderbilt Television Archives, I sample the entire population of nightly news stories on AIDS by ABC, CBS, and NBC between the years 1981 and 1993, looking specifically for trends regarding race and representation. I pursue a similar analysis of printed material, focusing on the *New York Times*.

The role of indigenous organizations, institutions, leaders, and norms in determining the political behavior of African-American communities is the focus of the rest of the book. Chapters 6–9 explore the ways in which indigenous players significantly structured the political understanding and response of black communities. As I have mentioned previously, this is not a historical exercise documenting all of the ways in which black communities did and did not recognize and respond to AIDS. I do, however, explore multiple institutions in African-American communities, attempting to identify patterns of response and resistance. Chapters 6 and 7 explore what I call questions of acknowledgement and consciousness. Specifically, I am interested in how institutions indigenous to black communities represented the impact of this disease on black communities and especially on the specific subgroups thought to be most at risk and living with AIDS. We must remember that because of the history of marginalization experienced by most black people, indigenous sources of information play a special role in shaping behavior. Accordingly, I examine the coverage of HIV and AIDS, in content and quantity, provided by major black newspapers and magazines. Throughout chapters 6 and 7, I explore whether black media sources constructed and communicated an image of AIDS that would enhance or constrain the activism of the black community. How did the representation of AIDS, in particular of individuals and groups with AIDS, in black media sources interact with internal ideologies and values thought to designate "community" issues?

Chapter 6 surveys the coverage of AIDS in traditional black newspapers such as the *New York Amsterdam News*. Chapter 7 focuses on alternative sources of information in black communities, including popular magazines such as *Essence, Jet, Ebony,* and *Black Enterprise,* printed material such as the Nation of Islam's paper *The Final Call,* and progressive newspapers such as the *City Sun*. Integral to this examination is an investigation of the representations of those African Americans most associated with this disease—gay men and drug users. Much of this discussion, therefore, takes up the portrayal of black gay men and injection drug users. If we recognize indigenous representation as significantly determining or at the very least contributing to ideas about AIDS in African-American communities, we must ask to what degree the black press challenged or reinforced dominant images and ideas concerning those with AIDS.

Chapters 8 and 9 concentrate on the actions of community leaders and organizations. I might call this section "Action versus Morality," since much of the discourse and many of the actions of established leaders seem to be constrained by concerns over morality. In chapter 8, I continue to explore the role of indigenous institutions and organizations, this time examining the response to AIDS on the part of traditional black organizations and "the black church." How did organizations such as the National Association for the Advancement of Colored People (NAACP) or the black church respond to AIDS as it increasingly devastated black communities? More generally, how have indigenous black organizations with some access to dominant institutions and resources handled the threat of AIDS in black communities? Again, the actions of indigenous institutions tell us a great deal about the ability and willingness of established, middle-class community organizations to incorporate cross-cutting issues and marginal segments of black communities into more visible and central positions in the politics of black communities. In chapter 9, I spotlight the actions of elected black leaders, in particular black congressional members. Under what political conditions were black congressional members willing to expend political resources on the issue of AIDS? What members of black communities were thought "worthy" and "black enough" to warrant congressional attention? The question of group membership, specifically indigenous constructions of membership, is especially important in understanding the actions and rhetoric of elected officials and appointed leaders.

Finally, I step back from my exploration of the political response to AIDS in African-American communities and revisit some of the questions outlined in this opening chapter. In particular, I bring back into focus some of the broader theoretical issues of power, marginalization, and resistance. Again, although I concentrate on the political responses to AIDS, especially those evidenced in African-American communities—a topic that alone has life-and-death significance—I also address issues of indigenous power, membership, identity, and representation. To what degree are internalized modes of marginalization working to stratify the black community, influencing who is represented and has access to the political agenda of the community? How do the concerns of marginalized groups find their way to the public agenda? Will the social and economic isolation in which marginalized individuals often find themselves be transformed into political isolation, where their most basic rights and needs are denied? Further, how does the continuous experience of marginalization transform the consciousness of groups? These are the questions that guide this examination of the politics of marginal groups, especially as they revolve around HIV and AIDS in African-American communities.

CHAPTER TWO

Marginalization: Power, Identity, and Membership

Quite often when trying to explain the slow, even negligent, response to AIDS in African-American communities, authors retreat to a familiar and substantively important list of barriers thought to prevent a more active response from community leaders and organizations (McBride 1991; Perrow and Guillén 1990). Regularly topping this list, for instance, is the claim that African-American communities control fewer resources than most other groups, and thus they cannot be expected to respond to AIDS in a manner similar to "privileged" (white) lesbians and gay men. Although there is truth to the assertion that most black people operate with limited access to resources, this explanation is based on a very narrow conception of resources and a very limited understanding of the history of black communities. As I argue more extensively in chapter 3, most of the cities hardest hit by this disease (New York, San Francisco, Los Angeles, Washington DC, Detroit, Chicago, Atlanta) have been or are currently headed by African-American mayors. Thus, while black individuals suffer from limited resources, black elected officials control or at least have significant input into decisions about how resources, albeit dwindling resources, will be allocated in their cities. Further, while individuals in black communities still suffer from marginalization and oppression, organizations like the National Association for the Advancement of Colored People (NAACP), the Southern Christian Leadership Conference (SCLC), and the National Urban League have all been able to gain access to national agencies and policy debates. I return to this topic in chapter 8. The claim, however, that African Americans have fewer resources than other groups, while accurate at the individual level, does not appropriately account for the institutional resources controlled or accessed by black elected officials and traditional organizations.

Another explanation for the poor response to AIDS in African-American communities centers on the numerous crises plaguing this group. Proponents of this view argue that members of black communities suffer from so many ailments and structural difficulties, such as sickle-cell anemia, high blood pressure, homelessness, persistent poverty, drugs, crime, and unemployment, that no one should expect community leaders to turn over their political agenda to the issue of AIDS. While we can agree that African Americans suffer disproportionately from most social, medical, economic, and political ills, I would argue that it is specifically because of the inordinate amount of suffering found in African-American communities that we might expect more attention to this crisis. AIDS touches on, or is related to, many other issues confronting, in particular, poor black communities: health care, poverty, drug use, homelessness. We might, therefore, reasonably expect black leaders to "use" the devastation of this disease to develop and reinforce an understanding of the enormity of the crises facing black communities. Rarely does an issue so readily embody the life-and-death choices facing an entire community, and rarely is an issue so neglected by its leadership.

Finally, many scholars and activists engaged in the fight against AIDS argue that homophobia in African-American communities is yet another important reason for the slow response to this disease by African-American elites and organizations (Cohen 1996a; Harper 1993; Dalton 1989; Hammonds 1986). Their concern is not just with homophobia among individuals, but also with the supposedly more pervasive homophobia (compared to that among whites) located and rooted in indigenous institutions like the black church, fraternal and social organizations, and some national political organizations. A more conservative and less informed variant of this argument suggests that the black community's homophobia and its aversion to anything gay or lesbian significantly structures its response to AIDS.[1] And while we must be aware of homophobia in black communities as one source of disinformation about AIDS, homophobia alone does not adequately explain the response to AIDS in black communities, nor does it capture the complex relationship of African Americans to issues involving and defined by sexuality.

For example, homophobia, as the fear or hatred of gay and lesbian people, cannot account for the slow response of black elites not only to black gay men with AIDS, but to others, such as black injection drug users stigmatized as "carriers" of HIV and AIDS in black communities.[2] This is not to say that homophobia, as a general process of socialization to which we are all subject, is not a part of black communities and has not influenced or slowed down the response to AIDS by African Americans. However, claims that homophobia alone defines the response to AIDS in black communities must be rejected and recast as part of a larger narrative about the role that sexuality—in particular, what is called deviant or non-normative sexuality—has played in justifying the marginalization of African Americans and motivating the internal policing or regulation of the public behavior and image of black Americans. We must remember that sexuality, or what has been defined by the dominant society as the abnormal sexuality of both black men and women (e.g., images such as oversexed black men in search of white women, promiscuous black women, and illegitimate baby producers), has been used to justify the implementation of marginalizing systems ranging from slavery to, most recently, workfare. Throughout the history of the United States, images and ideas of reckless black sexuality have been used to sustain the exploited position of black people, especially black women (Hammonds 1997; Cohen 1996a; Giddings 1992; Reed 1991; Carby 1987).

With such a history of marginalization in mind, we can begin to understand, yet never condone, how homophobia along with other systems of exclusion might be willingly deployed by black elites in an attempt to distance "the community" from blame and stigma and to retain their hopes of legitimacy and full incorporation. From such a perspective, it becomes clear that if we are truly to understand the response to AIDS and other cross-cutting issues by African Americans, we need a more complex theoretical model—one that not only makes central concerns over dwindling resources, or multiple crises, or community homophobia, but also incorporates the historical experiences of exclusion and marginalization that have so forcefully shaped the consciousness and actions of African Americans. Such a theory must not only highlight the past and current political, economic, and social location of African Americans, but must also pay strict attention to the internal processes of black communities, where group interests are constructed and power is deployed by indigenous elites and organizations. This desire to represent more accurately the multiple factors influencing the response to AIDS in African-American communities leads me to the broader theoretical framework of marginalization.

As stated in the last chapter, the theory of marginalization I develop for this analysis builds on traditional paradigms of power in political science. These theories explore how inequality in economic and, more generally, social resources influences and structures the political opportunities afforded to groups. At its core, the framework of marginalization expands our understanding of the places we must look to identify and understand the use of power. Quite often in studies of power, researchers become consumed with analyzing power as it is exercised by dominant groups "over" disadvantaged or "powerless" groups (Scott 1990; Gaventa 1980; Parenti 1978). Thus the power relationships and decision-making patterns situated within marginalized communities are often left unpursued. Such an oversight becomes particularly problematic when one considers the long history of de jure and de facto segregation that many marginal groups have encountered, resulting in the development of social spaces where indigenous institutions, organizations, and leaders, are relied upon for information, resources, and political support (Morris 1984). Thus, intracommunity patterns of power and membership can have a significant, if not overwhelming, impact on the political histories and approaching futures of marginal groups. The theory of marginalization, then, steps beyond the traditional dichotomy of powerful and powerless to examine the multiple sites where power is located, paying special attention to indigenous power relationships, or what Jim Scott calls the "hidden transcripts" (1990).[3]

Finally, this theory also tries to incorporate the reality of difference as it exists among marginal groups. For my purposes, a designation of marginal does not suggest, as it often does in traditional studies of power, that all resource-deficient groups can be summarily categorized as powerless. These groups cannot be understood to suffer from the same inequalities and the same strategies of exclusion, and to resist or struggle in similar ways. Instead, building on the assumed importance of internal community organization, this theory recognizes that the processes through which groups become marginalized and the options of resistance available to any specific marginal community vary, and must be addressed with attention to the particular context. Theories that focus only on general patterns of power and powerlessness ignore characteristics that are unique to a group, relying instead on simple categories that gloss over the specific status and history of a community.

The point is not to institute a ranking of marginal groups, with some "more" and some "less" marginal. Yet we must recognize that the processes that serve to marginalize, for example, Native Americans in the United States differ from those that marginalize gay men and lesbians. These varying processes uniquely shape the experiences of group members. Furthermore, within each of these groups are individuals with differential access to privileges and resources structured along, at the very least, the axes of class, sexuality, race, and gender. This more nuanced analysis of marginality does not deny the marginal experience of white gay men of upper-class backgrounds, nor does it deny the differing and multiple experiences with marginality of lesbians and gay men of color. Rather it provides a framework for understanding the differing experiences of marginality both *across* and *within* groups.

Throughout this chapter I attempt to sketch many of the components or ideas needed to operationalize an examination of marginalization. I begin by defining more concretely what is meant by the term *marginal group*. I then proceed to explore the processes or strategies of marginalization that support and enforce the relative exclusion of certain classes of people. There follows a discussion of some of the consequences of this systematic oppression. In particular, I highlight the development of indigenous structures, resources, leaders, and information as a response to the exclusion created by marginalization. The chapter concludes by briefly exploring four general patterns of marginalization that emerge from the history of African Americans.

The Making of Marginal Groups

The existence of marginal groups has long been recognized (Stonequist 1937; Dickie-Clark 1966; Buono and Kamm 1983; Hagendoorn and Hraba 1989). Whether we consider the political, economic, and social disempowerment of black Africans in South Africa under apartheid; African Americans in the United States; "undesirables" in India; or Palestinians in the Middle East, there exist clearly identifiable groups whose members have continuously been denied access to dominant resources, barred from full participation in dominant institutions, and defined as "others," living outside the norms and values agreed upon by society.

The framework of marginalization begins with the basic concept of marginal groups—those who, to varying degrees, exist politically, socially, or economically "outside" of dominant norms and institutions.[4] Denied access to the resources and skills that allow for substantial participation in decisions about the quality of life, these groups often find that their members lack access to resources such as political and social capital. A condition of marginality, therefore, is deficiency in the economic, political, and social resources used to guarantee access to the rights and privileges assumed by dominant group members. Several other processes or strategies contribute to the development or emergence of marginal groups, four of which I discuss below: identities and norms, ideologies, institutions, and social relationships.

IDENTITIES AND NORMS

Designation as a marginal group does not result solely from the historical and continuing resource-deficient position of those groups commonly labeled powerless. Rather, categorization as marginal is also directly tied to the stigmatized or "illegitimate" social identity that such groups have in the larger or dominant society. The stigmatization of an identity results from a process of social construction that defines certain behaviors, beliefs, or physical characteristics as abnormal and deficient. Marginal groups exist within a societal framework in which one or more of their primary identities has come to signal inherent inferiority. Dominant, and even indigenous, ideologies, institutions, and social relationships are used to create and maintain the definition of marginal groups as "other." Consequently, through the process of marginalization, a group's stigmatized identity works to constrain the opportunities and rights afforded community members, helping to solidify their secondary status.

This process has occurred repeatedly in the history of this country. Members of dominant groups, motivated by economic profit, social positioning, or political power, have used ascriptive characteristics or distinguishing behaviors to signal differences between themselves and "others." In the depiction of African Americans as uncontrollable savages requiring severe regulation through the Slave Codes of the seventeenth century; in the representation of Native Americans as hedonistic savages whose threat to white progress required the genocidal actions of the U.S. government during the Jacksonian period; and in the portrayal of Chinese workers as a primitive "yellow menace" whose inability to assume full democratic responsibilities required stricter immigration laws, we see that physical characteristics and behaviors have often been used by dominant groups to justify the exclusion and exploitation of other groups.

While social-constructionist paradigms reveal the created nature of identities, they also help us to recognize that the dominant norms, which often serve as a reference point in positioning marginal groups on the outside, are themselves constructed and quite malleable, with no definite borders (Opp 1982). For instance, there has been much discussion recently about how the natural sanctity of marriage is threatened by the idea of same-sex marriages. In truth, however, there is nothing inherent in some "natural" ordering of society to suggest that only individuals of opposite sexes should be allowed by the state to marry. Instead, systems of patriarchy, capitalism, and heteronormativity have structured both private and public relations as well as ideological narratives so that the institution of marriage is reserved only for those presumed to be heterosexual citizens.[5] The idea of stable, "natural," normative ways of being, taken as evident throughout history, masks a process of change in which dominant norms evolve to fit new political, economic, and social environments. This process only comes into view, however, when dominant norms are disrupted or contested. In truth, the construction of what is normal evolves over time, usually endorsing the dominant characteristics and experiences of whiteness, maleness, heterosexuality, and class privilege. For example, in the not-too-distant white supremacist past of state-sanctioned marriage, enslaved Africans and African Americans were not allowed to marry, and as late as 1967 interracial marriages were outlawed in some states (Cott 1987; Higginbotham, Jr. 1978). Far from being the codification of some natural law representing the "innate" standing of the heterosexual family, the institution of marriage has been used as a political tool to differentially benefit, punish, and regulate. The narratives associated with the institution of marriage have changed over time, which serves to explain why some populations had access to this privilege while others did not (Cohen 1996a; Duggan 1996).

In conjunction with a changing image of what is normal, there has also been an evolving notion of who or what constitutes the "other." Many groups have at different times experienced exclusion from dominant sectors of society, and many of these same groups have come to find themselves incorporated into conceptions of normal or dominant communities. Both David Roediger (1991) and Noel Ignatiev (1995) write persuasively about the transformation of Irish-Americans from a group that was once identified as racially marginal to a group of white Americans invested in and incorporated into dominant systems of power. We must therefore make a distinction between communities or groups like Irish-Americans or Polish-Americans, who in many urban areas maintain a self-imposed segregation by living in the same neighborhoods or reading community and ethnic newspapers, and marginal groups who are *forced* into patterns of segregation, relying on indigenous institutions for accurate or meaningful information about their groups (Massey and Denton 1993; Waters 1990).

Groups that experienced marginality at one point in their history may still claim as part of their identity that characteristic formerly used to justify their exclusion. For these groups, however, the formerly marginalizing factor does not carry the same significance or stigma today. So while Irish-Americans may have been marginalized at one point in their history in this country, George Bush would have been hard pressed, and found it strategically ineffective, to develop television ads that evoked negative and fearful feelings toward Irish men like those generated about black men by the Willie Horton ad.[6] Thus, while historical exclusion is central to identifying marginal groups, only those communities understood to *continue* to suffer from imposed, extralegal segregation, isolation, and exclusion are classified as marginal in this study.

The ostracized or stigmatized social identification of marginal groups makes them distinct from many of the groups studied by scholars concerned with group formation and behavior. For example, much of the work in political science that has paid any attention to group formation and behavior has centered around the study of formal interest groups (Walker 1991; Olson 1965; Truman 1958). The early work of group theorists concentrated on organizations and groups with a "significant economic aspect," formed most often by voluntary association. Truman, in particular, represented a mode of thought that centered around the propensity of individuals to come together *voluntarily* once they realized the commonality of their interests. In direct contrast to this process of development is the formation of marginal groups, brought together not by voluntary association in pursuit of shared interests, but instead defined by dominant groups into association based on some shared characteristic. Individuals from these groups have their autonomy severely restricted and thus increasingly depend on community structures and resources for group and individual advancement. The personal and collective survival of group members, or community linked fate, becomes the framework through which actions are evaluated, replacing the individualized calculus of dominant group members popularized by political scientists (Dawson 1994; Gurin, Hatchett, and Jackson 1989). Thus the shared experiences of marginal group members, as dictated in part by their subordinate identification, reinforces the importance of this identity in determining the common interests as well as the needed political activity of the group. In the case of AIDS, while there is little doubt that the stigmatized identities of those groups first thought to be associated with AIDS severely constrained the resources directed toward fighting the epidemic, these same identities would serve as the basis for much of the community mobilization witnessed in response to HIV and AIDS.

IDEOLOGIES

Ideology has long been recognized as a critical component of power, domination, and resistance. Philosophers from Destutt de Tracy to Marx and Gramsci have all theorized about the role of ideology in structuring hierarchical societies (Thompson 1990), but few agree on precisely what the idea involves. In this study the concept of ideology refers to the systems of beliefs that frame and guide our general understanding of, and interaction in, the world. While we all have different perceptions of situations, this analysis goes beyond the individual to locate ideas and behavior in a larger context. Ideologies, thus, presume to instruct and frame our understanding of what is "normal," what is "deviant," what is "right," and what is "wrong." Through the deployment of norms and values, ideologies confer legitimacy and authority and thus are directly tied to the distribution of power in society.

Ideology, as presented in the framework of marginalization, takes on a more "neutral" or progressive definition than did the concept of ideology presented by intellectuals such as Marx.[7] For instance, ideology in this analysis is not held to be an exclusive strategy of a dominant group or class. Oppositional ideologies, rooted in the experiences of oppressed or marginal communities, are also thought to exist. They challenge dominant systems of belief and provide marginal group members with a different framework through which to assess their secondary position in society. Underlying the recognition that numerous groups develop alternative and oppositional ideologies is the assumption that the context in which people find themselves significantly structures the manifestations of ideologies. A group's physical environment, material resources, and social position all help to shape the local manifestations of commonly held ideologies. To the degree that ideologies are manifested and reconstructed in ways that minimize the inconsistencies between the ideology and the specific context in which it comes to play a role, we can expect that general ideas—those thought to be held by the majority—will find different articulations in varying contexts. Barbara Fields (1982), in "Ideology and Race in American History," notes the impact of social relations on the concept and meaning of white supremacy:

> In any event, what might appear from a distance to be a single ideology cannot hold the same meaning for everyone. If ideology is a vocabulary for interpreting social experience, it follows that even the "same" ideology must convey different meanings to people having different social experiences. . . .
>
> The slogan of white supremacy was never sufficient to place the social and political ideology of the yeomen and poor whites at one with that of the planter class. From the democratic struggles of the Jacksonian era to the disfranchisement struggles of the Jim Crow era, white supremacy held one meaning for the back-country whites and another for the planters. (155–57)

Ideologies are thus understood to change as individuals and groups actively interpret the events around them, grounding the meaning of such ideologies in their social reality.

Further, just as patterns of power should be understood to be fluid, changing in response to effective strategies of resistance, so we should expect that ideologies justifying the exclusion of certain groups will change and adjust their emphasis when the validity of such ideas is effectively challenged; while the overall idea of exclusion remains intact, the specific justifications for that idea evolves. For example, while early historical justifications for the general oppression of African Americans centered around their inherent inferiority, as decreed by God, those myths of marginalization have evolved or been replaced by new narratives which highlight, for instance, the lazy or unproductive "nature" of black Americans.

Lawrence Bobo and James Kluegel (1991) in their examination of racial stereotypes found that whites, while exhibiting greater racial tolerance in some arenas of public opinion—overwhelmingly rejecting a divinely decreed inferiority among black Americans—still hold many stereotypic ideas about blacks. Their analysis of General Social Survey data indicated that nearly 59 percent of white respondents believed that blacks have a propensity to live on welfare, while only 4 percent believed that whites have a similar propensity. This disparity in the perceived abilities and values of blacks and whites was also reproduced in other areas, including investigations into the work ethic of racial groups. While 57 percent of white respondents believed that whites were hard-working, only 18 percent believed blacks to be hard-working. Similarly, 5 percent of white respondents believed other whites to be lazy, while almost 47 percent believed blacks to be lazy. These results support the proposition that, over the years, in response to information and action challenging the inherent, divinely decreed inferiority of blacks, whites have altered but not eliminated their specific explanations for the alarmingly consistent marginalized status of many African Americans.

This evolving yet consistently high level of negative attitudes toward black Americans on the part of whites suggests that ideologies of marginalization have great staying power. Over time these myths of marginalization become ingrained into society's core beliefs, as they are spread and recreated through dominant information and socializing institutions. Eventually certain observable characteristics and behaviors become commonly understood as markers of the inherent inferiority, subservience, and deviance of marginal group members. For example, in 1988, supporters of George Bush were able to tap into ideas of black violence and white vulnerability merely by running the Willie Horton ad. In 1995, Susan Smith was temporarily able to divert national attention from herself as the possible killer of her two young children by tearfully stating on television that a black man had hijacked her car and taken her children. In both cases it was the perpetuation of an ideology of marginalization—one that has continuously defined black men as violent and a threat, in particular, to white women—that gave credence to each suggested message. Marginal groups are thus distinguished by the pervasive way in which ideologies or myths that explain, justify, and recreate their secondary position become institutionalized throughout society. In the case of AIDS, ideologies and definitions of deviance and abnormality have been used to position many with HIV and AIDS outside not only the traditional health-care system but also the larger "moral fabric" of the country.

INSTITUTIONS

Institutional practices of marginalization include those embodied in organizations, policies, standard operating procedures, and laws that control or limit the full participation of marginal communities in dominant institutions. Historical analysis illuminates the ways in which the rules, structure, and general existence of an institution can work to exclude and regulate certain groups. In *The Wretched of the Earth*, Frantz Fanon (1963) discusses the wide-ranging strategies used by dominant groups to control oppressed or marginal groups. He discusses, in particular, the presence of two institutions, the military and the police, and their use of force to regulate and oppress colonized people:

> The colonial world is a world cut in two. The dividing line, the frontiers, are shown by barracks and police stations. In the colonies it is the policeman and the soldier who are the official, instituted go-betweens, the spokesmen of the settler and his rule of oppression. . . . In the capitalist countries a multitude of moral teachers, counselors, and "bewilderers" separate the exploited from those in power. In the colonial countries, on the contrary, the policeman and the soldier, by their immediate presence and their frequent and direct action maintain contact with the native and advise him by means of rifle butts and napalm not to budge. (38)

Marginal groups have always had their exclusion enforced by state-sponsored, as well as quasi-independent military organizations. And while force and violence are commonly used strategies of marginalization and oppression, other institutional practices center on the use of laws to exclude and regulate groups. Scholars such as Rogers Smith (1997) and Mario Barrera (1979) discuss the use of immigration policy to regulate groups. Barrera argues that while immigration laws were often constructed from a "racist reaction to the growth of immigration from areas other than northern and western Europe," they also resulted from the desire to guarantee employers a cheap, surplus, marginal labor supply (72). He observes that "the state has played a major role in the regulation of the labor supply for Southwestern employers. One way in which it has done this is through regulating the reserve role played by Mexican workers and other Third World groups" (167).

Along with public laws and organizational rules, which have been extremely useful in implementing measures of social control, less formal institutional mechanisms also limit access. Informal networks of recruiting and hiring, unspoken job segregation, as well as a hostile work or living environment can be just as effective as formal rules in limiting the participation of certain groups. Barrera discusses the many informal ways that government officials contributed to the regulation of Chicano workers. He calls attention, in particular, to the investigations by Paul Taylor (1929) that highlight the failure of school boards to explore the absenteeism of children of Chicano workers during harvesting periods. The reason for such negligence? These children were seen as "essential to prompt performance of beet labor operations" (Barrera 1979, 170).

Consider, for instance, a bank loan officer who believes that he is enforcing objective criteria when he reviews home loan applications. He may have no idea that many of the regulations he uses are biased to ensure that relatively few loans will end up in communities populated by people of color or poor people. By effectively performing his job, he participates daily in the continued marginalization of groups, denying them access to resources controlled by a dominant institution. The consequences of such marginalization are clear from a simple review of statistics on loan approval to poor people and people of color. To prove intentional malice on the part of our bank loan officer, however, would be difficult, if not impossible. Marginalization occurs, probably more often than not, systematically and efficiently, without observed intent. Iris Marion Young (1990), in *Justice and the Politics of Difference*, makes a similar argument:

> In this extended structural sense oppression refers to the vast and deep injustices some groups suffer as a consequence of often unconscious assumptions and reactions of well-meaning people in ordinary interactions, media and cultural stereotypes, and structural features of bureaucratic hierarchies and market mechanisms—in short, the normal processes of everyday life. (41)

Through the control of institutions, dominant groups (and more privileged marginal group members) not only constrain access to dominant resources, but also disseminate ideologies of marginalization that seek to explain the exclusion of certain groups. Over and over we find examples of the ways in which institutional resources, structures, and policies work with ideological strategies of marginalization to initiate and maintain the exclusion and oppression of certain groups. Whether the institution be the prison or the mental hospital, as detailed by Foucault (1979), or the educational system, as explored by Paulo Freire (1972), such structures embody the ability to monitor and restrict the behavior of less powerful, resource-poor, marginal group members. In assessing the role that institutions have played in defining AIDS activism, we must examine not only the overt actions of dominant institutions such as the Centers for Disease Control (CDC), but also the everyday practices and standard operating procedures of these institutions that have worked to facilitate or prevent mobilization.

Social Relationships

The final set of practices of marginalization I want to deal with in this section concerns the informal, interpersonal relationships of individuals and groups. Long after institutional barriers of exclusion have been torn down and the norms or beliefs supporting exclusion have been *formally and publicly* rejected, conflict between groups continues. Informal interactions often provide the basis for lasting exclusion. In the absence of state-sponsored institutional marginalization, individuals and groups often continue to judge marginal groups as inferior and deviant. Within the framework of race, this intergroup conflict is presently manifested in the United States through such behaviors as the outward residential migration of whites, the increased popularity of private schools, the development of closed or gated communities, and the separate racial seating evident in school and work cafeterias.

One example of the lasting effects of marginalization after formal barriers have been removed is found in the history and treatment of the Burakumin people in Japan. The Burakumin (formerly called the Eta) are an indigenous minority who have historically suffered marginalization. The ideology "explaining" their marginal position is not entirely clear, but some have suggested that the Burakumin were slaves and have historically been associated with unclean occupations. The result of their stigmatized identity has been a permanent position at the bottom of the social ladder in Japan. Anthony Head (1985) explains in his article on Japan's Burakumin that the Eta have a history of living with formal institutional marginalization:

> Discrimination was enforced. The "Eta" were required to live in designated ghetto communities and in some areas had to hang an animal skin from their homes to indicate identity. They were forbidden to marry outside their caste, deviants being forcibly divorced and punished. They could not wear colorful clothing, nor traditional wooden "clogs." Their urban movements were restricted, and in many areas they were forbidden to own land, or to farm and fish commercially. Being "non-people," they were usually excluded from the population census. (75)

Even after formal institutional barriers were removed, the Buraku-min continued to live a marginal existence. Exclusion, in this case, persisted through the social relationships and informal interactions of groups. No longer were formal institutional mechanisms of marginalization necessary; instead, exclusion had already taken root in the identity of the Burakumin and was evident in the everyday social interactions that structured the society:

> In 1871 the Emancipation Edict was issued, declaring equal status for the "Burakumin" and prohibiting use of the term "Eta." But it did little to erase deep-rooted prejudice and was unaccompanied by essential economic reforms. . . . Although some "Burakumin" have shaken off their socio-economic shackles through intermarriage . . . the majority still live in ghettos on river-banks. The squalor is appalling. (75)

Head cites as another example of the Burakumin's continuing marginalization the existence of informal "Buraku Lists" as late as 1975:

> The self-styled "Association for the Protection of Industries and Business" published, promoted, and sold the book, a 600-page compilation of the names and locations of "Burakumin" ghettos, the number of households, and the main occupations of the inhabitants, who were portrayed as militant troublemakers. The lists were purchased by about eighty companies, including heavyweights like Toyota, Nissan, Kubota, Daihatsu, and the Yasuda Trust Bank. (76)

The history of the Burakumin is just one example of the lasting impact of an ideology of marginalization in conjunction with institutional sources of socialization. When institutional and formal ideological practices of oppression have been banned, marginalization often continues through the informal interactions and prejudices of individuals.

Examining informal social relations is especially important for understanding AIDS activism. In attempting to explain the political response to AIDS, it may be easier to identify formal laws, rules, or institutional structures that prevented organizations and individuals from responding than the informal social practices that reinforce the exclusion of already marginal groups. The real work of marginalization, however, happens systematically through the daily actions of individuals, many of whom seem to be nice people who are simply doing their jobs and have no obvious plan to actively participate in the exclusion of certain groups. Thus we should be clear that intent or malice is not a necessary condition for marginalization to occur.[8] Take for instance, the informal social pressures faced by Billy in the opening narrative of chapter 1. The fear that family and friends might recognize him at a meeting or protest sponsored by the local AIDS or gay organization prohibited him from participating in activities that have direct relevance to his HIV status. The possible negative judgment of his family by those in his hometown community effectively disempowered Billy more than any formal rule might have. Whether through the words of the local minister or the actions of the community funeral director, these localized sites of marginalization often represent the intersecting point for normative, ideological, institutional, and social practices of marginalization. Only through identifying and examining the multiple sites and practices of marginalization can we begin to see how marginal groups view the world and how they react to the formal and informal rules that significantly structure the conditions of their existence.

Marginalization and Its Consequences

In response to processes of marginalization, groups develop strategies to address their needs and to challenge those structures that constrain their life choices. Many of these strategies focus on developing alternative resources, different ideological frameworks, and oppositional institutions and organizations. Because of the excluded or outsider status of marginal groups, the development and functioning of these alternative structures are usually grounded in the indigenous or communal relationships of marginal groups. As we might expect, the response to marginalization varies across groups. More importantly, it varies in response to the stage or pattern of exclusion that is most prominent. The next section examines four patterns of marginalization that characterize the evolution of such strategies encountered by African Americans. In this section I briefly explore the link between marginalization and the mobilization or resistance of marginal groups. Specifically, I focus on three consequences of marginalization which affect the political actions of these groups: (1) an altered world; (2) the development of indigenous organizations, information, and leaders; and (3) a comprehensive framing of mobilization.

ALTERED WORLDVIEW

Marginal groups, living most of their lives on the outside of the dominant society, are likely to develop an alternative or oppositional
worldview. In much the same way that ideologies provide the framework for interpreting and providing meaning to our daily interactions,
worldviews can be thought of as maps of our understanding of the
world, developing from a specific position or status in society (Luker
1984). In the case of marginal groups, a worldview develops from the
position of an outsider: one who is fully acquainted with the workings
of dominant society but denied access to full participation. When information is processed through such a framework, one comes to understand the central components of the dominant society, but usually
approaches its institutions, organizations, and leaders with distrust
and skepticism. In this way marginal group members recognize their
position: not fully outside, but marginal participants in the norms,
rules, and practices of dominant society (Scott 1990). In her book *Feminist Theory: From Margin to Center* (1984), bell hooks writes of marginality and its impact on how marginal group members "see reality":

> To be in the margin is to be part of the whole but outside the
> main body. As black Americans living in a small Kentucky
> town, the railroad tracks were a daily reminder of our margin-
> ality. Across those tracks were paved streets, restaurants we
> could not eat in and people we could not look directly in the
> face. Across those tracks was a world we could work in as
> maids, as janitors, as prostitutes as it was in a service capacity.
> We could enter that world but we could not live there. We had
> always to return to the margin, to cross the tracks, to shacks
> and abandoned houses on the edge of town.
>   There were laws to ensure our return. To not return was to
> risk being punished. Living as we did—on the edge—we de-
> veloped a particular way of seeing reality. We looked both
> from the outside in and from the inside out. We focused our
> attention on the center as well as on the margin. We under-
> stood both. This mode of seeing reminded us of the existence
> of a whole universe, a main body made up of both margin and
> center. Our survival depended on an ongoing public aware-
> ness of the separation between margin and center and an on-
> going private knowledge that we were a necessary vital part
> of that whole. (preface)

These feelings of alienation and distance result not from a one-time,
or single-domain, experience of marginalization, but instead are

rooted in a historical experience of exclusion across domains. Integral to understanding the consequences of marginalization, then, is the recognition that historical experiences of exclusion inform and influence the framework through which marginal groups currently view other groups, political issues, and their ability to mobilize around critical concerns. Gaventa (1980), in his work on quiescence in an Appalachian valley, emphasizes the importance of historical precedence in understanding the current behavior of communities. He argues that "power serves to create power":

> Powerlessness serves to re-enforce powerlessness. Power relationships, once established, are self-sustaining. Quiescence in the face of inequalities may be understood only in terms of the inertia of the situation. For this reason power in a given community can never be understood simply by observation at a given point in time. Historical investigation must occur to discover whether routines of non-conflict have been shaped, and, if so, how are they maintained. (255)

History provides the context in which issues are defined, interpreted, and pursued. In the case of AIDS activism, it would be difficult to understand the current mistrust of the medical establishment exhibited by black Americans without knowing the history of exploitation and blame that has been directed toward them under the guise of health and medicine. For instance, community members do not have to reach far back into their collective memory to recall the racist blame placed on them as the originators of diseases such as tuberculosis and syphilis (Hammonds 1998; McBride 1991). Even more ingrained in the minds of black Americans is the medical exploitation of black sharecroppers during the Tuskegee Syphilis Study (Jones 1981). Recently, early AIDS coverage through the mainstream media included a number of stories claiming that Africa, in particular the "African green monkey" or the "African swine," was the source of AIDS. Once again "the" black community, in its diasporic form, received blame for the creation and spread of a devastating disease: this time AIDS. Thus, living through a history of alienation and blame, marginal groups naturally develop a different analytical framework for evaluating their position in society—one that views as suspect the actions of and information from dominant groups and institutions and embraces those ideas and individuals seen as indigenous and authentic. I return to this topic in chapter 6.

INDIGENOUS INSTITUTIONS, INFORMATION, AND LEADERS

Possibly the most recognized consequence of marginalization is the limited material resources available to marginal groups. Marginal groups find themselves unable to accumulate the resources and skills that allow them to substantively participate in general quality-of-life decisions. Resource deficiency, as defined in this analysis, is recognized as being cumulative, extending across social, political, and economic domains. As Michael Parenti (1978) explains,

> Inequalities tend to be compounded for the haves as well as the have-nots. The possession of one power resource often creates opportunities to gain access to other resources, as when celebrity and money bring opportunities for political leadership. . . . [I]f indeed resources can be compounded, then they tend to be *cumulative* rather than noncumulative. Power resources are accumulated over time and are not up for grabs with each new issue. (76; emphasis in original)

Cumulative inequality thus assumes that outcomes in one domain are tied to the group's status in some other domain. For example, the economic marginalization of the majority of African Americans significantly affects the availability of resources necessary for the mobilization and participation of individual African Americans in political decisions where money plays a substantial role in determining who gets heard.[9] Groups unable to obtain resources and develop skills needed for basic organizing and education around issues find their chances for effective mobilization drastically diminished. The lack of access to institutional resources and information also affects the responsiveness of dominant groups and institutions. Thus, in conjunction with the resource-deficient state of marginal groups, their secondary or inferior status negatively affects the responsiveness of dominant institutions that control the distribution of information and resources needed by marginal group members.

Recognizing the inaccessibility of dominant systems, marginal groups often turn inward, redirecting their resources, trust, and loyalty toward community-based institutions and relationships that more directly address their needs. They rely upon indigenous organizations, leaders, networks, and norms to provide some version of the resources and information that are unavailable from dominant institutions and relationships. These indigenous structures and relationships provide not only material resources and information but also the sites and networks for developing the skills necessary for effective decision making and participation (Barkley Brown 1994).

The political activity of marginal groups, therefore, must be understood in a context in which indigenous sources of information and resources take on an expanded role in building a base for mobilization. Indigenous structures are a primary source for materials, skills, and cognitive resources needed for political activism. Marginal group members, who individually have little political power, are able to pool their resources and thus gain greater collective power. Central, then, to understanding the relationship between marginalization and resistance is a recognition of the role of indigenous institutions, information, and leaders in building a base for the development of political activism (Morris 1984).

Closely associated with the provision of indigenous resources for mobilization is the role that indigenous organizations, elites, and networks of communication play in structuring the political outlook and group consciousness of the community (Miller et al. 1981). Marginal group members, having been conditioned to look upon dominant institutions with distrust, turn instinctively to indigenous sources of information—community leaders, newspapers, organizations, social networks—for new ways to understand and process their experience. Such leaders and institutions can encourage group members to view their deprived social position as a question of political entitlement, providing the basis for mobilization. Richard Shingles, in his article "Black Consciousness and Political Participation" (1981), writes,

> The realization that the reason for black deprivation does not lie squarely on them has allowed many poor blacks to transfer the responsibility for poverty from themselves to society and to the most visible symbol of society, government. The result is a mentally healthier and politically more active black citizenry. (89)

Indigenous sources of information, from local newspapers to videos, music, and organizers speaking on street corners, are able to transform and redefine issues in ways that make mobilization more feasible. Further, information structured around the community and the specific conditions of marginal group members reduces information costs for marginal group members. Through indigenous sources of information, marginal group members begin to develop a political consciousness

that can potentially transform an alternative worldview into an oppositional ideology. Doug McAdam (1982), in his analysis of black political
mobilization, discusses the role indigenous structures play in creating
cognitive liberation among oppressed group members:

> The existent organizations of the minority community also
> figure prominently in the development of this insurgent con-
> sciousness, lending added significance to their role in the gen-
> eration of insurgency. . . . [T]he importance of indigenous or-
> ganizations stemmed, in part, from the fact that they afforded
> insurgents an established interaction network insuring the
> rapid and thorough diffusion of social insurgency throughout
> the minority community. (49)

Through formal and informal networks, marginal group members
learn which issues are important to the group. How group members
think about issues is often created, maintained, or challenged by indigenous sources of information, as constrained by the norms of the community (Cohen 1996a). Here, the political meaning of an issue is at
least minimally structured and communicated. Group members are
encouraged to think of issues in terms of the rights and entitlements
of the community, concepts that are more easily linked to group mobilization. Thus, being a segregated group promotes a process that ele-
vates the role of indigenous structures and provides the basis of group
consciousness needed for collective mobilization.

COMPREHENSIVE MOBILIZATION

A final consequence of marginalization manifests itself in the form and
breadth of political activity among marginalized communities. Experiences of severe deprivation and cumulative exclusion may lead marginal groups to specific types of political mobilization, where the strategies of resistance employed challenge the fundamental assumptions
of the political system beyond the boundaries of any specific grievance
or issue. Thus marginal groups, experiencing individual issues as tied
to the larger context in which their group is defined and exists, may
pursue strategies that confront the overall marginal status of the group.
Moreover, group members who view themselves as outside the dominant society may more willingly engage in nontraditional methods of
resistance toward perceived injustices. Finding it ineffective and irrelevant to delineate the boundaries of specific issues, they may instead
focus on strategies of resistance that are broad in their approach and

tied to the overall identity and condition of the group. In *City Trenches* (1981), Ira Katznelson argues that blacks in the 1960s, excluded from city decision making, waged campaigns of resistance that raised numerous issues confronting the marginal status of the community:

> For blacks, the invocation of any one issue—whether welfare, police, health care, housing, job discrimination, unemployment, or political underrepresentation—invoked all the others. The combination of being excluded from the system of city trenches and being preponderant in the secondary work force drove blacks to raise issues through different channels (or, in a real sense, nonchannels) from those that white ethnics used. These issues, though raised at the physical level of the community, exploded the community boundaries—they were not just about community control and neighborhood services, but also about wages and jobs and many other aspects of the black condition. (115)

In a stage of advanced marginalization, however, where significant numbers of African Americans have secured relative privilege and mobility through dominant institutions, there may be some reluctance on the part of privileged leaders and officials to make systemic or transformational demands of dominant groups and institutions. Having acquired some level of access to and control over state apparatuses and private resources, black officials may choose to distance themselves from stigmatizing and socially damaging issues as well as from segments of black communities that are in need of a more comprehensive or system-altering approach. Concern with protecting the respectability and legitimacy of the community, in particular of its middle-class members, may lead to conflict within marginal groups over which issues to embrace and which strategies to pursue. The next section explores this topic more fully.

Patterns of Marginalization

As stated earlier, marginalization takes many different forms. In this section I sketch four general patterns of marginalization, which may overlap: categorical, integrative, advanced, and secondary. Paying close attention to the latter two, I briefly detail these four patterns to highlight the role that varying processes of marginalization can play in exaggerating and manipulating differences within marginal groups. In particular, I am interested in the way indigenous leaders and organizations are positioned relative to dominant structures as patterns of exclusion change. I contend that African-American communities currently find themselves in a state of advanced marginalization, where stratification and cross-cutting issues increasingly define the political landscape. In such a state, traditional linked-fate approaches to black politics may be limited by the diverging interests and identities of group members. Furthermore, as traditional black leaders perceive certain stigmatized segments of African-American communities as threatening the progress, via respectability, of the group as well as their own personal mobility, indigenous processes of distance and exclusion may increasingly come to characterize public politics in black communities. I outline these four patterns of marginalization, therefore, in an attempt to understand the evolving configurations of power, leadership, and politics in black communities.

I offer two final points of clarification. While the theory of marginalization developed in this chapter is a general model applicable to the conditions of numerous oppressed groups, the examples in this section are drawn specifically from the experiences of African Americans. Thus, these four categories are not the only patterns of marginalization which might be identified. Second, patterns of marginalization change over time in response to both resistance on the part of excluded groups as well as the evolving and diversified interests of both marginal and dominant group members. Thus, as discussed earlier, the relationship between power and resistance as it has existed and continues to exist between marginal and dominant groups as well as *among* marginal group members, is both dialectical and dynamic in nature, evolving in response to different political, economic, and social practices and conditions. Thus each pattern detailed below encompasses multiple and changing configurations of identities, ideologies, institutions, and social practices for the purpose of marginalization.

Categorical Marginalization

Categorical strategies of marginalization include practices that seek to exclude an entire class or group of people from any central control over dominant resources and institutions. This form of marginalization deploys numerous practices involving identities, institutions, ideologies, and social relationships to enforce the complete exclusion of some group. A central component of successful categorical marginalization involves the manipulation of ideological concepts—norms, values, and attitudes—in an attempt to explain and legitimize the exclusion of, and developing domination over, marginal communities. Such strategies are mobilized when some belief, characteristic, or behavior shared by all targeted group members (e.g., race, gender, religion, or sexual preference) is used to signal the "inherent" inferiority or "natural" deviance of a group, promoting the idea that these individuals are somehow deserving of their marginal or secondary status. Secondary status does not, however, mean the negation of interaction between marginal and dominant group members. In fact, the successful implementation of categorical marginalization often necessitates some form of daily observation and direct regulation of marginal group members by the less privileged of dominant groups. It is, however, the categorical exclusion of the entire group, making indigenous differences largely inconsequential, that defines this pattern of marginalization.

In the history of African Americans the "peculiar institution" of slavery most clearly demonstrates the categorical exclusion of black Americans from any formal control over dominant resources and institutions. Slavery, as experienced in the United States, epitomized an institution based on, structured around, and maintained by marginalizing practices, insisting, in this case, on the complete domination and dehumanization of black Africans brought to this country. Ideological practices of marginalization defined black Africans as inferior, less than human, and animal-like, arguing that such status was signaled by their black skin. This discourse sought to justify the exploitation and oppression of all blacks as southern and northern whites sought economic profits. The preservation of this economic structure, however, served as the catalyst not only for the development of a separate and distinguishable ideology of race as it applied to black Africans, but also for institutional and social practices guaranteeing the total oppression of enslaved black people.

The twenty black Africans who stepped ashore at Jamestown in 1619 were not legally defined as slaves; their status was similar to that of white indentured servants (Higginbotham 1978; Jordan 1968). Not until 1661 would Virginia "legally" establish slavery. Within this time span Virginia's colonists would come to recognize that neither Native Americans nor white indentured servants could satisfy their need for cheap, accessible labor. To fulfill this need, they would eventually adopt a model seen in the Caribbean—that of enslaving black Africans for the provision of labor and profit. Fundamental to the success and longevity of this system of slavery was the eventual development of a marginalizing ideology. Barbara Fields (1982), writes that the practice of enslavement had "lasted for some time before race became its predominant justification" (152). The questioning of the morality of slavery by significant numbers of the white populace, she argues, motivated the development of an ideology of race supportive of slavery. A justification of slavery, therefore, had to explain what was different about Africans that necessitated their complete domination during an "age of freedom." This ideology based its reasoning on their "non-Christian, hedonistic and inferior ways," corresponding, of course, to their black skin. Thus the ideology of the "other," associated with an observable ascriptive trait, allowed Africans to be controlled and contained under a harsh and debilitating system of profit and oppression.

Southern slavery, implemented through the oppressive and severe actions of whites, was structurally codified through elaborate legal statutes devised to regulate blacks in the colonies. The Slave Codes, a legal attempt to restrict and control the actions and thoughts of every enslaved black person, provided the institutional backbone of slavery. These codes represented the formal institutional practices that reinforced the marginal status of black slaves and supported the status of dominant whites, in particular white planters. Historian Eugene D. Genovese (1976) discusses the use of such laws to ensure the relative positions of both blacks and whites:

> In southern slave society, as in other societies, the law, even narrowly defined as a system of institutionalized jurisprudence, constituted a principal vehicle for the hegemony of the ruling class. . . .
> The laws of Virginia and Maryland, as well as those of the colonies to the south, increasingly gave masters the widest possible power over the slaves and also, through prohibition of interracial marriage and the general restriction of slave status to nonwhites, codified and simultaneously preached white supremacy. (26–33)

The Slave Codes ensured that the marginalization of enslaved black people would govern nearly every domain of their lives. They prohibited blacks from having access to courts and thus to due process. They denied blacks the right to own property; they prohibited their assembly without the presence of a white person; generally they restricted the actions and interactions of blacks throughout the South.

Finally, whites, in addition to imposing their domination through legislative, ideological, or legal strategies, relied on and emphasized the emotional and physical torture of black bodies to enforce marginalization. The social degradation that black women, men, and children encountered during (and after) slavery has been documented by numerous historians (Blassingame 1972; Jordan 1968; Bennett, Jr. 1966). The disruption of family, friends, and community relationships through the buying and selling of black people was also an important factor in the categorical marginalization of blacks. However, the cruelty of lynching, rape, beating, burning, and other forms of physical brutality as complementary practices of marginalization may be the distinguishing feature of southern slave society.

Categorical marginalization, whether evidenced through southern slavery or other periods such as the Jim Crow era, attempts to implement a system of total disempowerment and control. It is important to recognize, however, that marginalization not only imposes barriers but motivates resistance. Just as a shared characteristic can be used as a basis of exclusion, this same characteristic or shared experience of marginalization can be used as a unifying element among marginal group members. The group cohesion that results from such extreme isolation, segregation, and exploitation can be an important element in successful strategies of resistance. Thus, categorical exclusion from dominant society often facilitates the development of indigenous networks and institutions mentioned earlier. With no possibility of, nor interest in, participating in an oppressive, unresponsive, dominant society, marginal group members work toward the development of their own indigenous community—"a nation within a nation." Here, in a segregated and hidden indigenous community, acts of resistance often develop and find support.

INTEGRATIVE MARGINALIZATION

Practices of integrative marginalization work to maintain the relative power of dominant groups over marginal communities. Instead of the all-encompassing control over the quality of life and life choices of marginal group members exerted by categorical marginalization, integrative strategies provide control by unequivocally regulating the *majority* of marginal community members while allowing *a chosen few* to have limited access to dominant institutions and resources. I want to be clear on a couple of points. First, access to dominant resources does not mean, for instance, the use of black workers during a labor shortage. I am referring, instead, to those few individuals who gain, either through the indigenous resources they control or through their relationships with dominant group members, special status among dominant group members and in dominant institutions. Second, access to dominant resources and the limited participation in decision-making achieved through practices of integrative marginalization does not mean that these marginal group members are viewed as equals within dominant communities. More privileged marginal group members, while holding a unique position in and outside of the marginal community, are still understood as inferior or subordinate to most dominant group members. Those provided access are expected to live out, in some sense, a "double status." We might call their social location a more privileged subordination, with great range in the degree of subordination. Katzman (1973), writing of the black elite in Detroit before the turn of the twentieth century, notes, "The city's upper-class blacks were a marginal group whose relative position in the social system was at some point between the white caste and the general black caste. Their life style and values incorporated characteristics of each of the two distinct castes, and they interacted with both groups" (83).

Practices of integrative marginalization often develop in conjunction with, or in response to, deficient or ineffectual strategies of categorical marginalization. When categorical marginalization is no longer feasible or can only be imposed on a segment of the marginal group, due in part to the resistance and resources of some marginal group members as well as the actions, beliefs, and needs of dominant group members, then a strategy of integrative marginalization may evolve. Again, the access provided to certain marginal group members is both limited and expected to serve the needs of dominant group members while tangentially providing benefits and status to selected marginal group members. For example, dominant groups wishing to maximize the benefits of regulating marginal groups while minimizing the threat that results from direct control may attempt to create a stratum of marginal group members who can act as a buffer or bridge between marginal and dominant groups. To facilitate the development of this stratum, dominant elites provide schooling, jobs, and housing to certain members of the marginal group. In return, the new stratum of integrative indigenous elites are expected to promote (and enforce) compromise and conformity to dominant norms within marginal communities.

Integrative marginalization alters dominant ideological practices previously used to justify the total exclusion of marginal group members in order to account for the limited integration of some oppressed group members. The adjustments made in the ideological explanations of exclusion stress the ability of certain oppressed group members to assimilate and take on dominant group characteristics and values. The success of their assimilation is rationalized as being facilitated by biological, social, or material characteristics differentiating them from the majority of marginal group members.

Modifications in the original dominant ideological discourse also have internal consequences, illuminating issues of stratification in marginal communities along such lines as class, education, gender, and skin color. Such differences, which are always a part of marginal communities, are used to determine and justify the existence of an indigenous elite. While these distinctions are recognized and affect one's status within the segregated spaces of marginal life, under categorical marginalization they have little opportunity for *formal* articulation. Integrative marginalization, however, rewards marginal group leaders willing to conform to and replicate dominant hierarchies of power with limited access to dominant institutions, resources, and social networks. Through their actions and writings, many of these leaders espouse the norms and values of dominant whites, promoting what has been labeled a self-help ideology. Kevin Gaines (1996) writes in *Uplifting the Race*, "Elite African Americans were replicating, even as they contested, the uniquely American racial fictions upon which liberal conceptions of social reality and 'equality' were founded" (3).

As Gaines notes, the access that integrative marginalization provides is not without contradictions. For example, those allowed mobility are most often those who already have some grasp on power within marginal groups. The internal power or resources controlled by indigenous elites may either be used to mobilize marginal group members against dominant forces or directed internally toward the regulation and control of marginal group members. Thus it is in the interest of dominant groups to provide incentives such as limited mobility to coax or force indigenous leaders down a *general path of collaboration*.[10] I deliberately use the phrase "a general path of collaboration" because no single strategy is entirely monolithic. Some indigenous leaders, while generally choosing strategies of cooperation with dominant groups, may on occasion resort to more confrontational practices of resistance, mirroring dominant groups that utilize both physical terror and limited mobility as complementary practices of marginalization.

E. Franklin Frazier, in his book *Black Bourgeoisie* (1957), details one process of integrative marginalization in his description of the development of a black, upper-class elite during the mid-to-late nineteenth century. Living under a system of categorical marginalization in the slave-owning South, free blacks in the North and the South developed separate segregated communities. In these indigenous spaces, consti- tuted most often in southern and northern cities, a black or "mulatto" elite developed. These elites gained their status primarily through a mixed family ancestry which included white parentage, as well as by their sporadic interactions and relationships with dominant whites. Such interactions often came in the form of personal service to white clients through such activities as barbering. This small status group of mulatto elites was often set apart from the rest of the black community, choosing to live and socialize among themselves. Frazier writes, "In this segregated world, especially in cities, a class structure slowly emerged which was based upon social distinctions such as education and conventional behavior, rather than upon occupation and income. At the top of the social pyramid there was a small upper class. The superior status of this class was due chiefly to its differentiation from the great masses of the Negro population because of a family heritage which resulted partly from its mixed ancestry" (23). Landry (1987) fur- ther informs us that these elites embraced their special and differenti- ated status, creating exclusive clubs, churches, schools, and housing arrangements (34). "Whenever possible, black elite families sought to live in white neighborhoods, if only on a single block of a street occu- pied by whites" (33).

In contrast to the few mulatto elites, Landry details the development of a true middle class in early twentieth-century, segregated black com- munities. This leadership or elite stratum arose largely through its po sition in and control over the indigenous institutions and resources of segregated black communities. Landry (1987) underscores this point, writing that "beginning around the turn of the century, an emerging new elite began to replace the old elite within the black community. What especially distinguished this new elite of realtors, insurance agents, undertakers, bankers, newspaper editors, politicians, and pro- fessionals was their orientation to, and dependency on, black commu- nity patronage" (39). Thus, this elite's location in and among the major- ity of black people established and facilitated its power. This is not to suggest that this stratum of black community members was not also interested in distinguishing themselves from the masses of people. In fact, as Landry notes, they too set up their own exclusive social clubs as well as benevolent societies geared toward educating and regulating working-class and poor blacks. However, it was their control over the indigenous resources and structures of marginalized black communities that secured their position as leaders both in and outside of the group. "Middle-class blacks also provided the leadership needed by the black community. In the North, some members of the black middle class were elected to public office from black districts and were able to represent the interests of blacks in a formal capacity. . . . Theirs was a moderate orientation, satisfied with a gradualist approach through an appeal to the goodwill and reason of whites" (66).

Indicative of the contradiction inherent in patterns of integrative marginalization were the dual goals of personal *and* community advancement that motivated the actions of this elite stratum. For example, some scholars have suggested that black integrative elites promoted a vision and rhetoric of self-help primarily to advance their own status. Gaines (1996), however, contends that it was not purely out of greed or ambition that black elites pursued a strategy of "uplift." He argues that many of these individuals believed that a framework of uplift was in fact in the best interests of the community, since it would allow group members to reconstruct a "positive black identity":

> It is crucial to realize that uplift ideology was not simply a matter of educated African Americans' wanting to be white. . . . On the contrary, uplift, among its other connotations, also represented the struggle for a positive black identity in a deeply racist society, turning the pejorative designation of race into a source of dignity and self-affirmation through an ideology of class differentiation, self-help, and interdependence. What was problematic about this was not African Americans' quite understandable desire for dignity, security, and social mobility. Rather, the difficulty stemmed from the construction of class differences through racial and cultural hierarchies that had little to do with the material conditions of African Americans, and less to do with the discrimination they faced in a racially stratified southern labor market, with the active complicity of the state and opinion-making apparatuses of civil society. (3)

Whatever the contradictions faced by these black elites, the access they secured under integrative marginalization resulted largely from their position of leadership in structured, indigenous black communities. From their positions of power in black institutions, this stratum of upper-class and middle-class blacks performed their role as internal regulators of the majority of poor black people. Although this delineation is just one example of the process of integrative marginalization, it does begin to underscore the substantial and often decisive role that indigenous structures, leaders, and resources play in shaping what we only later come to recognize and understand as the politics of black communities, especially when the society is segregated.

ADVANCED MARGINALIZATION

The pattern of marginalization I call advanced marginalization focuses on the heightened stratification of marginal communities. In response to continued resistance on the part of marginal groups, and occasional resistance from segments of dominant groups, the display of power under advanced marginalization looks radically different from other patterns of exclusion. Advanced marginalization signals at the very least a symbolic opening of dominant society. Where once formal exclusion was the law of the land, legal segregation and institutional subordination of marginal groups is removed under advanced marginalization. Ideological myths justifying the exclusion and oppression of marginal communities are also modified (at least publicly), emphasizing instead the *inclusion* and *legitimization* of marginal group members, especially those conforming to dominant norms and behavior. Further, social practices of segregation, intimidation, and physical violence are also professed to have been abandoned in favor of a more just system in which everyone has the same rights and responsibilities. On its surface advanced marginalization should be understood as a truly progressive step toward eradicating the inequality and oppression that have defined the histories of marginal and dominant groups.

Looking below the surface, however, we find that advanced marginalization is fraught with contradictions, manipulating, in particular, the social cleavages that exist within marginal groups. For example, under advanced marginalization far more integration and access to dominant resources are made available to significantly more marginal group members. Dominant elites, refiguring the process of regulation of and service to marginal groups, come to depend on a stratum of marginal group members expected or allowed to staff those dominant institutions that directly affect the quality of life of the most vulnerable in marginal communities. And while the increased mobility available to some marginal group members is a positive development, indigenous leaders risk assimilation or cooptation through such a process. Thus we may witness a gradual transformation in the purpose and goals of many of the most successful indigenous organizations and institutions in marginal communities. Largely due to their access to dominant resources and networks, these new strata of indigenous leaders and bureaucrats become connected to and identified with dominant groups, institutions, and ideologies. Further, as indigenous institutions increasingly involve themselves in the political, social, and economic activities of dominant groups, the goal of maintaining and expanding integration into the dominant society often becomes the primary concern of such institutions. This may come at the expense of more radical transformation and redistribution of dominant institutional resources.

Advanced marginalization also entails expectations of inclusion. New ideological narratives that emerge under advanced marginalization highlight the formal equality achieved by marginal groups, while actual inequalities are overlooked and avoided. Marginal groups looking for formal recognition and rights under advanced marginalization must embrace a model of inclusion premised on the idea that formal rights are to be granted only to those who demonstrate adherence to dominant norms of work, love, and social interaction. Marginal group members are forced, therefore, to demonstrate their normativity and legitimacy through the class privilege they acquire, through the attitudes and behavior they exhibit, and through the dominant institutions in which they operate.

As marginal group leaders pursue the goal of expanded access and integration, part of their strategy may become portraying their community as representing and adhering to values and norms as defined by dominant groups.[11] It is difficult for these indigenous leaders, who gain part of their authority and legitimacy by conforming to dominant values, to continually and actively challenge those same norms and values as unfair criteria upon which to judge individual merit. Thus, by accepting the dominant discourse that defines what is good, normal, and acceptable, stratification among marginal group members is transformed into an indigenous process of marginalization targeting the most vulnerable in the group. This process, which I label *secondary marginalization*, is explored in the next section.

Again, while there is clear evidence of the substantial progress of certain marginal group members under advanced marginalization, also central to this pattern of exclusion is the conflicting nature of mobility and power. For example, in the case of African Americans, many would contend that the late 1950s and early 1960s signaled the beginning of a period of substantial advancements. During these years, for instance, we witnessed the passage of the 1964 Civil Rights Act and the Voting Rights Act of 1965. This legislation paved the way for the election of black representatives across the political spectrum, including the election of black mayors in many of the nation's largest cities. It was also during this era that the development of a new and expanded black middle class took hold (Landry 1987). The economic prosperity of the 1960s and new legal guarantees against job discrimination combined to produce a doubling in the percentage of middle-class blacks between 1960 and 1970. Landry (1987) reports that the black middle class grew "from about 1 in 8 to 1 out of 4 black workers . . . the gain experienced by the black middle class during the 1960s exceeded their total increase during the previous fifty years" (70). Additionally, an ideological shift in whites' attitudes toward African Americans was said to be evidenced in public opinion polls and political discourse during this period as whites became more tolerant and accepting (Schuman, Steeh, and Bobo 1985).

Despite such strong indicators of the apparent progress of African Americans, additional measures suggest that the advancement of African Americans has been limited and contradictory, as we might expect under advanced marginalization. For example, in the area of income distribution, some black families have benefited from the greater access afforded under advanced marginalization, while other sectors of black communities have sunk further into poverty, part of an expendable surplus labor population. Using 1992 dollars, the number of black families making over $50,000 has grown from 10.2 percent in 1970 to 16 percent in 1992 (still less than half the percentage of white families in this same category in 1992, which was 37.5 percent), while the number of working-class black families has decreased over those same years. In 1970, for instance, 17.4 percent of black families made $25,000 to $35,000 per year, while an additional 24.1 percent made between $15,000 and $25,000. In 1992 the percentage of black families in both of those categories had decreased to 13 percent ($25,000 to $35,000) and 18.8 percent ($15,000 to $25,000). Undoubtedly, some of those families moved into higher income brackets; however, many also dropped into poverty. So, unlike the pattern to be found among whites, where the number of families making under $15,000 fell between 1970 and 1992 from 14.2 percent to 12.3 percent, the number of black families in this same category increased during this period. In 1970, 34.3 percent of black families (one out of three) made under $15,000. In 1992 that number had increased to 38.2 percent of all black families (Hacker 1995, 104).

Jennifer L. Hochschild (1995), referencing slightly different numbers, also discusses the increasing polarization evident in black communities:

> [F]irst, rich blacks have always held a larger share of their race's income than have rich whites, and poor blacks have always held a smaller share of their race's income than have poor whites. Second, the disparities within both races are increasing. Third, and most important here, the income disparity among blacks is increasing at a faster rate. . . . By 1992 the poorest quintile [of African Americans] had lost 30 percent of its meager 1947 income, and the richest quintile had gained 8 percent over its comparatively high 1947 income.
>
> Other indicators of well-being show the same pattern of growing polarization between well-off and poor African Americans. Consider housing, for example: in 1980 the index of residential dissimilarity between classes was higher among blacks (.50) than among whites (.39). Residential separation by class had increased slightly among African Americans during the 1970s, even though it decreased slightly among whites, Asians, and Latinos. Or jobs: white employers penalize black applicants for low-skill jobs for being black even after all of their specific traits are taken into consideration, but they reward black applicants for high-skill jobs for being black. . . .
>
> African Americans are becoming more disparate politically and demographically as well as economically and socially. (48–50)

While I cannot agree with Hochschild that highly skilled black applicants are rewarded for being black, I do concur with her on the increasing polarization evident in black communities. Again, the contradictory nature of social mobility is an essential component of the advanced marginalization of African Americans. Roger Waldinger, in *Still the Promised City?* (1996), discusses the limits to the increased mobility available to some African Americans, using New York as his case study:

> In the 1970s and 1980s, black New Yorkers built up and consolidated the niche they had earlier established in government work. Public sector employment offered numerous advantages. . . . But convergence on government employment had

the corollary effect of heightening the skill thresholds of the chief black economic base. To be sure connections helped in gaining access to municipal jobs. . . . However, civil service positions held promise only to those members of the community with the skills, experience, and credentials that government required—qualities not shared by the many African-American New Yorkers who have found themselves at economic risk. (5–6)

Waldinger continues, more explicitly detailing the different paths of opportunity and despair experienced by the middle-class and poor segments of New York's African-American communities under conditions that indicate advanced marginalization:

While the black middle class largely works in government, the black poor are its dependents. The interests of civil servants, regardless of ethnic stripe, leads them to push for higher wages and ever greater public jobs. The record shows that government has been extraordinarily responsive to these demands. Civil servants found that the 1980s were good times indeed, reaping more than half of the considerable increases in municipal expenditures that occurred during the 1983–1989 period. By contrast, the poor did a good deal less well, with public assistance payments actually declining and much of the increase in redistributive spending going to organizations designed to serve the poor. . . .

Public sector concentration thus pits the interests of the city's black middle class *against* the interests of its black poor. (252; emphasis added)

Waldinger's account of the tension that exists between the black middle class and the black poor in New York seems especially illustrative of the larger inherent tensions regarding social mobility and internal stratification experienced by all black communities under advanced marginalization.

In addition to the contradictory nature of black progress, there is also widespread disagreement among researchers over how to interpret increased tolerance in white racial attitudes evident under advanced marginalization. Some scholars suggest that the changes measured represent real progress in race relations that can be evidenced in the everyday lives of white and black Americans (Sniderman and Hagen 1985). Others, however, argue that the progressive trends of tolerance may instead represent a changing norm, one that has diminished the acceptance of public statements of racism and intolerance

(Sears 1988). Still other scholars hold a moderate position, suggesting that, while there has been real movement in certain racial attitudes of white Americans, race and black identification in particular still have significant negative meaning for many white Americans. The National Research Council, in its published work on the status of black Americans, reports as follows:

> The foremost conclusion [in their section on racial attitudes] is that race still matters greatly in the United States. Much of the evidence reviewed in this report indicates widespread attitudes of societal racism. This is not to gainsay convincing evidence of improving racial attitudes: a transformation of basic racial norms in the United States is the clearest finding from the survey trend data. . . . There are reasons to believe that this change extends beyond mere lip service or token and transitory forms of social contact. . . .
>
> Yet, a reluctance to live in racially mixed neighborhoods and interpersonal awkwardness and racially differential treatment across many situations all point to the persistence of race as an important factor in American society. (Jaynes and Williams 1989, 155)

Kinder and Sanders, in *Divided by Color* (1996), also comment on the continued and significant differences in public opinion to be found between black and white Americans around issues of race:

> To us, the most arresting feature of public opinion on race remains how emphatically black and white Americans disagree with each other. . . . Whites tend to think that racial discrimination is no longer a problem, that prejudice is withering away, that the real worry these days is reverse discrimination, penalizing innocent whites for the sins of the distant past. Meanwhile, blacks see racial discrimination as ubiquitous; they think of prejudice as a plague; they say that racial discrimination, not affirmative action, is still the rule in American society. . . .
>
> The racial divide is as apparent among ordinary citizens as it is among elites. It is not a mask for class differences: it is rooted in race itself, in differences of history. (287)

As noted earlier, continuing research on racial attitudes among white Americans suggests that while whites may be more publicly accepting of blacks, they still hold stereotypes of blacks that contradict dominant norms of hard work, intelligence, and self-sufficiency (Gilens 1996; Bobo and Kluegel 1991). These stereotypic images of black-

ness, rooted in historical ideologies of marginalization, continue to affect the economic and political power of blacks. Thus, although most
of the racially explicit legal barriers constraining the life choices of
African Americans have been removed, black Americans in 1993 suffered more than double the unemployment of their white counterparts;
black households, in 1992, had per capita incomes averaging 54 percent
of those of white households; black families in 1992 were more than
four times more likely to be in poverty than were white families; the
percentage of whites who had completed four or more years of college
was double that for blacks in 1993 (26 to 12 percent); the black infant
mortality rate in 1991 was 2.21 times that for whites; the expected life
span for black Americans in 1993 continued to be less than that for
whites (70.2 to 76.6); and residential segregation is still a fact of life for
all classes of black Americans and is more common for blacks than
for other marginal groups such as Asians and Latinos (Hacker 1995;
Farley 1989).

Despite the individual success of some African Americans, black
men and women as a group still find that race continues to significantly affect the quality of their lives. However, at the same time that
certain group members struggle to maintain their economic and social
position, a stratum of indigenous elites has emerged with unprecedented access to and ability within dominant institutions. These marginal group members have acquired such relative privilege in part
because of their connection to and authority within marginal communities. In a changing world where demographic characteristics are
evolving in conjunction with economic and political changes, privileged marginal group members, claiming authenticity within marginal
communities as well as familiarity with dominant practices, find themselves positioned as necessary components for the continued functioning of dominant institutions. They are the diversified workforce touted
by private businesses and institutions such as IBM and Harvard. They
are the new black police recruits in urban cities such as New York and
Los Angeles. They are the case workers helping to implement workfare
in inner cities across the country. Thus, marginal group members
under advanced marginalization are provided mobility, but in return
they are expected to police, both literally and figuratively, the most
resource-poor and alienated of their communities. In this sense, advanced patterns of marginalization should not be understood as the
final breakdown of systematic exclusion, but instead as a process of
further refining the mechanisms of power.

SECONDARY MARGINALIZATION

Traditionally, when researchers have included African Americans or black politics in their scholarly investigations, they have examined the struggles over the regulation or control of marginal group members by outside dominant sources—in an "us versus them" framework (Kinder and Sanders 1996; Hacker 1995; Myrdal 1944). However, scholars more intimately familiar with black communities know that the power to deny group rights, define group membership, and regulate group behavior is not exercised only by dominant sources (Reed 1994; Higginbotham 1993; Drake and Cayton 1993). Secondary processes of marginalization can be exercised by the more privileged members of marginal groups, as the "management" of marginal group members is negotiated daily by those they would call their own.

The exercise of power by relatively more privileged marginal group members over others in their community is not a new phenomenon. In the past, these power relationships were generally predicated on the exclusion or segregation of marginal groups from dominant society. Today, in contrast, these relations are based to varying degrees on more privileged marginal group members' access to and mobility within dominant groups and institutions. Thus, as dominant players attempt to remove themselves or are removed from the direct regulation of marginal communities, newly elected officials, traditional leaders, public intellectuals, and other members of marginal groups are *given* or *take on* the role (and some of the power) of policing their community.

I use the term *policing* here to mean the regulation and management of the behavior, attitudes, and more important, the public image of the group (Carby 1992). The indigenous construction and policing of group identity and membership serves as the site for local power struggles within the pattern of secondary marginalization. As I stated earlier, marginal communities faced with dominant definitions of themselves as inferior and "other" construct an indigenous and often oppositional group identity—redefining themselves for their group members and the larger public. These attempts at redefinition highlight the characteristics and contributions of marginal group members thought to be positive or in accord with dominant values. Through this process of demonstrating their "just as good as you" qualities, working-class, middle-class, and generally more privileged members of marginal communities build what Bourdieu (1986) has called the cultural capital of the group.

For example, in the case of African Americans, systematic degradation, stereotyping, and stigmatization have all but dictated that attempts at incorporation, integration, and assimilation on the part of
black people generally include some degree of proving themselves to
be "just as nice as those white folks." Thus leaders, organizations, and
institutions in black communities have consistently attempted to redefine and indigenously construct a new public image or understanding
of what blackness would mean. This process of reconstructing or (im)-
proving blackness involves not only a reliance on the self-regulation
of individual black people, but also includes significant indigenous
policing of black group members.

The writings of academics consistently refer to the black middle
class as an example for and regulator of appropriate behavior by the
black masses. Hazel Carby (1992) discusses the moral panic and threat
to the collective respectability of black communities attributed to uncontrolled, migrating black women that generated a system of indigenous policing by black institutions and organizations during periods
of northern migration:

> The need to police and discipline the behavior of black women
> in cities, however, was not only a premise of white agencies
> and institutions but also a perception of black institutions and
> organizations, and the black middle class. The moral panic
> about the urban presence of apparently uncontrolled black
> women was symptomatic of and referenced aspects of the
> more general crises of social displacement and dislocation that
> were caused by migration. White and black intellectuals used
> and elaborated this discourse so that when they referred to
> the association between black women and vice, or immoral
> behavior, their references carried connotations of other crises
> of the black urban environment. Thus the migrating black
> woman could be variously situated as a threat to the progress
> of the race; as a threat to the establishment of a respectable
> urban black middle class; as a threat to congenial black and
> white middle-class relations; and as a threat to the formation
> of black masculinity in an urban environment. (741)

As Carby demonstrates, the regulation of the black masses was often
pursued not only by individuals, but also by an extensive network of
community groups and organizations. James R. Grossman (1989) details how the Urban League in conjunction with black and white institutions worked to help black migrants "adjust" to urban standards
of behavior.

> The Urban League and the *Defender,* assisted by the YMCA,
> the larger churches, and a corps of volunteers, fashioned a va-
> riety of initiatives designed to help—and pressure—the new-
> comers to adjust not only to industrial work, but to urban life,
> northern racial patterns, and behavior that would enhance the
> reputation of blacks in the larger (white) community.... The
> Urban League, through such activities as "Stranger Meetings,"
> leafleting, and door-to-door visits, advised newcomers on
> their duties as citizens: cleanliness, sobriety, thrift, efficiency,
> and respectable, restrained behavior in public places.... Un-
> der the tutelage of the respectable citizens of black Chicago,
> migrants were to become urbanized, northernized, and indis-
> tinguishable from others of their race. At the very least, they
> would learn to be as inconspicuous as possible. (145–46)

Evelyn Brooks Higginbotham, in *Righteous Discontent* (1993), also details how middle-class and working-class black women engaged in a
"politics of respectability" through the black Baptist church club movement. She emphasizes how for these black women the regulation of individual behavior was a strategy for refuting the racist stereotypes that
shaped their lives:

> Respectability demanded that every individual in the black
> community assume responsibility for behavioral self-
> regulation and self-improvement along moral, educational,
> and economic lines. The goal was to distance oneself as far as
> possible from images perpetuated by racist stereotypes. Indi-
> vidual behavior, the black Baptist women contended, deter-
> mined the collective fate of African Americans.... There could
> be no transgression of society's norms. From the public spaces
> of trains and streets to the private spaces of their individual
> homes, the behavior of blacks was perceived as ever visible to
> the white gaze. (198)

It is important to remember when considering the response to AIDS
in African-American communities that a tradition of indigenous policing has constantly sought to manage what would be represented as
the public image of black people. As mentioned earlier, integral to such
public representations has been the domain of sexuality. Community
leaders and organizations, fighting for equal rights, equal access, and
full recognition as citizens, have struggled to "clean up" the image of
sexuality in black communities. Often, as numerous black feminist
scholars such as Evelyn Higginbotham (1992) and Evelynn Hammonds
(1997) have argued, this has meant silence around the topic of sexual-

ity, especially for black women, even when discussion is needed concerning crises such as HIV and AIDS.

Cornel West (1993) in *Race Matters* also discusses the unwillingness of most black institutions to engage in open discussions of sexuality in black communities:

> But these grand yet flawed black institutions refused to engage one fundamental issue: *black sexuality.* . . .
>
> Why was this so? Primarily because these black institutions put a premium on black survival in America. And black survival required accommodation with and acceptance from white America. Accommodation avoids any sustained association with the subversive and transgressive—be it communism or miscegenation. . . . And acceptance meant that only "good" negroes would thrive—especially those who left black sexuality at the door when they "entered" and "arrived." In short, struggling black institutions made a Faustian pact with white America: avoid any substantive engagement with black sexuality and your survival on the margins of American society is, at least, possible. (86)

Individuals who were (and are) thought to fulfill stereotypes of black sexuality as something deviant or "other" often had (and have) their morality questioned by leading institutions in black communities. For instance, sexuality thought to stand outside the Christian mores as set down by the black church was constructed and interpreted as an indication of the moral character of individuals and their families, as well as an embarrassment to the collective consciousness and cultural capital of the black community. Higginbotham (1993) notes, "In 1914, the church minutes of Shiloh Baptist Church in Washington, DC reveal that individuals caught dancing, imbibing alcoholic beverages, or engaging in other 'improper' behavior were literally delivered a summons to come before the church for censure" (201).

While the examples listed above may seem dated, we need only look around today to see the great efforts of many black leaders and academics to distance themselves from those perceived to participate in "inappropriate immoral sexual behavior." We see this not only in the absence of any sustained writing on black lesbians and gay men by black authors and academics, but in the proliferation of writing and policy attacks on the "inappropriate" and "carefree" sexuality of those labeled the "underclass," and more specifically black women on welfare (Wilson 1987; Reed 1991; Gates 1992). Keith Boykin, former director of the National Black Lesbian and Gay Leadership Forum, argues that policing has very real current consequences. He suggests that concern with the public image of black communities has slowed and often made ineffective the response to AIDS in black communities:

> I think what may be going on is that we have a tendency in our communities to want to impress other people or to live up to the expectations of other people. We therefore don't acknowledge the real problems we have in our communities at least not publicly. We don't want to deal with HIV and AIDS issues because the two principle groups of people affected by it in our country are IV drug users and homosexuals. And, of course, we don't want to talk about the fact that we have homosexuals in the black community. We don't want to talk about IV drug use problems in the community because we expect it to reinforce the perception that all black people are drug addicts and not productive working people.... I don't know how conscious it is—the idea that I don't want white people to know that we have IV drug users in our community. I do think that it is something that is eventually, subconsciously, ingrained into us as part of our identity.[12]

At the root of the process of policing is the idea that black communities can reconstruct themselves for the white gaze, formulating their own indigenous definition of blackness. These internally created, community-based definitions of identity, in this case blackness, center not merely on easily identifiable physical characteristics, but also use moralistic and character evaluations to appraise membership. While building on dominant ideas or definitions of who *is* black, indigenous definitions of blackness employ a more expansive, but at the same time often less inclusive, understanding of black group identity. Group members employ a "calculus" of indigenous membership, which can include an assessment of personal or moral worth, such as an individual's contribution to the community, adherence to community norms and values, or faithfulness to perceived, rewritten, or in some cases newly created African traditions. Thus indigenously constructed definitions of black group identity seek to redefine and empower blackness to the outside world by policing the boundaries of what can be represented to the dominant public as "true" blackness. Through the process of *public policing,* which communicates the judgments, evaluations, and condemnations of recognized leaders and institutions of black communities to their constituencies, the full membership of certain segments of black communities is contested and challenged.

Let me be clear: My concern here is not that these group members will be rejected by dominant groups as not being part of "the" black community. Racism in the dominant society functions with essentialist principles in its assessment of black people. Thus men and women who meet basic dominant ideas of how black people look and act, rarely have their "blackness" evaluated, except to have it negated as a reward for assimilation into dominant white society (e.g., Michael Jackson, Clarence Thomas, and formerly O. J. Simpson). Instead, my concern is with the process employed by other marginal group members to evaluate someone's blackness. Will certain group members be rejected by other marginal group members because of their inability to meet indigenous standards of "blackness"? Are there processes through which the full "rights," or empowerment, of group members are negated or severely limited within black communities because of a stigmatized black identity? Specifically in the matter of AIDS, does the sexual identity of out black gay men and lesbians threaten their standing or membership in black communities, and thus impede the community's response to issues such as AIDS, which have been framed by discussions of "deviant" sexuality?

Policing the visible or public boundaries of group identity threatens the status of those most vulnerable in marginal communities. Through such a process, those members of marginal communities most in need and reportedly extreme in their "nonconformist behavior" are defined as standing outside the norms and behavior agreed upon by the community. Because of their outsider position, these individuals confront the denial of access not only to dominant resources and structures, but also to many of the indigenous resources and institutions needed for their survival. Thus in most cases those individuals deemed to be on the outside of "acceptable blackness"—because of their addiction, their sexual identification, their gender, their poor financial status, or their relationship to the state—are often left with two choices: either find ways to conform to "community standards" of membership or be left on the margins where individual families and friends are expected to take care of their needs. In this case, the shared primary identification of group members, while still active, is mitigated by other identities such as underclass, homosexual, drug addict, or single mother. Further, these intersecting identities are used as signals, imparting judgments about the indigenous worth or authenticity of certain group members. Targeted members of oppressed communities are thus confronted with a *secondary process of marginalization*, this time imposed by members of their own group.

Increasingly, as marginal communities stratify and employ processes of secondary marginalization, the prospect of a meaningful, unified group response is called into question. This circumstance is of special significance for at least two reasons. First, because the political gains of marginal groups are often won through the coordinated efforts of the community, any threat to a unified group mobilization puts at risk the advancement of all members of the community except those most integrated into the dominant society. Second, the loss of group resistance strategies takes on added significance for unprotected members of the community. If the social isolation in which these members operate becomes translated into political isolation, where even other marginal group members are unwilling to take up their cause, we can foresee little prospect for them to find access to and representation within the political system.

Conclusion

Anyone familiar with the long evolution of the concept of power in American politics will realize that much of my definition of marginalization rests on the foundation laid by the earlier work of many scholars, both in and out of the discipline (Foucault 1980; Morris 1984; Rae 1988). In political science, however, more recent works on power have been most influential in directing the construction of marginalization as presented here. Scholars such as Lukes (1974), Gaventa (1980) and Scott (1990), among others, identify the multidimensional, subtle nature of power. These works, by demonstrating the numerous ways in which power relationships constrain the life chances of individuals and groups, encourage scholars to understand the systematic links between power and outcomes in numerous domains. They also instruct us to recognize the ever-present consequences of domination and exploitation of groups in our society. Finally, analyses such as these provide a more realistic image of oppressed groups, one which identifies the means of oppression as well as the sources and strategies of resistance from dominated groups.

While following in the tradition of other scholars of power, I attempt to take our understanding of power and mobilization one step forward, focusing primarily on marginal groups and the indigenous and exogenous factors influencing their political activity. Such a focus on the indigenous structure of the community follows the work of recent social movement theorists like McAdam (1982) and Morris (1984), as well as the work of political scientists such as Scott (1985), who have increasingly recognized and made central the role of indigenous structures in their models of mobilization and resistance.

The theory of marginalization suggests that without paying significant attention to the internal processes of monitoring and creating political information, opportunities, and behavior, researchers will never fully grasp the multidimensional nature of power. In this analysis, much of the activism or inactivity around AIDS in African-American communities is directly connected to indigenous systems of information, mobilization, and identity. Only by understanding these indigenous norms and structures can we begin to explore the political activism of African-American communities in response to AIDS and other cross-cutting issues.

CHAPTER THREE

Enter AIDS: Context and Confrontation

Throughout most of this book, I explore the reasons why many of the institutions indigenous to black communities, those that shape and influence the political attitudes and actions of black Americans, were unable or unwilling to own AIDS, making it a primary issue for African Americans and their politics. I engage in this project not to shame or expose these institutions and their leaders (well, maybe just a little), but to explore the processes associated with "black politics." Specifically, I want to understand how an issue comes to be deemed important to black communities and a part of "the black political agenda." For example, must a disproportionate number of African Americans suffer severe loss before an issue receives attention? Or is it enough for prominent organizations like the National Association for the Advancement of Colored People (NAACP) or well-known leaders like the Reverend Jesse Jackson to label such concerns important to the survival of "the race?" Further, what role do the masses of black people play in developing or ratifying "the" black political agenda?

Before examining the limitations of many black institutions and leaders in responding to AIDS, however, I want to look briefly at those community organizations and activists who were more forceful in challenging the development of this epidemic. As the political landscape becomes more divisive, producing cross-cutting issues which enhance differences between black Americans, we must take every opportunity to examine all attempts at group mobilization, whether they be successes, failures, or successful failures (Weinbaum 1997). This chapter, therefore, focuses on those black organizations, leaders, and activists that did attempt to address the needs of those with AIDS in their communities. Leading such battles, in what I call the first stage of the response to AIDS in black communities—the early years of the epidemic—were black gay activists. More traditional black leaders would find their way into the fray by the mid-1980s, engaging in less stigmatizing struggles during the second stage of the response. The early 1990s witnessed what I loosely call the third stage. During this period we witnessed the development of a professional AIDS infrastructure targeting black Americans. Members of this new AIDS bureaucracy included service providers rooted in black communities as well as other organizations seeking to serve a wider group than white gay men. Throughout this chapter I use these three loosely configured stages to map out the response to AIDS in black communities, paying special attention to evolution in the response to this crisis among African Americans. I begin by describing the political and economic context of black communities in which AIDS emerged.

Black Communities and the Emergence of AIDS

It was in the summer of 1981 that reports of a strange disease affecting gay men began to appear in a few newspaper articles. The first stories on AIDS in 1981 and 1982 paid little attention to its impact on African-American gay men, African-American injection drug users, or other members of African-American communities. Instead, these initial pieces highlighted the emergence of AIDS in primarily white, gay male communities, with a few stories in 1982 on AIDS among Haitians. The absence of a specific focus on AIDS in African-American communities led many in this group to believe that this disease was not about them. Black activists turned their attention, instead, to new and old crises plaguing black communities, not the least of which was the election of Ronald Reagan as the president of the United States in 1980. As noted in the last chapter, black Americans can point to, at best, a mixed record of economic, political, and social progress under advanced systems of marginalization. The 1980s during the Reagan administration were just such a difficult period, where few if any gains were made at the national level.

As with most Republicans in recent history, Reagan was elected to the White House without significant support from African Americans. In fact, Katherine Tate (1993) notes that "in the 1980 presidential election, Ronald Reagan was elected with the lowest percentage of Black votes of any previous Republican presidential candidate. Fewer than one out of every ten Blacks had voted for him" (60). African Americans apparently viewed Reagan's presence in the White House as a threat to their progress. The impact of Reagan's election on blacks and other marginal groups has become legendary (Amaker 1988). Believing that tax breaks and budget cuts were the way to stimulate the economy, President Reagan, through the Omnibus Budget Reconciliation Act (OBRA) of 1981, proposed massive cuts to several of the social service and welfare agencies on which many poor and black Americans depended for assistance. Manning Marable (1991) recounts some of Reagan's proposals and their devastating impact on black communities:

> Included within Reagan's broad assault upon the legacy of social centrist liberalism were numerous proposals: the abandonment of the Comprehensive Employment and Training Act program, . . . and the elimination of its 150,000 federally funded jobs; . . . a $2 billion reduction in the federal Food Stamps Program by fiscal year 1983; the elimination of the $2 billion Guaranteed Student Loan Program; the reduction of $1.7 billion from child nutrition programs sponsored by the federal government by fiscal year 1983; the closing of the Neighborhood Self-Help and Planning Assistance programs, which allotted $55 million in fiscal 1981 to aid inner cities. . . . Reagan also reduced "both eligibility and levels of support" for poor women to receive food stamps and Aid to Families with Dependent Children [AFDC] payments. By August 1981, Congress had ratified most of these proposals, and began to contemplate even more stringent restrictions in the areas of human needs. . . .
>   In one year, Reagan had succeeded where Nixon had failed: he actually expanded poverty in America. . . . In a single year, "much of the progress that had been made against poverty in the 1960s and 1970s" had been "wiped out," according to the *New York Times*. (181–83)

The Reagan administration's budget cuts were not confined to poverty programs such as AFDC, but were evident across a range of programs and departments, in particular those of the Department of Housing and Urban Development (HUD). For example, Moore and Hoban-Moore (1990) find that while the percentage of the population classified as poor increased from 11 to 15 percent during the 1980s, the budget at HUD decreased from 36 billion in 1980 to 15 billion in 1988 (14). This cut in HUD's budget was especially damaging to poor Americans, as Charles Perrow and Mauro F. Guillén (1990) find. While the housing budget at HUD was cut nearly 66 percent, programs promoting housing for "upper-income" citizens were largely left intact.

Nationally, funding for housing under the Department of Housing and Urban Development (HUD) fell by two-thirds between 1981 and 1986, the largest cut for a cabinet-level department in the Reagan Administration, and HUD-subsidized housing starts went from 144,348 to only 17,080 units (and much of even this small effort benefitted ineligible people because of corrupt administration). Meanwhile subsidies in the form of tax deduction for mortgages, which greatly favor those at the upper income levels, totaled $42.4 billion in 1986, when all HUD housing programs were only $10 billion. (166–67)

What made this attack on the housing of poor, often black, Americans even more troubling for many African Americans was the fact that it was led by conservative black Reagan appointee Samuel R. Pierce, Jr. (Perry, Ambeau, and McBride 1995, 120). The appointment of conservative blacks to attack social welfare agencies and progressive redistributive policies, both of which had benefited many black Americans, was a strategy used very effectively by President Reagan. Examples of this tactic include the appointment of black conservatives such as Clarence Thomas to chair the Equal Employment Opportunity Commission (EEOC) and Clarence Pendleton to head the United States Civil Rights Commission (Perry, Ambeau, and McBride, 121). The feelings of betrayal felt by many African Americans are further underscored when one realizes how few of Reagan's full-time appointees were black—4 percent compared to 12 percent in the Carter administration (Jaynes and Williams 1989, 243).

Again, the threat posed by the Reagan administration was understood and experienced among most blacks and other marginal groups, not just among poor black Americans. For example, one area in which Reagan's policies had a wide and lasting effect was in the domain of civil rights, especially as such agendas were pursued through the courts. Lani Guinier (1994) argues that the Reagan administration was especially effective in redirecting the country's civil rights agenda, shaping uniquely the composition of the federal judiciary:

> Under the leadership of its Department of Justice the Reagan Administration identified race-conscious civil rights policies which it considered inherently suspect. Reagan proposed the repeal of affirmative action, the end to many effective class-based remedies, and the abandonment of most racial discrimination cases except those filed on behalf of "identifiable" victims of racism. Propelled in part by the philosophic engines of New Right cost-benefit analysis, the Administration attempted

to drive civil rights laws out of the marketplace for being more costly than they are worth. . . .

Reagan has left an enduring mark on national civil rights policies. Before offering prospective nominees appointments to the federal bench, his advisers tested them by using ideological litmus tests on civil rights issues such as school desegregation, affirmative action, and other race-conscious remedies. The 366 Reagan appointments made to the bench now represent over half the federal judiciary, yet only 7 were black, proportionally fewer than were appointed by Richard Nixon from a pool of available minority talent one-seventh its present size. (23–24)

In examining the specific civil rights and social welfare policies initiated or destroyed by the Reagan administration, we should not lose sight of the larger ideological warfare waged especially against poor people of color by Ronald Reagan and his appointees. Reagan's presidential campaign began with and was fueled in part by targeting vulnerable and stigmatized groups. From his initial embrace of states' rights in Meridian, Mississippi to his construction of the "welfare queen" and his attack on "the underclass," Reagan's strategy of blame and punishment was a central component of his success (Tryman 1995, 71 n. 48). Manning Marable (1991) argues that the rhetoric of the Reagan administration was decisively threatening to African Americans, with his promise to defend states' rights serving as an early signal to most black Americans of the central role racism would play throughout his administration:

The "ideological glue" of Reaganism was racism. The 69-year-old conservative made this clear in August 1980, at a speech delivered in Philadelphia, Mississippi. Before a cheering white crowd, Reagan pledged that his administration would defend the principle of "states' rights." Given that the town was the site of the brutal murders of three desegregation workers in 1964, and that the phrase itself was [taken] by many southern whites to mean "white supremacy," the gravity of Reagan's speech could not be lost upon most blacks. (180)

Adolph Reed (1994) points to the ideology of "the underclass" as yet another essential component of Reagan's effort not only to dismantle many social welfare programs, but also to reorient the ideological framework of the country away from "big government" toward the ideal of individual effort and responsibility. Reed suggests that such a move allows the government to mask its responsibility for creating and maintaining the sub-par living conditions of marginal groups while also encouraging the demobilization of aggrieved groups. It was Reagan's use of black elites to disseminate a message of self-help and middle-class superiority and to promote the internal policing of behavior in black communities that is of particular concern to Reed:

> In Reagan's second term the administration apparently opted for a different posture as a new group of its black supporters, led by [Glen] Loury and Robert Woodson of the National Center for Neighborhood Enterprise, stepped into the spotlight. Although this wave of black Reaganauts (Woodson especially) also could be pugnacious with adversaries, they were far more inclined than their predecessors to make overtures to the entrenched race relations elite. Those overtures, moreover, disarmed partisan skepticism by emphasizing a transcendent ideal, the black middle class's supposedly special responsibility for correcting the black underclass and the problems associated with it. This message has both flattered black petit bourgeois sensibilities and meshed with, no doubt also helped to solidify, the increasingly hegemonic view that non-punitive government action on behalf of black and brown poor people is by definition ineffective and impolitic, if not misguided. Thus the stage was set for propagation of self-help ideology—at least vis-à-vis blacks—across the ideological spectrum. (11–12)

It is important to understand that ideological attacks on race-specific policies and poor people of color in inner-cities, mirrored similar attacks on other marginal groups, including gay men and injection drug users, in relation to and independent of AIDS. The administration's ideological attacks were most often joined with or augmented by the political agendas of conservative groups. Charles Perrow and Mauro F. Guillén comment on the success of conservative forces in blocking AIDS legislation and funding during the Reagan era: "AIDS victims are highly stigmatized; any administration would face obstacles in mobilizing government and private groups. But this [Reagan] administration was particularly beholden to the moral majority and thus particularly unenthusiastic about taking action. Conservative groups reportedly were successful in blocking educational programs and limiting counseling services; it is possible that they even blocked appropriations for research, education, and treatment programs" (52). As we might expect, Reagan's general attack on the budget priorities of the poor and people of color coincided with, and in many cases paved the way for, an underfunding of AIDS. Perrow and Guillén, along with other researchers such as Randy Shilts (1987), describe an administration that was not only willing to request fewer funds than were needed to harness a growing AIDS epidemic, but was willing to let allocated funds from Congress go unspent if they were to go to an "immoral" gay community:

> Each year Congress voted substantially larger budgets for research, education, and treatment in the AIDS area than the Reagan administration requested, and the administration sometimes failed to spend all the funds. For example, Congress earmarked $5.6 million dollars for AIDS activities in fiscal 1982 and $28.7 million in 1984; neither the president's budget proposal nor any Public Health Service (PHS) agency request for those two years allocated any money to AIDS. In 1984, Congress obligated $61.5 million to AIDS (54 percent more than the president's request) and $97.4 million the following year (61 percent more). More telling, Congress had to resort to the threat of legal action to get the data to confirm the widespread suspicion that officials were lying about the extent of their requests. Congress found that even as officials in the CDC [Centers for Disease Control], the National Cancer Institute (NCI), and other health agencies were testifying that they had all the funds they could wisely spend, they had been writing strong memos to their boss pleading for more funds to meet the seriousness of the problem. (Perrow and Guillén 1990, 18)

Whether it be Reagan's "policy of constructive engagement" with the Apartheid government in South Africa, or his support for tax-exempt status for segregated private schools, or his ideological and policy-based attacks on poor families, there was something in the Reagan presidency to draw the attention and concern of most segments of African-American communities (Jaynes and Williams 1989, 252; Guinier 1994, 23; Sirgo 1995, 91). Thus, in the early 1980s, it was the perceived threat posed by Ronald Reagan, not AIDS, that consumed the energy of many black organizations and leaders and acted, as Michael Dawson (1994) suggests, as a catalyst to mobilization in black communities:

> An excellent example of the process by which black elites and institutions can quickly inform and mobilize the black community at times of great perceived risk (during the Reagan administration) or opportunity (Harold Washington's 1983 mayoral campaign) was the rapidity and near-unanimity with

which black religious, civil rights, and other leaders responded to the Reagan administration's perceived hostility to blacks and sought to mobilize the community congregations and constituencies to the "danger" that the administration, its policies, or both posed for the black community. (59)

I detail the impact of the Reagan administration on black communities not to excuse the lack of action regarding AIDS by black leaders, but to highlight the complex political environment confronting black activists as AIDS emerged into their consciousness. As noted earlier, this was a period of contradictions and advanced marginalization. For instance, while African Americans during the post–civil rights era of the late 1970s and early 1980s made important electoral gains, they also faced increasing economic and social bifurcation (Wilson 1987). There is no disputing the fact that the civil rights era has had a lasting impact on the political and economic condition of black Americans, but to portray the impact as exclusively positive would be to distort this period. Even in the election of black officials we encounter limits to the progress of African Americans (Walton 1972).

Since the mid-1960s, through the passage of the 1965 Voting Rights Act, black communities have come to focus much of their political energy on the electoral system. Changing demographics of inner cities, determined in part by the massive in-migration of blacks from the South and the continuous out-migration of whites to the suburbs, facilitated the election of black mayors and representatives in many urban areas during the 1970s and 1980s (Williams 1987; Tate 1993). Linda Williams, using data from the Joint Center for Political Studies' (JCPS) *National Roster of Black Elected Officials,* finds that the number of black elected officials has increased dramatically since 1965: "When the Voting Rights Act was passed in 1965, it was estimated that there were fewer than 500 black elected officials in the United States. In 1970, when the Joint Center for Political Studies began its annual survey of black elected officials, there were 1,469 black officials. By January 1985 blacks held 6,056 elective offices, an increase of 312 percent during the 15-year period since 1970" (111). Even with the constant increase in the number of black elected officials, currently they still only account for 7,552, or 1.5 percent, of the nearly 500,000 elected officials in the United States.[1]

Those blacks elected to office were especially successful in securing municipal and educational government positions. For instance, between 1970 and 1985 the number of black mayors jumped from 48 to

236 (Williams 120). Under the governing regimes of these early black mayors, African Americans saw real improvements in areas such as police and community relations, social service expenditures, and affirmative action policies (Conyers and Wallace 1976; Jones 1978; Karnig and Welch 1980). The policies of black mayors made available to many middle-class blacks extended job opportunities in an expanding governing structure (Eisinger 1982, 1984). Black elected officials serving as mayors, city council members, or national representatives fought to improve the quality of life for their constituents, using their new-found control of state resources and power. These same elected officials, however, found their efforts severely constrained by the numerous economic crises that confronted their administrations (Reed 1988). The recessions of the 1970s and early 1980s, the retreat of the federal government from support for inner cities, and the tax incentives demanded by corporate entities to keep their factories and headquarters in financially strapped urban areas, for example, limited the resources available to deal with the many ills confronting central cities, including the emergence of a new disease called AIDS (Peterson 1981).

Thus, in spite of the political advances witnessed during the post–civil rights period, economically vulnerable black and Latino urban communities found themselves the victims of a changing economic structure. The late 1960s and the 1970s saw the deindustrialization of central cities, with many manufacturing jobs becoming obsolete (Wilson 1980). Those jobs that did not disappear due to technological advances moved out of the reach of urban workers, as factories followed government-supported highways out of the cities to the suburbs, or South to "right-to-work" and union-free regions, or out of the country in search of even cheaper labor (Rifkin 1995; Weinbaum 1997). These industries took with them not only a substantial inner-city tax base, but also stable, moderately paid, low-skilled jobs—the type of employment crucial to black communities systematically denied access to educational opportunities (Wilson 1980). In the place of manufacturing jobs, there developed a service economy comprised of low-skilled, often menial, low-paying jobs that provided no opportunities for advancement and lacked the stability of manufacturing jobs. Such jobs, along with incredibly high levels of unemployment, defined the economic environment for the majority of black workers in the 1970s and 1980s. Ira Katznelson (1981) describes the diminishing presence of manufacturing jobs in New York City during the 1970s and 1980s:

The composition of employment in the city changed dramatically. The gain of 450,000 new jobs mainly in headquarters employment in the private sector and in government masked the loss of about half that number in manufacturing. Private sector manufacturing jobs declined from 30 percent of the total in 1960 to 24 percent by 1970. . . .

These changes in the economy of the city affected in an especially powerful way black and Hispanic New Yorkers, who by 1970 constituted approximately one-third of the population—and one-half of the economically active population. Virtually two in three were in non–white collar jobs. (95–96)

These changes in the economic fortunes of the most vulnerable must be understood as part of the contradictory patterns found in advanced systems of marginalization. In this case the collapse of manufacturing jobs in the 1960s and 1970s was accompanied by a proliferation of high-skilled, middle-class jobs (Landry 1987; Wilson 1980). A number of factors contributed to the expansion of middle-class jobs for black Americans, including the passage of laws in the 1960s guaranteeing African Americans equal opportunity in employment. These laws provided "greater access to a wider range of middle-class occupations than had historically been the case" (Landry 1987, 76). Further, the transformation of many cities from goods-producing markets to service- and information-based economies also brought with it an additional source of skilled jobs that would come to be filled, in part, by black Americans. However, the most important development may have been the expansion of public employment opportunities. As government bureaucracies continued to swell, in part to meet the needs of those excluded or marginalized through the changing economy, there developed a pool of skilled, bureaucratic jobs requiring higher education levels (Waldinger 1996). Jeremy Rifkin argues that the public sector "saved" the economic fortunes of many black Americans:

The only significant rise in employment among black Americans in the past twenty-five years has been in the public sector: more than 55 percent of the net increase in employment for blacks in the 1960s and 1970s occurred there. Many black professionals found jobs in the federal programs spawned by the Great Society initiatives of President Lyndon Johnson. Others found employment at the local and state levels, administering social service and welfare programs largely for the black community that was displaced by the new forces of automation and suburbanization. In 1960, 13.3 percent of the total employed black labor force was working in the public sector. A decade later more than 21 percent of all black workers in America were on public payrolls. By 1970 the government employed 57 percent of all black male college graduates and 72 percent of all black female college graduates. (76–77)

Thus, while significant numbers of African Americans found the economic restructuring of the 1970s devastating to themselves and their neighborhoods, the expansion of skilled employment allowed for the evolution of what has been called the "new Black middle-class" (Landry 1987). Wilson (1987) notes that this pattern was most evident in northern cities where an increasing black middle class, through patterns of advanced marginalization and effective resistance, was able to gain limited access to the resources of the dominant society: "The figures show that all the major cities had consistent job losses in industries where [worker] education averaged less than a high school degree and consistent employment growth in industries where workers on the average acquired some higher education. For example, in New York City the number of jobs in industries with the lower education requisites decreased by 492,000 from 1970 to 1984, whereas those with higher education requisites increased by 239,000" (40–41).

The economic, political, and social dynamics of the post–civil rights era worked to exaggerate differences in the lived experiences of African Americans. While the middle-class found expanding opportunity, the majority of blacks found themselves facing fewer substantial job prospects and generally losing economic ground.[2] In response to the increasing stratification and the economic decay of many urban centers, municipal authorities, including black mayors, abandoned radical redistributive plans and instead implemented corporate strategies for economic development (Stone 1987). These policies generated varying degrees of success during the 1980s, and many inner-city residents found themselves facing a shrinking tax base and an economic structure redefining itself to make a large black labor pool irrelevant or only tangentially important (Rifkin 1995). Not surprisingly, at the same time that blacks were experiencing electoral success in urban areas, white residents were continuing to flee from cities increasingly populated by blacks and Latinos (Massey and Denton 1993). Consequently, in response to a depleted tax base, many basic city services in the areas of education, housing, health care, and community protection were left in disarray. Perrow and Guillén, commenting on New York City, describe a health care system and city in financial crisis not long before the emergence of AIDS:

> Experts writing in the late 1970s routinely discussed the fragmentation of New York's health care sector and its exploding costs. . . .
> It did not help matters that during the 1970s both New York City and New York State had greater budget deficits than most other cities and states. Thus, the city appeared to be at fiscal risk when AIDS arrived in 1982. . . . In addition, city hospitals were eliminating beds in the 1980s even as the growing AIDS burden demanded more. (68–69)

In light of these difficulties, it is an interesting and ironic observation that blacks would play a significant role in leading, politically, many of the cities that would eventually become the epicenters of AIDS in the United States: New York, Los Angeles, Newark, Atlanta, Chicago, and Detroit. As stated earlier, this fact makes it difficult to accept the argument that it was because of a lack of resources that African-American leaders mounted, at best, a slow response to AIDS in black communities. While individual black Americans continued to struggle to identify the resources necessary for their families and themselves, across the country black candidates were being elected to positions where they controlled the budgets, as limited as they may have been, of major urban areas. These officials were also becoming significant players in the state apparatus of local and national governments responsible for responding to this crisis. At the very least, these officials had access to their local "bully pulpits," so that they could make AIDS a priority for their constituencies.

Again, increased access provided to some African Americans, in conjunction with the limited economic and social mobility provided most black Americans, confronted black communities as AIDS emerged. It was also during this period, as manufacturing jobs were disappearing from inner cities, that other troubling social indicators began to appear. For example, there was an increase in the number of African Americans who were both arrested for and the victims of violent crime; an influx of drugs such as heroin and later crack cocaine into black neighborhoods; the expansion of concentrated inner-city poverty; the persistence of residential segregation; and a corresponding explosion in the number of black men and women incarcerated (Wilson 1987; Marable 1991; Massey and Denton 1993). Moreover, the outside demonization of certain more vulnerable segments of black communities continued, shaping the context in which AIDS would develop and be ignored. Ideological attacks, specifically on poor black communities, persisted throughout the 1980s, simultaneously promoting a discourse of law and order and one of individual responsibility. These narratives served to further stigmatize and marginalize those members of black communities already on the edge, such as young black men, poor single mothers receiving assistance, and unemployed black workers. Constructed images of a black community in disarray were used to legitimize the neglect of state and federal governments and the flight of corporations, individual whites, and some economically successful blacks from black and brown urban cities.

This was the environment in which many African-American leaders initially ignored the development of AIDS in black communities. And as the indicators of AIDS' devastation on African-American communities became more public, many black leaders pursued a more aggressive program of denial and distance, employing strategies of secondary marginalization to negate the relationship between those black people with AIDS and the larger black community. For instance, a number of black media sources ran stories on the need for members of the black middle class to take their rightful place as leaders and help those "other" blacks suffering from AIDS. Attempting to purify the reputation of the group and hold on to their hard-won cultural capital and social mobility, African Americans with relative privilege made their own distinctions between "good and moral" black people and those deemed unworthy or "tainted" by outside evils. Code words like *junkie, faggot, punk,* and *prostitute* were deployed both inside and outside of black communities to designate who was expendable. In the early years of the epidemic black leaders focused more energy and attention on detailing the "faulty and inferior" norms, culture, and behavior of those segments of black communities thought to be most at risk for AIDS than on dominant systems of marginalization contributing to the spread of this epidemic in black communities.

These patterns of response changed over time as some established organizations and leaders were forced into action, realizing there was nowhere to run from AIDS. As the disease progressed, traditional black institutions were often pushed into the fray by activists and group members. In most cases, their work focused on education and largely symbolic acts. Little was done by traditional leaders to make AIDS a priority and a political issue for African Americans. Instead, the more inclusive political and transformative work was pursued, at least initially, by black gay men and lesbians. In what follows, I briefly review the three stages of response to AIDS in African-American communities. The first stage consisted primarily of the actions of black gay men and lesbians in the early years of the epidemic. Much of this activity corresponded with, and in some cases produced, an increasingly visible presence among black gays. The second stage began around 1986 and centered on the response to this epidemic in black communities by traditional social service agencies and established black leaders and organizations. The final stage began in the early 1990s and included the continuing professionalization of black AIDS organizations as well as the development of new organizations pursuing AIDS work. I offer this categorization not as a definite model, but as a road map to help orient the reader to many of the arguments I present in the rest of the book.

Stage 1: The Emergence of AIDS and a Visible Black Gay Identity

The perceived importance of a unifying group identity cannot be overstated when trying to explain the structured politics of black communities. Systems of oppression from slavery to redemption, legal and informal Jim Crow segregation, and other more recent forms of deprivation have created an environment in which most African Americans share a history and current existence framed by oppression and marginalization. The resistance generated by African Americans in response to patterns of exclusion has also been structured around racial unity. Whether with regard to civil rights institutions, black liberation organizations, or even the electoral campaigns of black candidates, one primary identity—"blackness"—was understood to be the underlying factor joining all these struggles. Each organization espoused its own commitment to the liberation of black people. Anything thought to detract from this goal was dismissed and in some cases denounced. However, even as a unifier, "blackness" has always been mediated or contested by other identities that group members hold.

As discussed previously, during the 1960s and 1970s black communities experienced increasing stratification. Across the country African Americans witnessed the continuing bifurcation of black communities, illustrated most noticeably in the intensified division between an expanding black middle class and expanding numbers of black poor.[3] Aside from economic segmentation, other social cleavages were activated among African Americans during this period. Individuals increasingly began to recognize and acknowledge the multiplicity of identities upon which their oppression was based. Black women, the black poor, and other segments of black communities articulated publicly, and in numbers not seen before, demands specific to the conditions under which they struggled (Beale 1995; Piven and Cloward 1979).[4] At no time have both the primacy and the fragility of a unified group identity been more evident than in the liberation politics and social movements of the late 1960s and early 1970s. Thus, it is not surprising that in this changing environment the visibility of lesbian and gay people and the movement for lesbian and gay rights began to take shape in black communities and in the country at large (Duberman 1994; Seidman 1993; Vaid 1995).

It is important to recognize that while black gay men and lesbians have always existed and worked in African-American communities, they were often forced to be invisible, silent contributors (Garber 1990; Katz 1992). Their acceptance of this conditional black membership is not irrational when we consider the threat of racism faced by many black lesbians and gay men outside of black communities. The cost of silence and invisibility seemed a willing payment from black lesbians and gay men who in return received the support, care, and protection of African-American communities and, more important, the love of immediate family members. In *Talking Back* (1989), bell hooks discusses this dilemma:

> The gay people we knew did not live in separate subcultures, not in the small, segregated black community where work was difficult to find, where many of us were poor. Poverty was important; it created a social context in which structures of dependence were important for everyday survival. Sheer economic necessity and fierce white racism, as well as the joy of being there with the black folks known and loved, compelled many gay blacks to live close to home and family. That meant however that gay people created a way to live out sexual preferences within the boundaries of circumstances that were rarely ideal no matter how affirming. (120–21)

Thus, if you were willing not to "flaunt" your sexual orientation in front of family members and neighbors (although many would secretly suspect that you were "that way"), the repeated verbal abuse—taunts of "punk," "faggot," or "bulldyke"—and the periodic physical abuse were generally kept to a minimum. Again, I do not want to minimize the importance of even such conditional support on the part of family, friends, and community. The prospect of facing continuous residential, occupational, and social exclusion as a manifestation of widespread racism, even in primarily white lesbian and gay communities, underscores the importance of securing, often at very high stakes, feelings of safety and familiarity. However, the willingness and ability of black lesbians and gay men to remain quiet and invisible has radically changed.

Changes in the visibility of black lesbians and gay men have resulted from numerous factors connected to the development of new identities, as well as the politicization of old ones. Again, one major catalyst was the proliferation of liberation and social movements demanding access and control for groups long pushed out of dominant society. Cornel West (1990) speaks of this situation, arguing that "during the late '50s, '60s and early '70s in the USA, these decolonized sensibilities fanned and fueled the Civil Rights and Black Power movements, as well as the student anti-war, feminist, gray, brown, gay, and lesbian movements. In this period we witnessed the shattering of male WASP cultural homogeneity and the collapse of the short-lived liberal consensus" (25). A second factor facilitating the increased visibility of lesbians and gay men was the more formal establishment of an institutionalized, socially connected, and in many cases monetarily secure gay community in several of the nation's urban centers. These "ghettos" provided a space in which ideas of rights and political strategies of empowerment could be generated and discussed. John D'Emilio (1983a) contends that these enclaves, as well as dominant institutions such as universities, were integral in creating space for the exploration of gay independence away from the local communities and families who imposed conditions of silence and conformity. And while many black lesbians and gay men did not live in these gay enclaves, either because of choice or affordability—gentrified property can be very expensive—they developed their own social networks through writers' groups, political organizations, house parties, drag balls, and dance clubs (Chauncey 1994; Katz 1992).

In this context, then, we find not only the emergence of AIDS, but also the emergence of an outspoken and brave black lesbian and gay leadership—a new "vanguard" who openly claimed and wrote about their race *and* sexual identities. Individuals like Audre Lorde, Cheryl Clarke, Barbara Smith, Pat Parker, Michelle Parkerson, Joseph Beam, Essex Hemphill, and Marlon Riggs were intent on creating not only new cultural voices, but also a political analysis which made central the connections between homophobia and other forms of oppression. When these and other "queers of color" were denied the right to speak openly through traditional avenues in black, Latino, Asian, and Native communities as well as through newly formed organizations in white lesbian and gay communities, they established their own vehicles like Kitchen Table, Women of Color Press to affirm their presence in, and bond with, communities of people of color. Publications like *This Bridge Called My Back, Home Girls, Brother to Brother, In the Life*, and more recently videos such as *Tongues Untied, Black Is/Black Ain't* and *Black Nations/Queer Nations?* all detail, from various perspectives, the struggle to constantly mesh one's black and gay identities (Moraga and Anzaldua 1981; Smith 1983; Beam 1986; Hemphill 1991).

In conjunction with the more visible presence of cultural work embracing black *and* gay identities during the late 1970s and 1980s, political and social organizations such as SALSA Soul Sisters, Sapphire Sapphos, the Bay Area Black Lesbians and Gays (BABLG), the DC Coalition of Black Gays (DCCBG) and the National Coalition of Black Lesbians and Gays (NCBLG) emerged with a commitment to affirm the lives of black lesbians and gay men. These groups all helped create an environment in which the silence that had structured the lives of many black lesbians and gay men could now be escaped. Again, I want to emphasize that for many black lesbians and gay men, attempts to silence them and make their presence invisible came not only from black communities but also from racist white lesbians and gay men. Under such conditions black "queers" faced a dual process of secondary marginalization—one originating within black communities and the other rooted within white lesbian and gay institutions and space.

The conditions listed above did not lead to a massive coming out process in black communities. In fact, the level of silence among black lesbians and gay men is still an immediate and pressing concern for those organizing in African-American communities. Further, while more individuals choose to organize around their black gay identity—establishing groups and pursuing cultural and political work—the developing infrastructure in black gay communities did not approach in numbers or resources that found in many white gay communities. Nonetheless, the increased politicization of most black people, including lesbians and gay men during the 1960s and 1970s, did create a situation in which some black women and men chose to identify publicly as black *and* gay. The choice, or in many cases the perceived need, to embrace openly a black gay or lesbian identity undoubtedly escalated with the emergence of AIDS. In AIDS, black gay community members confronted an issue which demanded either recognition and resistance or death. Thus, after spending years affirming themselves, building consciousness, and contributing to black communities that had too often refused to embrace their particular needs, gay brothers and lesbian sisters faced a crisis that threatened to wreak havoc throughout black communities if they did not speak out and fight this growing epidemic.

In spite of the developing public activism among black gay men and lesbians as AIDS emerged, we must remember that many of these organizers came to this issue with great reluctance and fear. Gil Gerald, former executive director of the National Coalition of Black Lesbians and Gays, recalls both his first realization that AIDS was a disease that affected black gay men and the denial exhibited by other black gay activists. In the spring of 1983, while hosting a meeting of black gay activists working to ensure that there would be an openly gay speaker at the march to commemorate the twentieth anniversary of the March on Washington, Gerald received a visitor. He reported to me in an interview that the visitor said, "You might want to bring this [CDC report] up in your discussions with the national march organization." Gerald continues:

> Here is the report from the Centers for Disease Control, and it is the *Morbidity and Mortality Weekly Report.* I had never seen one in my life. This was in the spring of 1983 and [it] showed that blacks were disproportionately affected by HIV and by AIDS. I don't know what the terminology was at the time. I looked at it and just as a lay person it jumped off the page at you. I knew that as blacks, we were only 10–12 percent of the population, but [here] we were disproportionately affected. I think we were 20 percent. Like it was crazy at the time, and so that became the first real evidence to me personally. And the first thing I did was I took the report into the living room. And there were about ten other men from the, you know, prominent in the gay community—people like Mel Boozer and Dr. James Tinney. And I went to them and I said you know I think we need to change, there is something I need to tell you about with this health crisis, this health thing. I said you know this has got to stop. And they all chastised me. "This is typical." "Oh Gil, this only happens to people who slept with white men." And Dr. James Tinney, who is dead of HIV, says to me

this is all a plot, a government plot to hit us. I can't quote him directly. It's been so long, but basically there is an attack on our sexuality. So I mean I was ignored. But I really continued to take the issue seriously.[5]

The initial instinct to deny the impact of AIDS on black communities, even among black gay activists, was not a pattern unique to Gil Gerald. Phil Wilson, a longtime AIDS activist and one of the founders of the National Black Lesbian and Gay Leadership Forum as well as the National Task Force on AIDS, also remembers that his first reaction to AIDS was something that he is not proud of now because it was based in denial and fear. "My first reaction to AIDS was 'Thank God this is happening to them and not to us,' because I believed as everyone else did that this was about white gay men."[6] Shaping Wilson's initial response to AIDS is an "us versus them" framework where a unifying racial identity is the barrier which biologically and psychologically separates him from white gay men, in this case protecting him from AIDS. Ironically, it was the breakdown of Wilson's framework, as manifested in the rejection of AIDS as a central issue for black communities, and especially the rejection of black gay men with AIDS as community members we should care about, that motivated further activism on his part:

> I can remember exactly where I sat. I was outside the ballroom for the conference [the CDC conference on AIDS in Minority Communities], and I was in tears because I was so upset. I remember saying to myself, "You know they are going to let us [black gay men] die." And the thing for me was that *black folks* are going to let us die because I was still in that place that AIDS is about black gay men. AIDS in the black community is about black gay men. And do you know the only way that we are going to be saved is if we come together and decide that we are going to save ourselves. That is when I decided that there needed to be a meeting of black gays and lesbians. . . . I came home, and the gay and lesbian March in Washington was in October. So I went to Washington with these boxes and boxes of flyers to promote a conference [of black gay men and lesbians].[7]

It was this heightened political, social, and economic environment, where black gay men in particular were experiencing the destruction of AIDS, that produced many of the early pioneers of the response to AIDS in black communities. Ernest Quimby and Samuel Friedman

(1989) document much of the early organized activity around AIDS among people of color:

> In the epidemic's early days, media reports that AIDS was a disease of white gay men reduced the attention blacks paid to it. In general, blacks denied AIDS was a problem that affected them and blamed white gay men for it. According to Gil Gerald (personal communication, April 6, 1988), the National AIDS Network's former director of minority affairs, during this early period there was a dominant heterosexual view that "We don't have gays in our community," an attitude of some black gay men that "You only get AIDS if you sleep with white men," and a belief held by some other black gays that "Only whites who slept with whites got AIDS."
>
> By 1985, however, some leaders of the minority gay and lesbian community began to challenge this denial, and helped set up some of the first minority-focused AIDS events. (405)

The work of black gay men and lesbians largely defined the formal organizing—conferences, community education, and service provision—during this first stage of response. When traditional black organizations and leaders refused to step forward and deal openly with the escalation of AIDS in black communities, black gay men in particular provided leadership. In fact, two of the earliest national conferences on AIDS among people of color were organized by lesbians and gay men of color. The Third World Advisory Task Force, a primarily gay group out of San Francisco, organized a western regional conference in the early part of 1986 (Quimby and Friedman 1989).[8] The National Coalition of Black Lesbian and Gays, a progressive national organization structured around local chapters, organized the "National Conference on AIDS in the Black Community" in Washington, DC, in 1986. This conference, which was cosponsored by the National Minority AIDS Council and the National Conference of Black Mayors, was funded in part from a grant from the United States Public Health Service (Weston 1986, 13–15).

In such spaces—conferences planned and controlled by black gay activists—open and constructive contestation over the role of black institutions and leaders in the response to AIDS could take place. For instance, in his welcoming remarks at the "National Conference on AIDS in the Black Community," Gil Gerald, then executive director of the National Coalition of Black Lesbian and Gays, highlighted the absence of national mainstream black organizations. "You have come here [from] over 23 states in the Union and from Brazil. No, not the

Urban League, or the NAACP, or the National Medical Association, or the National Association of Black Social Workers, none of them are here as they should be to openly join in the call for more action and involvement by the Black community in the issue of AIDS."[9]

It is important to remember that prior to, and often in conjunction with, the formal response of black gay activists during the very early years of the epidemic, families—most often mothers, lovers, and friends—took on the task of caring for their loved ones. In the early 1980s there was no community-based AIDS industry—except the one developing in white lesbian and gay communities—to deal with the problem of AIDS among African Americans (Patton 1990). Instead, black gay men, injection drug users, members of Haitian communities, and black women living with AIDS found themselves dependent on their previously established systems of support—a familiar tradition in black communities (Stack 1975; Gutman 1976; Martin and Martin 1985). Thus a significant portion of the response to AIDS in black communities during this first stage (as well as among most groups) came from the support networks of individuals, long before traditional social service organizations thought to care about this issue (Ostrow et al. 1991).

It was primarily in the later phase of this initial period of response that black gay men and lesbians facilitated the establishment of a formal infrastructure, working to build some of the first AIDS service organizations located in black communities and more broadly targeting minority communities. Organizations like the Minority AIDS Project in Los Angeles, the Black Coalition on AIDS in San Francisco, the Kupona Network in Chicago, Blacks Educating Blacks About Sexual Health Issues (BEBASHI) in Philadelphia, and the National Task Force on AIDS Prevention owe much to the initiative and leadership of black gay men like the Reverend Carl Bean, Gil Gerald, Reggie Williams, A. Billy Jones, Lawrence Washington, David Naylor, the Rev. Charles Angel, and Phil Wilson. In New York City, black gay activists like Dr. Billy Jones, Craig Harris, and George Bellinger Jr. helped establish and expand the Minority Task Force on AIDS (MTFA). This more formal, organized response to AIDS in black communities, provided largely by black gay men, concentrated on educational activities and service provision. This is not surprising, since the predominant activities during this first stage were increasing recognition and acceptance of AIDS as a disease affecting black communities and obtaining basic services for those in need. Thus, one of the goals of these new organizations was to provide AIDS information and education in a manner that resonated with black Americans. The idea, as Gil Gerald notes, was to produce culturally relevant information that could be disseminated in black communities across the country:

> We created a brochure that was funded originally by the District of Columbia. Our issue was that all of the brochures that were being produced by places like the Gay Men's Health Crisis [at] first did not have any black images. People could not relate to them. Second, they were not informative, and the language that was used was not a language that was usable or accessible to people of color, particularly black men who were at risk for this disease. So we created one, "AIDS in the Black Community." . . . Our concept was to basically make a camera-ready copy that people would request. They would pay for just a camera-ready copy, and they would have a place where they could put their organization's name and address on it. And they could go and take it to the printer and reproduce it by the thousands.[10]

In pursuing this work, the Minority Task Force on AIDS, like a number of other AIDS service organizations in which black gay men played a crucial early role, while it was gay-sensitive, never focused exclusively on AIDS' impact on gay men of color. Instead, MTFA defined itself as "a community-based organization that was founded in 1986 to respond to the effects of HIV infection and AIDS in the people of color communities of New York City" (MTFA guide, 1). In part, the choice of black gay activists to build organizations which had as their mission serving all parts of African-American communities was motivated by the obvious need for services across the boundaries of sexuality to multiple populations within black communities. However, Colin Robinson, former executive director for Gay Men of African Descent (GMAD) and current director of the Community Partnership Initiative at Gay Men's Health Crisis (GMHC), suggests that such an inclusive framework also came from an internalized hierarchy in which black gay men viewed their black (male) identity as primary in defining their social location:

> At that time the mainstreaming of a black gay male identity that emphasized both blackness and gayness hadn't happened yet. People were black first and gay second. There was very much a consciousness of that hierarchy within folks' identities. People saw race as the more important, for political identity, strategic identity, and also the identity that had the most im-

pact, the structure they realized most. So I guess it was the most important cultural identity. We hadn't yet developed the kind of black lesbian and gay culture that exists now, that sort of sustains the community. . . . Also because there weren't any models, I mean there wasn't any gay infrastructure in our communities—there were a few small organizations—partly people weren't visible. I mean AIDS precipitated a lot of that culture. You know, creation of a culture and a consciousness and community as people became ill—the risk of coming out becomes moot.[11]

Although AIDS, according to Robinson, helped solidify a growing infrastructure in black gay communities and made coming out "moot," a number of other factors helped to lay the groundwork for the response to AIDS from black gay men and lesbians. For instance, this group received extremely helpful information from white gay AIDS activists. Also, the limited access and economic privilege possessed by some black gay men and lesbians proved to be useful in developing contacts and pooling resources. The personal experiences of loss which brought together and raised the consciousness and anger of black lesbians and gay men were also instrumental in motivating their response. Additionally, the increasing numbers of "out" black gays and lesbians created a pool of potential activists less vulnerable to the moral judgments of traditional institutions in black communities. Because of their public identity as black lesbians or gay men, these individuals already stood outside (often voluntarily) the ideologies and institutions which sought to regulate their behavior through a secondary process of marginalization. They, more than anyone else, were able to challenge both the dominant and indigenous marginalization associated with AIDS. This positioning, of course, was accompanied by great sacrifice and loss, yet as black gay activists engaged in dialogues with multiple segments of black communities about the dangers of this growing epidemic, it became clear that the silence and invisibility that had been a part of their conditional membership could no longer be honored if lives were to be saved.

In this first stage of response, black gay men and lesbians, families, and friends all stepped forward to care and sometimes empower those with AIDS in black communities. They provided the beginnings of an AIDS infrastructure in minority communities that would expand as the epidemic progressed. Although not always starting from a position of power, these individuals, groups, and organizations worked past their denial, fear, and at times internalized homophobia to lead the first battle in the war against AIDS in black communities. And while black gay men and black men who sleep with men composed the majority of documented AIDS cases in black communities during those early years, the organizing and activist efforts of black gay men extended beyond the black gay community. These early AIDS organizations and activists sought to provide education and services to all in need in black communities, while still holding on at least minimally to their open and visible identity as black and gay.

Stage 2: Social Service Agencies and AIDS in Black Communities

The second stage in the black community's response to AIDS ran from about 1986 or 1987 to the early 1990s. During this period traditional institutions, both political and social, began to attend to the issue of AIDS. Drug treatment programs, civil rights organizations, popular black magazines and newspapers, as well as "the Black church" demonstrated increased interest in the spread of AIDS in African-American communities. This heightened concern was directly tied to the work of black AIDS activists who fought to make AIDS a central community issue. In addition, of course, these institutions finally began to see sizeable numbers of their clients or members living with, suffering, and dying from AIDS—making their continued denial nearly impossible and visibly negligent. Furthermore, the increased government and private funding available for "culturally sensitive" AIDS programs also seemed to open the eyes, and possibly the pocketbooks, of a number of these organizations.

Whatever the motivation for this new interest in AIDS, the response by traditional black leaders and organizations during this second period was not one of acceptance and mobilization. Instead, many of the organizations and leaders of black communities, while elevating the importance they assigned to the disease, held onto old beliefs about those living with HIV and AIDS. For instance, a number of black ministers, even as they started AIDS ministries, still preached against what they believed to be the "sinful" behavior involved in the transmission of HIV. Rev. Calvin Butts, executive minister of Abyssinian Baptist Church in Harlem, in a 1988 *Amsterdam News* article, stated that while the church has a "divine responsibility " to those who live with AIDS, drug addiction and homosexuality are still "against the will of God" (Cooper 1988, 36).

Black elected and public officials also became more involved in dealing with AIDS and its manifestation in African-American communities during this period. After largely ignoring AIDS in the first few years of the epidemic, black elected officials could no longer discount the reports coming from the CDC, state and local health departments, and their constituents of the rampant spread of HIV and AIDS in their communities. It was in this context that black officials like David Dinkins began to speak out and take limited action. For example, at the end of 1986 David Dinkins, then Manhattan Borough President, sponsored a meeting of minority elected officials to apprise them of the impact of AIDS on their communities.[12] In 1987 he continued such efforts, fighting for more money for AIDS programs in the city budget, while also cosponsoring the "Helping Hand" rally at St. Mark's Church in Harlem (Anekwe 1987). Much of the progress of black officials, however, resulted from quiet negotiations with and continual education from AIDS activists in black communities. So while David Dinkins is to be applauded for his work regarding AIDS, Dr. Billy Jones, former head of the Health and Hospitals Corporation under Mayor David Dinkins, reminds us that some of Dinkins's actions came at the direct urging of black AIDS activists:

> One of the things that we [board members of the Minority Task Force on AIDS] did to some degree was to get the then borough president [David Dinkins] to convene a meeting. [We wanted to] get the black leadership in the city at the meeting and say, "Look, it's time we pull all this together and address this." I was at that meeting that the borough president had. At that point there was then a kind of two-day symposium that was held. You know, a retreat kind of thing. And out of that grew the Black Leadership Commission on AIDS. So I can't really say that black leadership didn't get involved. I mean it took some doing to move them to the point of, you know, action.[13]

During this period other black elected officials also sought to act, at least symbolically, holding public hearings, conferences, and community meetings. Congressman Charles Rangel, New York State Assemblymen Ed Towns, Al Vann, and Roger Green of Brooklyn were just some of the black New York officials who either sponsored or added their names to AIDS events, attempting to become more visible around this issue without expending substantial political resources (Quimby and Friedman 1989). In response to developments such as the death of Max Robinson and the increasing evidence of "innocent victims," namely women and children under attack from this disease, indigenous leaders such as Representative Louis Stokes, organizations such as the National Urban League, and social service organizations such as Reality House, a drug prevention and education program, all sought or were forced to become involved in the "AIDS business."

Although numerous indigenous leaders and organizations became involved in the fight against AIDS during this period, it was not always to protect the interests of all black people living with, or at greater behavioral risk for, AIDS. A glaring example of this tension between the interests of those blacks thought to be at higher behavioral risk for AIDS and those thought to be at no or little risk is found in the controversy surrounding a proposed needle-exchange program for New York City. In 1987 and 1988 many black and Latino/a leaders responded in force to oppose a plan by the New York City Health Department to distribute, on a severely limited basis, clean needles to injection drug users. These leaders, calling the proposal everything from an embarrassing misstep on the part of Health Department officials to a genocidal plot meant to destroy black and Latino communities, argued that the distribution of clean needles would lead to the further degeneration of black communities. Community leaders warned that the proposed program sent the wrong message about drug use and encouraged African Americans and Latinos/as, especially children, to become addicted. Rev. Butts, continuing his earlier comments, argued that "passing out needles and condoms is like saying you can't do anything about drugs, so you might as well pass out cocaine and crack. . . . We know it's difficult to get people to do what's right. But that doesn't mean we should stop trying" (Cooper 1988, 36). Thus, in a classic example of the victories to be won with "moral" and political clout, the majority of black elected officials and traditional black leaders, after evaluating the possible lifesaving benefits from a needle-exchange program to a largely black and Latino/a drug-using population and the minimal threat posed to nonusers in these same communities, sided with their black, nonusing, *voting*, and *morally upstanding* constituents. Consequently, one of David Dinkins's earliest acts as the first black mayor elected in New York City was to dismantle the small needle-exchange program run by the City Health Department (Joseph 1992, 230).[14]

While the majority of black and Latino/a leaders who weighed in on the needle-exchange controversy voiced their disapproval, a few leaders registered their support for the program. These leaders and activists struggled to move black and Latino communities to what they considered a more enlightened and inclusive position on this issue. In particular, they attempted to challenge the popular framing of those supporting needle exchange as condoning and promoting drug use. Yolanda Serano, then director of the Association for Drug Abuse Prevention and Treatment (ADAPT) commented, "We support it [needle exchange]." She continued, "ADAPT does not condone drug use. We say it is not the needle that gets people to use drugs—it's the drugs, the high" (Dobie 1989, 82). And Benny Primm, director of the Addiction Research and Treatment Center was quoted as saying that "you [black officials] may call people racist now if they adopt this policy; but if they do not do it, in five years you will accuse them of racist genocide" (Friedman et al. 1987, 492). In the same article, the authors (of which Mr. Primm is one) attribute much of the negative reaction to the needle-exchange proposal by black and Latino officials to the negative feelings and experiences that members of these communities have had with drug users. Thus standing in opposition to needle exchange meant standing with and for the majority of black New Yorkers who saw drugs as destroying their communities and often their families— a winning situation for any politician:

> Minority communities bear a disproportionate burden of crime by drug users seeking money for drugs, and a disproportionate loss of access to neighborhood facilities that are taken over by drug users. Thus, many blacks and Hispanics are unfriendly to drug users or to any proposals that seem to offer aid to drug users. One indicator of this attitude is a poster that was plastered on many lamp posts in Harlem in 1986. It says: "When will all the junkies die so the rest of us can go on living?"; on many occasions, we have seen approving graffiti added to these posters. (491)

Dr. Billy Jones takes this same argument one step forward, suggesting that the majority of black and Latino/a leaders in New York City opposed the needle-exchange proposal in part because their personal experiences made it difficult for them to separate the issue of intravenous drug use and AIDS from the devastation of black communities by drug use:

> I think, and this is a guess, that most of the black leadership in this city has grown up in the midst of either the black community or the poor black community. And they have been either very close to people who turned out to be substance abus-

ers or ripped off by substance abusers. They have in one way or another had to manage their lives so that didn't happen to them. I don't know that one makes the movement very easily from that [point of view] to—[one which understands that] this is really a disease, rather than this moral issue.[15]

Thus, as black elected officials and indigenous black leaders tried to enter into the debate on AIDS during this second stage, often their efforts were layered with the class politics and social complications evident in African-American communities and noted in the quotations above. The image of a split black community, with one group composed of poor drug users and black gay men engaged in behaviors that transmit HIV, and the other group dominated by middle-class and professional blacks burdened with the responsibility of taking care of the "other" group, was a familiar frame for reporters who wrote about this disease. That story line, however, ran only a close second to the numerous articles and essays written about the innocent victims of this epidemic in black communities: children and the unsuspecting female sex partners of HIV infected men. It was these less stigmatized individuals living with HIV and AIDS that black leaders gravitated toward. Urged to respond to this burgeoning crisis, indigenous black leaders sought out ways to distance themselves from the more stigmatized aspects of AIDS and the populations associated with it. Theirs was a limited engagement; they wanted to test the water before diving in.

Similar to the reluctant and often symbolic entrance of black elected officials into the AIDS arena, the response of social service organizations, especially drug treatment programs, was slow. This delay was especially harmful to black and Latino communities, since it is estimated that "by the late 1970s, the nation . . . [had] about one million IV drug users, about a quarter of them in New York City. Some 80–90 percent were males and mostly black or Hispanic" (Joseph 1992, 221). By the mid-1980s the seropositive rate among this population was estimated to be 50 percent (Des Jarlais, Friedman, and Sotheran 1992, 280). Many drug treatment programs, however, were hesitant to become directly involved in the provision of AIDS services because they viewed this crisis as outside their domain of expertise. The staff at these organizations, while recognizing that AIDS posed a serious problem for the drug-using community, viewed the disease as a health issue, not an issue of addiction, and saw their mission as focused on addiction, not health (Oppenheimer 1988).[16] Perrow and Guillén discuss the initial unwillingness on the part of drug treatment organizations to confront the issue of AIDS, defining it as an issue outside the sphere of addiction:

> In addition to the warnings from medical experts, evidence of AIDS in the communities most affected by drug use was available from state and city agencies. The New York State Division of Substance Abuse was very well organized (even though, unlike some gay groups, the drug users were not), and it had methadone clinics and other drug treatment centers in place well before AIDS. . . . The Substance Abuse Division, tiny and underfunded as it was, had many routes into the minority community; but like most organizations, it virtually ignored the problem for the first few years. Its mandate was to fight substance abuse, not the disease that was killing the abusers. (75)

The substance abuse industry would eventually come to realize, as did black elected officials, that the need for services among those living with HIV and AIDS was so great that denial was no longer feasible. Des Jarlais, Friedman, and Sotheran, in their article "The First City: HIV among Intravenous Drug Users in New York City," call this period of adjustment, when organizations began to integrate AIDS services into their regular programs, the "coping stage." The authors comment that "the *coping stage* has been occurring since 1986, and involved incorporating AIDS issues into the day-to-day operation of drug treatment programs" (1992, 286). Quimby and Friedman also remark that "by 1987, some black medical and substance abuse personnel who had not been activists on these issues became more interested and involved. Emerging CDC evidence of black heterosexual transmission and pediatric AIDS cases heightened this concern and made continued avoidance difficult" (1989, 407).

Thus, during this second stage, drug users, their advocates, and substance abuse program staff began to see AIDS as an issue just as fundamental to their mission as addiction. As one staff member explained, "You can't deal with someone's addiction, if you don't keep them alive first." Other social service agencies initiated new programs to respond to AIDS during this stage, motivated perhaps by the information they received at national conferences on AIDS in minority communities, such as the one sponsored by the CDC in August of 1987. At these events public health officials would report the official numbers describing the disproportionate impact of AIDS on communities of color. More important than the numbers, however, was the funding made available to community groups after such functions. Agencies like the CDC, hearing the demands of community activists, would on occasion identify new, although insufficient, funding initiatives targeting organizations that served communities of color. These programs provided added incentives to traditional social service agencies contemplating a role in the response to AIDS.

With new funding incentives emerging, traditional social service agencies and drug treatment programs increasingly added AIDS education, prevention, and support to the list of services they provided. And the increased participation of traditional social service agencies in the provision of AIDS services, seemingly in response to funding opportunities, did not go unnoticed or unremarked by many black gay AIDS activists involved in the first stage of response. Phil Wilson suggests that a common practice was to use AIDS funding to replace other dried-up funding sources:

> I think that a lot of money was diverted. There was a time when a lot of drug money that was funding some social service agencies was drying out. And so a lot of folks whose funding stream had been drug money realized that they could continue their funding streams by switching to AIDS money. But they didn't have any commitment to changing the work and certainly no commitment to kind of focusing on the population.

Wilson continues, noting that some of the funding opportunities through the CDC were made possible by the controversial compromises of black gay activists:

> The other thing we did out of our naïveté, is that we came up with this phrase, "men who have sex with men." Quite frankly it was a phrase that was created by black gay men, and we created it because we knew that the CDC would not fund black gay men. So we wanted to create a phrase that was palatable to them. In the beginning we created it out of the air. There was no statistical work done to quantify the magnitude of this population of black men who were having sex with other men but didn't identify. Now intuitively we knew that they were engaged in homosexual behavior. However, the way that behavior manifested itself was not, or did not mirror the way it manifested itself in white gay men. But now the implica-

tion that there are no black gay men out there who identify as gay is absurd. And so there for the longest time all the programs were, like, targeted to this group of folks who may or may not be gay. And I used to say, what are we doing? We're marching over the dead bodies in hopes of finding a people who may not be there. And how many dead bodies do we have to march over looking for this theoretical body? Besides who are these men who have sex with men fucking anyway? They are fucking men who identify with being gay, that's who they are fucking. How else do they connect? Somebody has to have a clue about what is going on.[17]

As we can imagine, one consequence of the influx of human services professionals into the AIDS arena was that, while possibly marginalized through any number of identities, many of these people had no understanding of the political struggles that had so informed the work of black gay men. These workers saw AIDS as a crisis to be cured or serviced, not as an issue to be fought politically. Thus, as these professionals worked to provide more services in black communities, the importance of internal political struggle around issues associated with AIDS, such as homophobia, was lost or minimized. Also increasingly shut out by this crop of new AIDS service providers were members of those groups, namely black gay men, who had been so instrumental in fighting the early political battles necessary to get a number of these organizations established and funded. Undoubtedly, the decreasing presence of openly black gay men in leadership positions was also a manifestation of AIDS. Some of the most outspoken black gay activists in the AIDS community died during this period. Others chose to leave AIDS work, burned out from the loss of too many friends and too many clients. Still others, no longer willing to deal with insufficient and inconsistent pay, training new bosses with a lack of knowledge about grassroots organizing around AIDS, and the constant reminder that many in "the" community saw them and their life choices as "antiblack," either chose to leave or were driven out of AIDS work.

One especially unfortunate consequence of this influx of different AIDS service providers was the presence of identifiable levels of homophobia among this new professional staff. Joe Presley, a former staff member of the New York AIDS Council (NYAC) and a current staff member at Harlem United, describes having dinner at a conference with a black heterosexual woman who worked on the staff of another AIDS organization. During the dinner the woman explained to Mr. Presley that it was time for "you black gay men to let go, move over, and let the rest of us [heterosexuals] decide the agenda for a while."[18] And while some might applaud the willingness of black members of the new AIDS bureaucracy to claim this disease as a crisis for all those in black communities, including heterosexuals, it is the zero-sum approach represented in the comments of Mr. Presley's dinner companion that cause concern. Far from sharing in and learning from the work of black gay men, this advocate seemed to believe that the concerns of black heterosexuals living with AIDS are significantly different from those of black gay men, and thus cannot be represented by this group. Again, we need to remember that members of this new AIDS bureaucracy had their roots in the provision of services, not in struggles for rights and empowerment, at least not struggles around gay and lesbian rights, or the distribution of condoms in the high schools, or needle-exchange.[19]

In the midst of this change, however, there were some positive developments. For example, while it became increasingly clear that the staff of traditional social service agencies would not lead the fight for a more inclusive and confrontational response to AIDS in African-American communities, these organizations did attempt to improve the quality of life for people of color with AIDS. Whereas initially the staff of these organizations had little knowledge specific to AIDS, such as the best available treatments or the best doctors for referrals, they were skilled in dealing with the many extenuating circumstances that accompanied AIDS in black communities. Homelessness, unemployment, mental health issues, and a lack of access to health care were just some of the familiar problems that distinguished the manifestation of AIDS in black communities, and traditional social service workers were most successful in tackling them.

Finally, a discussion of this second stage would not be complete without some mention of the growth in AIDS-specific organizations in black and other communities of color. With the continued spread of AIDS, particularly in communities of color, the need for organizations that could address the unique needs of African Americans with AIDS as well as develop and implement culturally "sensitive" education and prevention programs became more evident. In response to this need, new funding streams were initiated from sources such as the Public Health Service and the New York State AIDS Institute. The idea behind many of these new programs was to infuse badly needed resources into poor and marginal communities. However, due to the traditional structure of these programs, many community-based organizations pursuing the most innovative work in communities of color were either judged incapable of fulfilling contract requirements or were written out of contention completely as grants focused on national organizations and regional consortiums. Consequently, much of this early money designated for "minority" education and prevention programs ended up being awarded to well-known, national black organizations like the National Medical Association, the Southern Christian Leadership Conference, and the National Urban League (Bowles and Robinson 1989; Holman et al. 1991). Despite these difficulties, a wide range of new organizations like the Black Leadership Commission on AIDS, People of Color in Crisis, Stand Up Harlem, Housing Works, and the National Minority AIDS Council (NMAC) were established during this period.

The specific AIDS organizations begun during this second stage were not all that different from the black and minority AIDS organizations initiated in the first stage of response. Most of the new organizations were staffed, at least in part, by some of the most vulnerable members of black communities—black gay men and lesbians, poor women and injection drug users. Many were begun in response to neglect on the part of traditional black organizations and newly formed white gay organizations. However, a number of these new organizations expanded their mission beyond the provision of services to individuals and began providing technical assistance to smaller grassroots organizations working around AIDS in communities of color. Gil Gerald recounts that NMAC was begun for just such a reason and with just such an agenda:

> I think it was the fifth international conference on AIDS at the Washington Hilton in 1987. We did a workshop there and were so revolted by some of the things we had heard and seen that we returned to the NAN [National AIDS Network] headquarters office that night—myself, Carl Beam, Suki Ports, Craig Harris, Don Edwards, Norm Nikens, and Paul Kowatta. We had a meeting and said we have to go ahead and formally establish [something]. We have to have somebody in Washington that recognizes the significance of people of color organizations, the technical assistance that they need, and [is willing] to be an advocate for them.[20]

While these new organizations of people of color were not that different from AIDS organizations started during the first stage, they were different from AIDS organizations whose client and funding populations came primarily from white gay communities.[21] In primarily white gay communities the subject of AIDS had become a rallying cry and a standard of liberation for the entire group. Many black AIDS organizations instead walked a tightrope, trying to gently challenge indigenous ideologies which constructed gay and lesbian lifestyles, drug use, and premarital sex in general as wrong and immoral. Facing both ideological hostility and resource deficiency, black AIDS organizations took on additional responsibilities in trying to serve their constituencies. Although none of these organizations, I believe, saw their role as purely political, a few in this group knew that to truly change the development of AIDS in African-American communities, they had to engage in political battles over how to redefine in non-normative frames drug use and homosexuality. Several of these bold organizations had been started or were currently staffed by significant numbers of black gay men, lesbians, and current or recovering drug users. Organizations whose staff and clients consisted of the "contested members" of black communities often struggled to develop new ways to transform the meaning of the epidemic and their work, so that they might empower their clients without destroying the networks which linked them to support systems in black communities. Thus, as the second stage came to a close, the most marginal members of black communities—black gay men and lesbians, drug users, sex workers, poor women and men, homeless adults and teenagers—through their struggles for survival fought to ensure that those serving African-American communities responded to AIDS in a more comprehensive and political manner. Because of *their* work, the participation of indigenous black leaders, black elected officials, and traditional social service agencies was the defining development of the second stage of response.

Stage 3: The AIDS Bureaucracy in African-American Communities—Beyond Race?

The third stage of response to AIDS in black communities began in the early 1990s and continues today. Extending beyond the scope of this book, a few defining characteristics warrant comment. The first is the continued professionalization of AIDS work in black communities. Even more clearly than in the second stage, we can discern the shift that has occurred from the first stage, where there was an absence of formal AIDS organizations and a cadre of workers "staffed" primarily by black gay men. In the third stage, we find a process of professionalization that mirrors in significant ways the wave of professionalism experienced by primarily white AIDS organizations earlier in the epidemic and discussed by Cindy Patton in her book *Inventing AIDS* (1990). Prior to this trend in professionalization, those doing AIDS work in black communities seemed to have a dual focus. One goal was to ensure that dominant institutions would provide resources and services to black communities in response to this and other crises. The second goal centered on the work of activists, often black gay men, struggling internally with indigenous institutions. Here efforts were mounted to have indigenous leaders and organizations acknowledge and work in partnership with all segments of black communities affected by AIDS. Increasingly, in the third stage, professional social workers, policy wonks, and administrators have come to staff and head the few AIDS organizations centered in communities of color, especially those receiving significant amounts of state or federal funds. As mentioned earlier, these individuals have often come to their jobs devoid of any political focus except acquiring more funding for their agencies. Consequently, many organizations servicing people of color with AIDS pursue agendas structured around service provision and education, with little effort devoted to politics.[22] Struggles for gay and lesbian rights or the empowerment of the drug-using population beyond the issue of AIDS are seen as secondary or tangential to the work of the many traditionally modeled multiservice organizations that increasingly compose the AIDS bureaucracy in black communities.

A second defining characteristic of this period has been the institutionalization of an emphasis on community-based organizations. At the national level, government agencies have begun to demand at least the symbolic participation of local community groups in funding decisions. Such directives provide the opening into dominant institutions needed by smaller, grassroots AIDS organizations. Community-based organizations are finally able to secure a foothold in their efforts to change the discourse and distribution of resources around AIDS. For example, the CDC currently requires all states and municipalities receiving funds for HIV and AIDS programs to establish a planning group that includes community delegates. At the local level, numerous community groups, such as substance abuse organizations—which in the early years of the epidemic were seen as outside the AIDS bureaucracy—now have increased contact and interaction with other AIDS service providers. These organizations have become important players in the AIDS industry, and some of the more radical groups, such as those seeking to organize drug users, are leading important political struggles around issues such as needle exchange.

Additionally, as women come to constitute a larger percentage of those with HIV and AIDS, they have also become more integrally involved in the formal work of black AIDS organizations. More generally, there has been an increase in the number of service providers attempting to develop and implement programs aimed at the different issues women face regarding HIV and AIDS. This expansion has resulted not only from a desire on the part of AIDS organizations to respond to the needs of their female clients, but also from an attempt to enlarge the populations these organizations serve for funding purposes. Furthermore, lesbians and women with AIDS, many of them women of color, have been active, demanding that the different manifestations of HIV and AIDS in their lives be recognized and addressed. Interestingly, while black and Latina women are disproportionately represented among women with AIDS, the majority of women who work in the AIDS bureaucracy are white.

Third, the issue of funding or resource allocation also seems to have motivated new activity. The question of equitable funding through sources such as the Ryan White Care Act brought a number of black elected officials into the thick of political battles around AIDS. Sensing an issue which they could rally around without too closely linking themselves with the marginal groups associated with AIDS, black elected officials took up the fight for increased AIDS funding in black communities. Often this struggle for money has been framed as a battle between resource-rich and overly indulged white gay communities and poor and largely ignored black and Latino communities. Of course, a case can be made that white gay men have received and controlled the lion's share of available AIDS funding; this simple dichotomy, however, does little to advance the interests of any group working for more AIDS funding.

Despite this unfortunate competition for limited resources, the fight for funding has occasionally united AIDS organizations serving numerous communities. For example, in the summer of 1992, AIDS organizations from across the country came together under the banner "United for AIDS Action." The efforts of this coalition of over 425 organizations and groups was directed at both the Democratic and Republican presidential nominees, although the most visible action was a massive rally of nearly twenty-five thousand people in Times Square during the Democratic Convention in New York City. This campaign was centered around a five-point program calling for: (1) presidential leadership on the issue of AIDS; (2) AIDS care through universal health care; (3) increased funding for research; (4) expanded AIDS education; and (5) protection from HIV- and AIDS-based discrimination. In the end the coalition fell apart or disbanded, depending on one's perspective, due to the specific demands and interests of each member organization, as well as dissension over whether the Gay Men's Health Crisis, the initiators of this effort, had too much control. However, before its dissolution, United for AIDS Action made a substantial effort that mobilized the resources of multiple communities in the fight against AIDS.[23]

In the third stage, there seems to be an increased, although constrained, willingness on the part of "minority" AIDS organizations to work in coalition with "white" AIDS organizations on funding and policy issues perceived as benefiting all groups.[24] Frequently, the first request for coalition work is initiated by white AIDS organizations that increasingly need either contact with organizations serving people of color or minority clients to justify their expanding budget requests in the face of demographic changes in the distribution of AIDS cases.[25] Dr. Billy Jones suggests that as AIDS continues to take root in communities of color, white AIDS organizations will have to work with AIDS activists and organizations of color if they want to protect their funding:

> If those agencies and groups that already have a well-rounded foundation in this are going to be able to be funded federally, and otherwise if they are going to continue to be of service, then they are going to have to deal more and more with the minority patients. To do that; then, would bring them naturally much more into contact with the other groups that are basically the minority groups. And there has got to be some kind of give and take and some kind of compromise and some kind of coalition development for that to happen. The HIV Planning Counsel which I chair is a good example of that. I mean there are minorities on it and minorities stand up and say we're gonna make it happen. So there has to be a negotiating [process] that happens to kind of move everything forward.[26]

Again, social service professionals in communities of color who are focused on the delivery of services may have less stringent ideological standards which preclude them from working with white AIDS organizations. Also, AIDS organizations rooted in communities of color often do not have the resources available to assign staff members to non–service oriented work, such as lobbying and policy analysis. Under such circumstances, they may benefit from working with more financially secure white AIDS organizations. So for example, Gil Gerald has stated that the National Minority AIDS Council relies quite heavily on information it receives from the AIDS Action Counsel, an AIDS lobbying organization based in Washington and funded substantially by the Gay Men's Health Crisis, when trying to assess which political issues will be a priority for them.[27] I do not, however, want to minimize the degree of skepticism and hostility still felt by those working at black community-based organizations about primarily white, gay, community-based AIDS service organizations. A number of people serving the black community, like the woman in the second case history at the beginning of this book, repeatedly see white AIDS organizations being awarded government and private contracts, while their own organizations struggle to stay in business. Further, this tension is heightened by what is perceived to be the disjunction or inconsistency between the staffing patterns of many white AIDS organizations, whose staff members are often primarily white gay men and lesbians, and the public, almost preachy stances they take on issues such as needle exchange, condom distribution in the high schools, and the development of an AIDS curriculum—issues that black AIDS activists lament are experienced most severely in communities of color.

Finally, the fourth and last characteristic that I want to comment on is the development of organizations supporting specifically gay communities of color. Some of these organizations were purely political and focused on struggles around AIDS in communities of color; others were multidimensional and devoted attention to AIDS secondarily or in conjunction with other service, educational, and political programs. The important thing about these later groups is that their organizational vision and mission are broader than those of most AIDS organizations. These groups view AIDS as just one issue, albeit a critical one, shaping the quality of life for black lesbians, gay men, and other "queer" identified people. For example, black gay organizations like Gay Men of African Descent (GMAD) of New York City have been and continue to be essential in educational efforts seeking to reach large numbers of black men.[28] And while GMAD has been in existence for over ten years, it has only been recently, in the beginning of this third stage, that members have turned their attention to the formal provision of services and the development of education and prevention programs. Robert Penn, the former acting director of GMAD, explains that they see their mission as including, but not limited to, AIDS.

The Audre Lorde Project (ALP), a lesbian, gay, bisexual, two-spirit, and transgender (LGBTST) center for people of color, is another such organization.[29] Begun in 1993 through the efforts of Advocates of Gay Men of Color—a multiracial group of HIV policy advocates—the Audre Lorde Project seeks to develop "innovative and unified community strategies to address the multiple issues impacting LGBTST people of color communities."[30] While receiving their initial funding from a contract with the New York AIDS Institute to develop AIDS programming for gay men of color, this project alone does not define the entire agenda of the center. Instead, energy has been devoted to securing additional money that allows the organization the freedom to implement numerous programs, especially projects focused on organizing efforts by women, youth, and immigrants. Thus, in this third stage, government contracts to provide or coordinate AIDS services in communities of color are being used to provide services as well as establish and stabilize the financial base of community organizations. However, black gay and lesbian multiservice organizations seem unwilling to have their work restricted to just the domain of AIDS. These organizations from their inception have had a more expansive purpose in mind and are committed to pursuing a broad agenda aimed at the various issues confronting lesbian and gay communities of color. Unlike early attempts by black gay men to respond to the entire black community, these new gay people of color organizations focus their work specifically on gay men, lesbians, and other queer-identified community members believed to be neglected by traditional social service agencies and white AIDS organizations.[31]

In conjunction with the development of new gay people of color organizations and centers, a few political organizations of lesbian and gay people of color also developed that were centered around AIDS. The third stage included the emergence of organizations such as VOCAL (Voices of Color against AIDS and for Life) and BAM! (Black AIDS Mobilization). These organizations provided few if any direct services to those with AIDS; instead, they concentrated most of their energy on participating in political battles centered around AIDS in communities of color. Although not as resource- and membership-rich as ACT UP (AIDS Coalition to Unleash Power), these organizations worked within their limitations to draw attention to the spread of

AIDS in communities of color. In fact, many of the activists of color involved in both BAM! and VOCAL had previous connections to and maintained contacts with white AIDS activists in ACT UP; in fact, BAM! grew out of the black caucus of ACT UP. Individuals frustrated with what they perceived to be the racist actions of some in ACT UP and the narrow interests of many men in the organization who wanted to concentrate the group's resources almost exclusively on the process of drug approval decided to build an alternative organization.

Much like the black gay men and lesbians who responded to AIDS in the early part of the epidemic, these largely young "queer" activists of color saw their agenda as reaching beyond the specific issues of lesbians and gay men of color dealing with AIDS. And while this cadre of activists sought to involve themselves in many political issues shaping the development of AIDS in people of color communities—issues ranging from needle exchange to AIDS funding and the distribution of condoms in New York City high schools—they were most effective and generated more authority when responding to AIDS issues rooted in the intersectional experiences of black lesbians, gay men, and bisexuals. Thus, for example, when the *New York Post* accused black city council member Enoch Williams in 1992 of making extensive homophobic statements concerning AIDS and AIDS funding, members of both VOCAL and BAM!, but in particular BAM!, jumped into action, releasing their own press statements on the issue and organizing other gay and lesbian groups of color to respond as a unified entity. These organizations functioned primarily in a responsive mode, reacting to individuals and groups both inside and outside of black and gay communities that were perceived as inattentive to, or dismissive of, the needs of those with AIDS in communities of color. Eventually, both BAM! and VOCAL collapsed, but during the early part of the third phase they provided a small, yet mobilized group of individuals focused almost exclusively on the politics of AIDS in black and other communities of color. The emergence of these small political organizations, even for a short time, is a dynamic that has not been repeated in recent years. While the increasing professionalization of even people of color AIDS organizations undoubtedly has something to do with the dearth of activism from communities of color, I am sure that the absence of other political organizations such as ACT UP, signaling a "cycle of protest" and acting as a contagious element, is also a significant part of the explanation (Tarrow 1989).

Conclusion

Since the formal recognition of AIDS in 1981, the response to this epidemic in black communities has changed dramatically. Beginning largely from a base of activist black gay men, family, and friends to include the efforts of social service agencies, traditional organizations and leaders serving black constituencies, an AIDS industry has now emerged in black communities. However, to say that there now exists an infrastructure for the provision of services and the distribution of limited funding is not to say that we have arrived at a time when African Americans view AIDS as the most or one of the most important issues facing black communities.[32] We still have not arrived at a moment where all those with AIDS in black communities, including African-American gay men and drug users, are embraced and "owned" as essential members of the group. We are still far from the day when black organizations, leaders and elected officials define their success around AIDS as the ability to transform fundamental thinking in black communities about this crisis.

However, the response to AIDS as it has developed in African-American communities is not a failure; to read this chapter (and those that follow) as making that claim would be a mistake. Instead, I have tried to make two general points. First, to understand the response to AIDS requires identifying the context in which African Americans and their leaders acted. Attention to context does not excuse inaction, but provides a more complicated picture of the multiple institutions and individuals shaping and constraining politics in black communities. Second, while there has been substantial failure in the response to AIDS in black communities—a topic pursued throughout this book—there has also been change. It would therefore be unfair and disingenuous of me not to acknowledge that in a time of crisis some individuals and institutions were able to respond. And while often they were further marginalized, facing secondary process of exclusion, they mounted a response for black communities. Thus we must explore both the failures and the successes in the response to AIDS as we construct the political agenda and identities of African Americans for the twenty-first century.

Having laid out the general contours of how the response to AIDS in African-American communities unfolded, we can return to the beginning of this epidemic, when the CDC learned of a new infectious disease and set the wheels of response in motion.

CHAPTER FOUR

Invisible to the Centers for Disease Control

With over half a million (612,078) Americans classified as having AIDS and over three hundred thousand deaths from this epidemic, I can assert with confidence that by now most people have heard of AIDS.[1] In fact, survey results from as early as 1983 indicate that within two years of the first public notification of a "strange cancer afflicting gay men," more than a majority of whites and nonwhites were aware of AIDS (Singer, Rogers, and Corcoran 1987, 584).[2] Despite such high levels of general public recognition, there were substantial differences in awareness between groups. For instance, while 79 percent of whites indicated awareness of AIDS in 1983, only 63 percent of nonwhites indicated comparable awareness (Singer, Rogers, and Corcoran 1987). Similar differences between whites and blacks were also noted by researchers, not in general levels of recognition, but instead in respondents' ideas about transmission routes, perceived risk, regulation of those with AIDS, and willingness to alter personal behavior to prevent AIDS. Public opinion analysis and empirical research, while not conclusive, suggest that blacks (nonwhites in some surveys) tend to be less accurate in their assessment of actual transmission routes for HIV; more concerned about the possibility of contracting HIV; more supportive of regulatory measures purported to control the spread of AIDS; and they report more adaptive behavioral changes thought to prevent AIDS (Singer 1989; Herek and Capitanio 1993; Nicholas, Tredoux, and Daniels 1994). It is this phenomenon of different group understanding, conceptualization, and reaction to AIDS that frames the next few chapters.

Beyond observable differences in levels of awareness among communities, I am interested in how groups, in particular African Americans, came to conceptualize this epidemic and their relationship to it. Today it is commonly understood that AIDS is a disease that wreaks disproportionate havoc and death on gay men and their communities.[3] Male-to-male sex, as at least one form of possible transmission, still accounts for 55 percent of all those classified with AIDS.[4] But how many people, especially African Americans, see this as an equally dev-astating crisis for black communities? Further, how has an understand-ing of AIDS as something threatening black communities, but located in groups and behaviors thought to be inherently "outside" of black communities—in particular gay sex—directed the political responses of black leaders? Before Magic Johnson, before Arthur Ashe, before Rock Hudson, even before the picture of AIDS as a disease first and foremost of the gay community was etched into our collective con-sciousness, there was a time when we knew nothing of AIDS. Yet over the years, decisions were made, and images and narratives were mobi-lized that would frame our understanding of this epidemic. Chapters 4–7 explore this process of defining the issue of AIDS.

Starting from the framework of marginalization detailed in chapter 2, it is very clear that an examination of only dominant institutions as information providers would be inadequate and could not tell the complete story of how any group, let alone a marginal group such as African Americans, came to conceptualize this epidemic. Research in the area of AIDS education has previously demonstrated the impor-tance of culturally sensitive information, often produced indigenously, in increasing the retention and reception of this material (Stevenson and Davis 1994; Bowser 1992; Thomas and Quinn 1991). Thus I exam-ine community-generated news and the importance of credible sources in the communication of sensitive information later in the book. Still, it would be at best naive and at worst simply wrong to proceed as if dominant institutions played no significant role in shaping African-American thoughts about AIDS. Whether it be directly, through the information these institutions provide, or indirectly, through the suspi-cion that information from such sources generates, dominant institu-tions are major players in shaping black communities' understanding and response to this disease. For this reason, I begin by inquiring how the framing of AIDS by dominant or external institutions affected Afri-can Americans.[5] The next two chapters do not provide a complete his-tory of dominant institutional responses to AIDS; rather, they highlight general trends in dominant system responses to this crisis.

Specifically, I focus on two broad institutions of information devel-opment and transfer during the AIDS epidemic: the Centers for Dis-ease Control and Prevention (CDC) and the mainstream of corporate media. My sources on the media include the network evening news and the *New York Times*. I have chosen to examine these dominant institutions because each performed critical tasks in bringing AIDS to the public's awareness. The CDC—as the nation's public health institution responsible for promoting "health and quality of life by preventing and controlling disease, injury and disability"—served, in the early years of this epidemic, as the most important informant on the progression of AIDS.[6] The epidemiological work of CDC staff members constructed the "facts" of this disease. The CDC helped to define who was at risk, as well as the appropriate paths of research, reporting, and response that others would follow. The media, on the other hand, served as a critical "linking institution," transferring agency-specific information into more general ideological frames for the public's consumption. Different domains of the media facilitated the transformation of what might be considered private concerns into more generally understood public issues. Their actions and attention indicated the salience of AIDS to individuals' lives. I analyze the network evening news and the mainstream print media separately, since each contributes to our knowledge of AIDS in very distinct ways— for overlapping yet distinguishable constituencies. While print media such as the *New York Times* serve as an agenda setter for elites and presumably more informed individuals, the nightly news is in the business of producing headlines for mass consumption. And although each institution or media domain communicates general information on AIDS, their goals, methods, and perspectives are quite diverse.

Finally, I explore not only the descriptive question of how these institutions defined AIDS for the general public, as well as for specifically black communities, but also why elites in these institutions chose certain images, framings, and narratives instead of others. Researchers involved in the analysis of dominant institutional responses to AIDS have taken up a similar question, namely: Did the marginal status of those individuals and groups first thought to be at risk for AIDS—gay men and injection drug users—influence the epidemiology pursued by the CDC or the information advanced through the media? I extend this line of inquiry to pose a more specific question: To what degree did the marginal status of African-American communities influence the attention and information African Americans and other people of color received from both the CDC and the media?

I expect that this analysis will identify the absence of any significant and sustained attention to AIDS in black communities. And if, in fact, there is an absence of images about, or a silencing of information on, AIDS among African Americans, how do we explain this omission? Is the invisibility of marginal communities the result of intentional actions on the part of individuals working within these institutions? Does the absence of attention result merely from the institutional rules of both the CDC and the media, having little to do with common prejudices and preferences? Or is the absence of images and stories a manifestation of the systemic marginalization confronting these groups, reinforcing and reproducing their secondary status?

Much of the dominant institutional response to AIDS, as highlighted by these examples, can be understood through two distinct yet intersecting factors: one, the complicated marginal status of those groups first identified with the disease, including their secondary status within marginal communities; the other, the preexisting institutional biases under which dominant systems "normally" respond to new and evolving issues. I want to be clear that highlighting the role of systemic bias and the marginal status of groups does not negate the critical role race played in determining the early response to AIDS from dominant institutions. In fact, both of these intersecting factors are integrally tied to and work through race as it serves as a marker of marginalization, and racism as it structures and guides institutional bias. So while most individuals probably suspect that the social location of those first associated with this disease constrained and directed the activities of numerous dominant institutions, I believe empirical analysis of this frequently stated and under-researched hypothesis might be helpful. With this as a goal, we turn our attention to the work of the Centers for Disease Control in constructing the public's understanding of AIDS.

The Centers for Disease Control and Prevention

On 5 June 1981, the Centers for Disease Control (CDC) published the first official notification of a disease that would later be called AIDS in the *Morbidity and Mortality Weekly Report (MMWR)*. This report (which will be cited in the text) notes general health trends in the country as compiled by the CDC and is sent to thousands of hospitals and health agencies across the country. A short article on the second page of the report noted the occurrence of five cases of biopsy-confirmed pneumocystis carinii pneumonia (PCP) in the Los Angeles area. Of special note was that all five patients were men who were young, previously healthy, and homosexual. This first governmental reporting of the AIDS epidemic highlighted the common sexual identity of the patients, suggesting that some aspect of their gay "lifestyle" might be the underlying cause of the disease. "The fact that these patients were all homosexuals suggests an association between some aspect of a homosexual lifestyle or disease acquired through sexual contact and pneumocystis pneumonia in this population" (CDC, *MMWR* 5 June 1981).

The CDC was notified of the occurrence of this new disease when Dr. Michael Gottlieb, an immunologist at UCLA's medical research center, was treating a young gay man and recognized his symptoms as similar to the symptoms of another young gay man he had recently seen.[7] Believing that something unusual and medically exciting was happening, Gottlieb followed the procedures for notification of new and possibly infectious agents, as detailed by the CDC. When presented with a possible infectious agent, doctors are instructed to contact their local or state health department officials or the CDC directly.[8] If the threat seems serious enough, the CDC will send out an Epidemic Intelligence Service (EIS) officer to investigate. The critical component in this process that often goes unnoticed, however, is the doctor's ability to recognize a pattern of unusual occurrences for a specific population of patients. Dr. Gottlieb contacted the local health department and was connected to his friend, Dr. Wayne Shandera, who at the time was working as a CDC EIS officer on site at the Los Angeles Health Department. Shandera used his connections within the CDC to produce the government's first report on the AIDS crisis in the *MMWR* of June 1981.

With notification of these cases of PCP, the official tracking of AIDS had begun. A task force in the CDC, headed by Dr. James Curran, was set up by mid-1981 with the goal of providing surveillance of this disease.[9] As Gerald M. Oppenheimer (1992) notes, it was the early epidemiology pursued by the CDC, before the discovery of the reported cause of AIDS, the human immunodeficiency virus (HIV), that produced the initial "facts" of the disease—defining who was at risk and how the disease was spread:

> Epidemiology played a key role in the AIDS epidemic for at least two reasons—one institutional, the other scientific. The institutional link was the Centers for Disease Control (CDC) in Atlanta. . . . The CDC is responsible for monitoring morbidity and mortality trends in the United States and for responding to acute outbreaks of disease—infectious disease in particular. To fulfill its mission, the CDC depends heavily

on case reports, surveillance, and epidemiological investigations. . . .

Consequently, epidemiology bore the initial responsibility of
outlining the direction of research, generating hypotheses, and
synthesizing the results. (51–52)

Clearly, staff at the CDC played an enormous role in defining this disease: delineating those at greater risk (risk groups); deciding who
could be classified and counted as having AIDS (case definition); and
communicating to the public the progress of the epidemic. It was also,
however, the early actions of the medical profession—physicians, the
blood industry, and health care workers—when AIDS was seen as a
disease of "homosexuals" and "junkies," that helped signal the marginal position of those believed to be most at risk for this disease.[10]

In their initial investigations of AIDS, the CDC did not know the
cause of the immune deficiency experienced by patients. The suggested causes ranged from theories focused on repeated attacks on the
immune system leading to an overload, to ideas of a possible infectious agent, to the hypothesis that there existed a genetic defect among
gay men, to speculation that centered on environmental factors as well
as lifestyle or behavioral relationships (Oppenheimer 1988). The evidence and analysis of decisions made by members of the CDC task
force suggest that while pursuing all possible leads regarding the origin of the disease, the task force focused much of its attention on the
gay lifestyle hypothesis. The initial data indicated that the one common feature of this outbreak was that it had attacked primarily young,
white, gay men. In fact, in the 28 August 1981, issue of the *MMWR* the
CDC announced that it had registered 108 patients, of whom 94 percent were homosexual or bisexual. Thus it became the objective of
CDC staff members to identify what about "the gay lifestyle" led to
the onset of immune deficiency.

The importance of the CDC as a primary signaling institution in the
medical care and health policy industries cannot be overstated. Since
its beginning in 1946 as the Communicable Disease Center, researchers
at the CDC have been at the forefront of defining the causes, nature,
and importance of emerging medical crises.[11] As noted previously, the
CDC, as the main institution providing information and direction to
the rest of the country, had a very powerful rippling effect in constructing the public's understanding of the AIDS epidemic. Thus, as
the CDC pursued its investigation of what came to be known as AIDS,
focusing on the connection of this disease to the gay community, they

were, possibly unwittingly, sending a message to those who take their cues from this institution—physicians and health care systems across the country, scientific and lay media, as well as government and community leaders—that this was a disease primarily, and possibly exclusively, of gay men. The strength of this commitment to framing this disease as one exclusively located in gay communities is reflected in the early working names given this medical mystery by the press (including the gay press) and researchers—"gay pneumonia," "gay cancer" and the more official sounding "GRID" (gay-related immune deficiency).

The overriding focus of the CDC on the gay community has been documented by others studying this phenomenon. Gerald Oppenheimer (1988), in his article detailing epidemiological approaches to AIDS, informs us that almost all of the fieldwork initiated by the CDC focused on gay men. Further, one of the first case-control studies of AIDS initiated by the CDC in October 1981, as well as most other early case-control studies, used only gay men as the subjects. Dr. David Ostrow, a well-known AIDS researcher and one of the premier doctors dealing with hepatitis B, also states that much of the research generated through previous work in gay communities, investigating especially sexually transmitted diseases, was used as baseline data for research on AIDS.[12] I point out these practices not to deny the overwhelming numbers of gay men who suffered from this disease or to suggest that such attention was unmerited, but instead to highlight how "normal" institutional procedures can bias or limit the "objective" work of scientific analysis, influencing the social construction of a medical crisis.

For many researchers during the 1980s, the data showed conclusively that the first wave of AIDS was experienced by gay men—primarily white gay men. Other groups, such as injection drug users and women—primarily black and Latino/a—were often characterized as forming a second or later wave of HIV and AIDS, transmitted through blood, needles, and heterosexual sex (Joseph 1992). In retrospect, researchers in the 1990s have begun to rethink their characterization of the development of HIV and AIDS. Specifically, scholars are moving away from a model of phases or waves regarding the onset of HIV and AIDS in different communities to a model that emphasizes the parallel tracking or multiple sites of development of the epidemic among both gay men and injection drug users. For instance, Des Jarlais, Friedman, and Sotheran (1992), leading researchers on AIDS and drug-using populations, argue that HIV was clearly present and being transmitted among the population of injection drug users during the 1970s. Their research indicates that between 1975 and 1978 the seroprevalence rate of HIV among injection drug users in New York City was probably less than 20 percent.[13] However, between 1978 and 1982, reports suggest that seroprevalence rates among that population increased to 50 percent.

In part, this increase was due to an expansion in the supply of heroin and cocaine in the late 1970s and early 1980s. It is believed that readily available heroin led to more injections and thus increased transmission of HIV among injection drug users (Des Jarlais, Friedman, and Sotheran 1992). Additionally, Wallace and Wallace (1990) point to the fiscal policies of New York City officials during the late 1960s and early 1970s as contributing to the increase in seroprevalence among injection drug users. Specifically, the researchers argue that when New York City Mayor John V. Lindsay decided to cut fire-control services in order to save money, he may have inadvertently helped trigger "a contagious epidemic of building fires beginning in 1973." A number of these burned-out shells of buildings, located predominantly in poor communities of color, would eventually be used as shooting galleries by injection drug users. This argument builds on the work of other researchers, such as Friedman et al. (1987), that "the proportion of injections that one took in shooting galleries (clandestine commercial establishments whose 'owners' rent space, syringes, and needles to IV drug users to use in shooting up) was a risk factor in addition to drug-injection frequency" (482–83).

Other researchers, such as Cindy Patton (1990), have also discussed the prevalence of HIV and AIDS among injection drug users during the 1970s. Patton describes, in particular, an epidemic that some called "junkie pneumonia," thought to be the precursor to or manifestation of AIDS in injection-drug-using populations during the late 1970s. However, the most startling evidence to suggest the parallel development of HIV and AIDS among injection-drug-using populations and gay men is a study highlighted by former New York City Department of Health Commissioner Stephen C. Joseph. In *Dragon within the Gates* (1992), Joseph describes research conducted through the New York City Department of Health by Dr. Rand Stoneburner. Staff at the Department of Health reviewed medical records of all *drug-related* deaths in New York City between 1980 and 1986. The researchers found an additional twenty-five hundred deaths that seemed to be HIV- or AIDS-related but did not meet the federal (CDC) case-definition of

AIDS at the time and therefore were not recorded as AIDS-related deaths. (I will come back to the reason these diagnoses were never made.) Stoneburner et al., in a 1990 editorial review commenting on this and other findings, state that "surveillance in New York City based on the CDC AIDS case-definition has been shown to underestimate cases of fatal HIV-related disease in IVDUs by over 100 percent. The true proportion, therefore, of HIV-ill heterosexuals with a risk of intravenous drug use is much larger than that reflected in AIDS surveillance" (103).

Such significant undercounting is itself cause for concern, since it signals the inefficiency of current surveillance procedures. However, what may be of greater importance in these findings is the potential of these twenty-five hundred AIDS cases to redefine how we think and talk about AIDS, at least in New York City. Specifically, Joseph claims that if one readjusts the city's mortality figures to take into account these additional deaths among injection drug users, then the number of AIDS-related deaths among injection drug users would have surpassed those among gay men during the early phase of the epidemic. At the very least, this evidence seems to undermine the second-wave theory of AIDS among injection drug users. However, much more significantly, these findings underscore the importance of how certain narratives and assumptions construct our thinking and reasoning about AIDS. We can only imagine how the general public's understanding of and response to AIDS might have been even more negatively influenced, had the dominant image associated with the epidemic in its earliest advent been poor black and Latino/a drug users. More specifically for this project, we are left to wonder how the response of African Americans and Latinos/as in particular would have evolved if faced from the very beginning with the framing of AIDS as a disease of black and Latino communities.[14]

I focus on the undercounting in particular of black and Latino/a drug users because it is generally recognized that the escalating rates of HIV in drug-using populations disproportionately affect drug users of color. It is believed that racial differences in the conditions surrounding drug use put black and Latino/a drug users at greater risk for AIDS. For instance, the risk of being arrested for possession of hypodermic needles and syringes—clean "works" that could possibly save your life—is higher in black and Latino neighborhoods under greater police surveillance.[15] Black and Latino/a drug users, in response to this risk, are therefore more likely to use shooting galleries where needles and works can be rented with no risk of possession. The result of such differential conditions is that while estimates from the 1993 National Household Survey on Drug Abuse indicate that there are nearly two and a half times as many white drug users (320,000) as African-American drug users (133,000), African-American drug users are *five* times more likely to be diagnosed with AIDS (Day 1995).[16]

However, the problem is not simply that the CDC overlooked the development of HIV and AIDS among injection drug users and thus entirely mischaracterized the nature of this epidemic for the general public and more specifically for communities of color. There was unquestionably some awareness early on that this new disease was also appearing among injection drug users. In the 10 December 1981 issue of the *New England Journal of Medicine,* Dr. Henry Masur reported on the occurrence of AIDS among five drug users (Grmek 1990, 11). Further, by mid-1982 the mysterious new disease was beginning to be known less as GRID and more as the four-H disease: homosexuals, Haitians, heroin-users, and hemophiliacs (Grmek 1990, 31). My focus, therefore, is not on why the CDC did not know, in the first few years of the epidemic, that AIDS was emerging among injection drug users, but instead if and why, with infection rates nearing 50 percent in this population in urban areas like New York City, there seemed to be a severe, possibly systematic, undercounting of their cases of AIDS. Moreover, and perhaps most important, what was the impact of this undercounting?

There are, of course, numerous reasons why such undercounting may have occurred, but I want to focus on five factors that seem to have influenced the statistical portrait of AIDS: (1) access to health care; (2) the CDC's familiarity with certain subpopulations; (3) perceptions of health by providers; (4) the inability of the CDC to fully incorporate new information; and (5) the larger political context. On the question of access, if we take as an example the data available to CDC staff in the early years of the epidemic, we know that much of this information came from health departments and physicians across the country reporting cases of illness and disease among populations previously perceived as healthy. Thus, the ability of providers to notice and report irregularities in their patient populations was of critical importance in the first stages of identifying those subpopulations at risk. Without the cooperation and input of doctors and health officials, the CDC would never have understood the full range of this disease, even after the implementation of regulations making it mandatory to report AIDS diagnoses. Through this reporting mechanism, most of the initial cases classified by the CDC as AIDS or GRID were among gay men. The data on AIDS took this form in large part because this community was disproportionately affected by the disease. But the content of the data was also shaped by the access to quality medical care available to some members of gay communities.

Members of other groups facing HIV and AIDS were often under-represented in the initial data of the CDC due to their lack of access to adequate medical care. Injection drug users, poor women, and other economically marginal people at behavioral risk for AIDS rarely saw the same doctor twice. They rarely received services from providers who had the time and resources to closely follow developments in the health status of their "visits."[17] They rarely interacted with physicians who were consistently aware of the latest developments concerning AIDS. They rarely encountered specialists who were connected to the inner circles of the CDC. And when these people did meet specialists in infectious disease, it was often as they lay dying from what ap-peared to be some complication from pneumonia. This population most often received their care from "Medicaid mills" or the emergency rooms of teaching hospitals like UCLA or NYU—the same hospitals that were so critical in identifying this disease among referred and formally admitted gay patients. Keith Cylar, executive director of Housing Works, an organization dedicated to finding housing for people who are HIV positive and homeless, discusses the difficulties in finding medical care for poor, HIV-positive people of color:

> I spent three months trying to get my client benefits so that he could go to a medical clinic, but access to a clinic doesn't guarantee he will get *good* health care, it just guarantees he'll get *some* health care. I mean he won't have the same doctor following his case, his doctor won't know the latest treatment recommendations with regard to AIDS, and for all we know the way hospitals close in our neighborhoods, he may not even have a clinic to go to next year (emphasis added).[18]

The medical marginalization of, in particular, injection drug users occurs for a number of reasons. Most significant is their lack of access to the resources needed to guarantee medical care, whether those re-sources are money or health insurance. However, the insufficient medi-cal care received by this group is also an artifact of the illegal activity in which many in this population are engaged periodically, often as a means of securing their next hit. Most drug users deliberately avoid interacting with institutions where their drug use can be identified, curtailed, and possibly used to obtain their incarceration. This distancing from the medial establishment poses a concern, not only for their personal health and, in this case, the accurate counting of AIDS cases, but more generally for monitoring and controlling "the public health." If segments of the population are systematically outside the realm of health care surveillance, then we can expect that the diseases that plague these groups will be identified only after significant numbers of ostracized group members have been seriously affected by such illnesses—leading in some cases to their death—or when these same diseases reach those parts of the population with access to mainstream health care.

Ernest Quimby and Samuel Friedman (1989) comment specifically on this phenomenon of finding and identifying many injection drug users with AIDS after they had died. They suggest that many injection drug users were dying from HIV-related disease long before they could be classified as having AIDS (404). Randy Shilts, in *And the Band Played On* (1987), also reports that Mary Guinan, a member of the CDC's first task force on AIDS, found that most of the AIDS cases among intravenous drug users (IVDU) that she tried to follow were dead before they ever got reported to the CDC. Thus it seems that the marginalized status of poor people and injection drug users, who had limited access to the health care system, rendered them invisible to the CDC. If these individuals were invisible to the CDC, then the cause of their death was also invisible to the communities of color, like the African-American and Latino communities, to which many belonged.

In contrast to the exclusion and neglect experienced by injection drug users and poor people at behavioral risk for AIDS, the social and economic privilege afforded a sufficient number of gay men, independent of their stigmatized sexual identity, helped them in their fight against AIDS. In his autobiography, former Surgeon General C. Everett Koop (1991) suggests that by developing an indigenous set of doctors who were familiar with the health patterns of the gay community, gay men in the 1970s and 1980s may have "effectively *placed themselves* outside the mainstream of clinical medicine, making them difficult to reach and to help," adding to the delay of the Public Health Service in responding to AIDS (emphasis added, 197). While Koop may be correct in his assessment that those gay men who were able to did patronize physicians who were sensitive to and knowledgeable about issues specific to the gay community, his insight ends there. His assertion that gay men "placed themselves outside the mainstream of clinical medicine" demonstrates his lack of understanding of the causal direction and institutional practices of marginalization that necessitate that marginal groups such as gay men and lesbians develop community health organizations and networks of doctors that will be attentive to their needs. Further, Koop seems to ignore the ability of some of these same gay men to access not only the mainstream of the medical profession, but in some instances the best of the medical profession with respect to the diagnosis of AIDS.

Still, Dr. Koop's comprehension that there are those who exist outside the mainstream and are thus difficult to recognize through current institutional structures should not be lost. It was, after all, the severely marginalized position of many who were suffering from AIDS that would deny them access to "mainstream medical care" and perpetuate their invisibility in the official numbers of this disease. At the same time, some members of the gay male community, because of their access to both dominant resources and indigenous institutions, were able to gain the attention of staff at the CDC. This, of course, did not guarantee an adequate response from that agency, if in fact it guaranteed a response of any kind. Again, I am less concerned with the personal intentions of researchers and staff members at the CDC than with the structure and procedures of the CDC which served to bias the system, making some groups invisible to this institution.

A second factor contributing to the invisibility and undercounting of injection drug users is that of familiarity with the CDC. Specifically, institutional marginalization prior to AIDS resulted in the privileging of certain groups, individuals, and organizations with whom the CDC had a prior relationship and often some residual control during the early years of the epidemic. Having mounted numerous studies about sexually transmitted diseases (STDs), using in particular gay participants, the CDC had a familiarity with gay communities not replicated among any other groups thought to be at risk. This was especially true during the late 1970s and early 1980s, when the CDC and gay researchers completed a multisite study of hepatitis B. Dr. David Ostrow, who was intimately involved with the hepatitis B project, explained the CDC's relationship with gay communities:

In the mid-seventies people within the CDC began to steer parts of the organization to those communities connected to the increase in STDs (sexually transmitted diseases). Gay doctors and organizations after the liberation movement resembled the organizations (academic and public STD clinics) the CDC was used to dealing with, so we began to work together. Much of the hepatitis B research was done in collaboration with gay community clinics. In 1981 we finished the hepatitis B research just as AIDS was coming on the scene. It was this research, institutions, and relationships that laid the groundwork for much of the initial work on AIDS. They could use the stuff already set up from hepatitis B to pursue their work on AIDS.[19]

Note that it was not necessarily an acceptance of the "gay lifestyle" that led the CDC to work in gay communities. In some respects, it was the internalization of ideologies of deviance, extremity, and promiscuity that provided the basis for such relationships. Gay communities were regarded as opportune sites for the study of sexual diseases. Several of these studies were led by Dr. Jim Curran, the same man who was picked to lead the initial task force on AIDS. Thus there was a previous and well-established working relationship between Dr. Curran and many of the health leaders in gay male communities, which undoubtedly facilitated their new work around AIDS in gay communities.

In direct contrast to the CDC's previous work with the gay community was its lack of knowledge and association with medical and social issues found among injection-drug-using populations. Most of the institutional responsibility for issues concerning this population was traditionally delegated to the National Institute of Drug Abuse (NIDA). However, Oppenheimer (1988) suggests that NIDA decided early on to treat AIDS like any other disease and leave it to the direction of the CDC or the National Institutes of Health (NIH):

> NIDA's traditional focus, however, was only on drug abuse, eschewing investigations of diseases such as hepatitis B and endocarditis that were endemic or epidemic in their target populations. The leadership of NIDA decided that AIDS would be treated like any other disease, thereby leaving the research to other centers at NIH or the CDC. Unfortunately, the CDC, lacking previous experience and expertise, shied away from studying the drug-using population, leaving a lacuna. (279–80).

Again, institutional constraints, in this case structural familiarity with certain communities as well as territorial conflicts between government agencies, specifically inhibited research addressing the progression of AIDS in drug-using populations.

Not only did the structural division of labor identified above shape national research agendas, it also influenced the information about AIDS that drug users received at the local level. As discussed in the last chapter, Des Jarlais, Friedman and Sotheran (1992) found that "in New York City the drug treatment system is not integrated with medical treatment. The staff of drug programs had little experience in providing treatment for infectious disease" (282). Not until 1984 and 1985 did local drug treatment programs fully respond to the need to integrate their programs in such a way that AIDS would become a significant component. The authors continue: "The *coping stage* has been occurring since 1986, and involves incorporating AIDS issues into the day-to-day operation of drug abuse treatment programs" (286). We can only wonder how much earlier treatment programs would have reached the coping stage had the CDC revised and expanded its early research agenda by pursuing additional research and outreach among intravenous drug users.

The importance of institutional familiarity must also be placed in the context of a third factor affecting the undercounting of injection drug users: the attitudes of individual scientists and the perceptions of doctors regarding the perceived health of this group. The ideologies and myths of marginalization that researchers held regarding both gay community members and the population of primarily poor black and Latino/a injection drug users clearly influenced their interactions with these groups. For example, notwithstanding their familiarity with the gay community, many researchers used a conception of the group as deviant or sexually extreme to justify their inquiry into the lifestyle hypothesis of AIDS. Citing specifically the rise in STDs evident in parts of the gay community, researchers familiar with this group used this trend to justify the importance they attributed to "promiscuity" and drugs in understanding AIDS (Oppenheimer 1988, 272). Further, researchers unfamiliar with the gay community were also willing to pursue the lifestyle hypothesis, since their distance from the community allowed them to continue to view group members as "deviants" who engaged in behaviors that possibly produced this new disease. At the extreme, some scientists, knowing little if anything of gay sexuality,

discarded the belief that a virus could be transmitted sexually between men:

> Policy analyst Sandra Panem, reviewing charges that homo-
> phobia delayed federal research efforts, concluded that preju-
> dice against homosexuality per se would not have deterred
> ambitious scientists from initiating interesting and rewarding
> research projects. But ignorance, she suggests, does appear to
> have played a role, citing as evidence observations by James
> W. Curran, by then head of the CDC's AIDS task force, that
> among scientists there is little widespread research interest in
> sexuality of any kind and "not much understanding of homo-
> sexuality." Indeed, Curran went on to say that many eminent
> scientists during those early years rejected the possibility that
> AIDS was an infectious disease because they had no idea how
> one man could transmit an infectious virus to another; through
> what orifice could such a virus possibly enter a male body,
> lacking as it did the vaginal portal approved for the receipt of
> sperm. (Treichler 1988, 199)

Despite such obvious homophobia and ignorance of gay sexuality,
the attitudes of researchers and the ideological frames used by the
CDC to structure its research about injection drug users were much
less varied and much more severe than that for gay men. Dr. David
Ostrow again comments that "IVDU's were thought to get all kinds of
diseases, so many doctors just looked the other way."[20] On the same
subject, Oppenheimer notes that there exists "a feeling among many
clinicians and researchers (in this respect reflecting the attitudes of the
public at large) that addicts are of less social consequence than other
patients" (1992, 59). Dr. Helene Gayle, head of the AIDS/HIV Unit of
the CDC, also comments on this belief in the "unhealthiness" of injection drug users. "I guess I think that sickness in injecting drug users
is common. I mean it's not the same as sickness in a healthy gay man.
And so [the illness] was much more suspicious because the first reports were in gay men, I mean people called it GRID. People were so
focused on that, that when the same thing started happening for [injec-
tion drug users] who have such a myriad of other problems, I think it
just didn't hit."[21] Finally, in *Inventing AIDS* (1990), Cindy Patton also
writes about the presumed unhealthiness of injection drug users:

> The epidemic, noted at the time as "junky pneumonia," did
> not trigger public health investigators' interest because it was
> not considered remarkable that injecting drug users should

get sick and die from any number of illnesses as users were considered intrinsically unhealthy. The emerging syndrome [AIDS] was defined as immune malfunction in "previously healthy" people; the rapid and unexplained decline in health which set the Centers for Disease Control in motion was noticeable only because the gay men affected had previously been considered "healthy." That gay men were seen as "healthy" despite having a variety of treatable sexually transmitted diseases attested to the acceptance and positive valuation of gay men and their sexuality in the urban settings where these cases were under study. (27–28)

Thus, although some researchers perceived the gay community as marginal, weird, and perverted, the more comprehensive and cumulative marginal status of injection drug users—encompassing economic, political, and social domains—played a significant role in limiting their inclusion in research and made identification and treatment of their illnesses rare. Providers seemed uninterested in the sickness of poor drug users, many of whom were people of color. Ideologies of exclusion that defined their lives as expendable had become systematically integrated into a public health system purportedly responsible for their well-being. These individuals never received the attention they deserved from the CDC, in part because of systemic biases that made them invisible to the official record keeping of the CDC, but also because of the personal attitudes of researchers who viewed this population as merely disease vectors and unworthy victims.

This story is, of course, complicated because it's not just about the biases of providers; it is also about the empirical reality that injection drug users are usually sicker than the general population, and so recognition of disease is undoubtedly more difficult in this group. Still, we do not want to lose sight of the fact that many researchers were uninterested in the sickness of poor drug users. Thus, the suffering and deaths experienced by this group from AIDS often went unreported to the CDC. The consequences of such absence and neglect were manifested in a number of areas, including the exclusion of injection drug users and their distinct symptoms from research, prevention strategies and, possibly most important, the case definitions used by the CDC to track the development of AIDS. Prominent AIDS researcher Gerald Friedland suggests that early case definitions were

constructed without enough sensitivity to the already evolving demography of AIDS. So the definition excluded a lot of things that resulted in underreporting of the disease in drug users, and women, and people of color. . . . I really feel very strongly that the case definition inadvertently changed the perception of the epidemic because it undercounted very severely. So now when people started talking about a second wave, it's not a second wave, it was part of the first wave. It just wasn't seen because of the way things were counted. So when pressure was mounted for the CDC to change its case definition, they would say, "We're not seeing it in our data." And its true they weren't, because the data was flawed, because it wasn't capturing the disease where it was.[22]

The bias in the initial data generated by the CDC was not the only problem with its response. Having initial assumptions about the causes and associations of a disease is, of course, essential to any process of theory building and investigation. However, it was also the CDC's inability or unwillingness to revise its initial assumptions in the face of new evidence about AIDS that points again to the systemic impact of marginalization on the epidemiological process. AIDS activists have long struggled to force the CDC to expand its case definition, and such expansion has often been won only in response to the outcry of a coalition of activists, providers, and people with AIDS. Steven Epstein (1996) recounts the struggle waged primarily by female activists, many of them lesbians involved in ACT UP, to push the CDC to expand the case definition to include the diseases specific to women:

> The Centers for Disease Control's definition of AIDS, created largely with reference to the opportunistic infections contracted by gay men, systematically "exclude[d] the symptoms appearing exclusively in women," such as pelvic inflammatory disease. In very practical terms, this meant that women were not receiving the health and disability benefits that accrued from an AIDS diagnosis. . . . However, the definition couldn't be changed to include women's symptoms, the CDC maintained, because of the absence of data proving a causal link between those symptoms and HIV infection. But the necessary data *couldn't be generated* because "women of childbearing potential" had largely been excluded from clinical trials. (288)

Epstein goes on to note that "eventually, women activists pressed successfully for a change in the CDC case definition" (289). However, Maxine Wolfe of the Women's Caucus of ACT UP comments that to secure a meeting with NIAID officials, something men in ACT UP routinely did, women AIDS activists "had to stage a sit-in at the offices of Dr. Daniel Hoth, . . . make constant phone calls, send him several letters threatening a repeat sit-in, and 'zap' him in front of 5,000 of his colleagues at the Sixth International AIDS Conference." (289).

This rigidity of assumptions is the fourth factor I highlight as contributing to the invisibility of injection drug users and people of color in the early AIDS data. For example, early in the epidemic evidence began to emerge that this was not a disease strictly tied to the gay community. As was reported earlier, the first heterosexual cases were identified and written about only three months after the first public notification of this new threat. In an August 1981 issue of the *MMWR*, the CDC publicly reported the first case of a heterosexual with AIDS— a woman. However, Mary Guinan of the CDC states that she encountered resistance from within the CDC Task Force, as well as from physicians treating AIDS patients, early in the epidemic to viewing this disease as reaching beyond the gay community:

> Several of the cases, it turned out, weren't gay men at all, but drug addicts. At the CDC, there was a reluctance to believe that intravenous drug users might be wrapped into this epidemic, and the New York physicians also seemed obsessed with the gay angle, Guinan thought. "He says he's not homosexual, but he must be," doctors would confide to her. (Shilts 1987, 83)

Dr. Gerald Friedland also recalls the reluctance of staff at the CDC to see this new disease as extending beyond gay male communities. "Okay, well, so there I was in the Bronx having just returned to New York after working in Boston for quite a few years and there were these three guys dying of pneumocystis pneumonia. . . . So I contacted the CDC and told them we were seeing the same disease in injection drug users and the response was, 'No, no this must be a different disease and you are making the wrong diagnosis. This is a disease of gay men.' And it did take about six months—maybe even a little longer to convince them."[23]

In part the reluctance of the CDC to expand its own conception of AIDS, as well as the message it communicated to the general public, was tied to the lack of power and influence possessed by the heterosexual population thought to be at risk. Dr. James Curran, head of the initial CDC task force on AIDS, in trying to explain the reluctance of CDC staff members to expand their focus when researching and talking about AIDS, emphasizes the inability of the CDC to find conclusive evidence of a pattern of heterosexual transmission:

The point is that we couldn't establish a pattern that was convincing. I mean the pattern [transmission through injection
drug use] was certainly possible and plausible, and we always
said that was true that this could be spread through injecting
drug use but the skeptics would say, "How come all your cases
are in men? And how come you have eighty cases in gay men
and six cases in men who are injecting drug users? How do
you know those six weren't gay too, or they might have been
straight but they were selling themselves or they might have
had sex in prison."[24]

Eventually cases reported to the CDC and published in the *MMWR*
would make the claim of no conclusive evidence obsolete and confirm
the need for an expanded understanding of this disease. For example,
on 24 September 1982 the *MMWR* reported that 20 percent of the patients with KS and PCP were heterosexual, 60 percent of them injection
drug users, one-third of them women. This report was followed by an
article in the 17 December issue of the *MMWR* identifying an "unexplained" immunodepression and opportunistic infections in some infants whose parents were former or current intravenous drug users.
Three of the four infants were black. The 7 January 1983 issue of the
MMWR included two articles on AIDS among heterosexuals. The first
article detailed "immunodeficiency among female sexual partners of
males with AIDS." Two women were highlighted: one black, the other
Latina. The second report indicated that sixteen prisoners in New York
and New Jersey had been identified with AIDS: seven of the prisoners
were black, and two were Latino. This increase in AIDS cases among
heterosexual injection drug users came slightly before the clear identification of AIDS in the hemophiliac population. Further, these findings
should be viewed in the context of mounting examples of heterosexual
transmission in Central Africa, making it clear that there was a strong
case for the CDC to expand its recognition and research efforts with
regard to nongay cases of AIDS. But in spite of all the data and despite
a name change from the unofficial GRID to the official and more inclusive acquired immunodeficiency syndrome (AIDS), changes in the focus of research and the attitudes of researchers occurred slowly. AIDS,
even with its new name, was still seen as a disease of primarily one community, the gay community, and that connection became the underlying message from almost every institution dealing with this disease.

The consequences of this framing of the syndrome were manifested,
not only in the exclusion of injection drug users from research, prevention strategies, and general access and input into policy decisions, but

also in the distorted or missing information forwarded to members of African-American and other communities of color. Again, as discussed in chapter 1, marginal communities often use their primary identities, in this case race, as a cost-saving strategy to screen or evaluate the relevance of information to their lives (Dawson 1994). Without some initial identification with those thought to be at risk in the very first years of the epidemic, two unfortunate consequences were left to develop. One was that many African Americans came to see this disease as something they did not need to be concerned about, something completely outside of their communities. The comments of Gil Gerald and Phil Wilson in the previous chapter illustrate this point. The other effect was that even among those African Americans who understood the threat AIDS posed for community members, there was inadequate information, resulting in deficient and erroneous knowledge of the epidemic.

The inadequate handling of public information about black communities and AIDS is probably most infamously illustrated in the CDC's designation of Haitians as a risk group.[25] In contrast to the CDC's rigid limitations on the disease framework in the early 1980s, its seemingly haphazard and what Haitian political leaders called racist categorization of all Haitians as a "risk group" in 1982 infuriated many inside and outside of Haitian communities.[26] By the beginning of 1982, evidence of heterosexual Haitian emigrants with AIDS-like symptoms began to emerge. Based on thirty-four reported cases of Haitians with opportunistic infections and Kaposi's sarcoma, Haitians were designated a high-risk group in the 9 July 1982 *MMWR*. Over the next few years this designation would generate much controversy and outrage. Foremost was the concern that such a classification, highlighting demographic characteristics and not behavioral practices, targeted all Haitians and not the actions that put one at risk, making it inappropriate for the purpose of detailing and designating *transmission routes*. Eventually, the CDC came to understand, both through the lack of data to support this characterization and the response of Haitian communities, that such a designation was a mistake, and removed Haitians from its list of high-risk groups.[27] Note that the CDC's decision to take Haitians off its list of high-risk groups was not just a response to new data or better evidence, but arose more directly from dialogue or political actions, in particular mass protests of Haitians around this policy. On numerous occasions the Haitian community and its supporters took to the streets of New York to publicly demonstrate their opposition to federal policies targeting the entire group in response to AIDS. The most successful of these events occurred in April of 1990, when nearly fifty thousand people marched across the Brooklyn Bridge to protest the FDA's decision to ban all Haitians from donating blood, even to their family members. Dr. Curran argues that while the CDC and other federal agencies got "burned on" the Haitian issue, there was no conscious attempt to target this community unfairly:

> But see initially what we had were people fitting this case definition who didn't have an apparent mode of transmission, who happened to be recent Haitian immigrants. And they were different from other Haitians in that they had been in the country a short period of time. They were more likely to be in Florida than in New York. Most of the Haitian-Americans live in the New York-Northeast area, but 75 percent of Haitians with AIDS initially lived in Florida. . . . So the pressure from the Haitian organizations was to say that this was really no different from the Americans who had AIDS—that they were either drug users or gay. We couldn't say that they got it through heterosexual contact because there weren't partners [accessible to us in this country] who had it. . . . It had to all fit together. . . . The only thing was on the issue of Haitians we were kind of burned on that. I mean the Haitians were upset. And some people, African Americans were upset because we were saying something about Haitians. But it was related to Haitians; it wasn't related to black Americans.[28]

Thus again the CDC's behavior, in this instance concerning the Haitian community and AIDS, only reinforced already established beliefs among African Americans about the need to be skeptical of information from the government, including government-sponsored public heath agencies. In part, this distrust was generated and fueled by the history of the Tuskegee Syphilis Study (Herek and Capitanio 1994; Guinan 1993; Thomas and Quinn 1991). However, other rumors of government involvement in promoting social crisis in black communities, like those of government responsibility for the proliferation of drugs in black communities, also added to feelings of suspicion (Jones 1981; Thomas and Quinn 1991; Guinan 1993). Stephen Joseph, former Commissioner of Health for New York City, suggests that the series of incidents around the Haitian designation made the CDC extremely cautious and hesitant to communicate important and needed information about AIDS in racial terms. He argues that even when presented with the data on the disproportionate impact of AIDS in communities of

color, the CDC was unwilling to highlight the racial demographics of
this disease:

> The CDC's earliest public health reports noted only in passing
> the disproportionate numbers of minorities among the drug-
> associated, female, and infant cases. Nowhere was there a
> clear statement of the future implications of disproportionate
> rates of AIDS among racial and ethnic minority groups. Per-
> haps bruised by the controversy over the labeling of Haitians
> as a high-risk group and the subsequent charges against it of
> racism, the CDC was reluctant to head into a situation with
> similar potential again. (Joseph 1992, 118)

The CDC's wariness of discussions of race when talking about AIDS
is disputed by Dr. Helene Gayle. She suggests that early in the epidemic the CDC highlighted the disproportionate impact on black communities:

> I think in the early days the CDC was very clear in its reporting
> of the disproportionate risk to African American communities.
> Early on there was one of our *MMWR*'s, I can't remember
> which year, it was probably around 1986 or 1987, that came
> out stating the disproportionate effect. One could say that it
> should have been obvious before that, but if you see a disease
> where 70 percent of the folks, maybe even more, but about 70
> percent are white and then divided between minority groups,
> it didn't look so disproportionate early on because the large
> majority were among white, gay men.[29]

Dr. Curran reiterates Dr. Gayle's assessment that the CDC never attempted consciously to misrepresent the demographics of AIDS. He
also comments on the difficulty of trying to signal the right balance or
emphasis when dealing with race:

> I think the CDC always reported the truth, but the question
> was one of emphasis. Like when we reported cases, we never
> hid cases or didn't detect cases associated with race or gender
> or any other risk factor. . . . So even though they were mostly
> in whites, we never said that they only occurred in whites,
> although that was a distinct hope [for some people]. An awful
> lot of the public's views on AIDS have always been related to
> denial and wishful thinking. And how many times did people
> say, "It's a white, gay man's disease." It was never a white, gay
> man's disease, but a lot of people in the black community
> wanted it to be because they didn't want it to be them. So the
> thing is, we wouldn't say it was a black disease, because it

wasn't a black disease, it was a disease that affected a lot of groups. . . .

See, the epidemiological characteristic thought to be relevant was not race or ethnicity. In other words, if we said seven black people in New York City have AIDS, that wouldn't help, I mean, the real issue is seven injecting drug users had AIDS. So if we say seven black people have AIDS, then people say, "Oh, wait a minute here." . . . You'd have to say seven injecting drug users have AIDS, and they're black. And then you have to say which is the more important characteristic. Well, initially, the injecting drug use was. I'd say that the emphasis changed.[30]

It seems that while Dr. Curran's concern about only expressing the information that is important to understanding the transmission of the virus may be true for the scientific community, it is not accurate when we are also trying to construct an understanding of AIDS for the general population. Specifically, since most people want to know how they or those close to them might be affected by this new phenomenon, other characteristics beyond the mere description of the transmission routes seem important information to put forth, unless you want individuals to construct, independent of the actual data, their own versions and reasoning about who is at risk and why. What is interesting in the discussion recounted above is that Dr. Curran omits a concern about defining AIDS as a disease primarily of people of color that he commented on in an earlier discussion over the phone. Specifically, he raised the problem that if AIDS had been identified as a disease of "minority" communities, there would have been even less public and governmental support for fighting this crisis.

The role of the government, specifically with regard to limitations on speech, brings me to my fifth and final point: We must not forget the limitations imposed by the larger political context in which the CDC responded to this epidemic. For example, AIDS appeared only five years after the CDC had urged most Americans to get a swine flu shot for an epidemic that never really materialized. In 1976, expecting a major outbreak in response to the swine flu virus, the CDC had mounted a major vaccination campaign. However, instead of a major flu epidemic, the CDC encountered nearly five hundred cases of Guillain-Barré syndrome brought on largely by the vaccination (Grmek 1990). In the aftermath of that fiasco, through a process of institutional learning, the staff at the CDC was reticent to make overarching claims about the impact of AIDS on communities of color without what they considered to be substantial evidence.

In addition to the swine flu problem, officials at the CDC also encountered AIDS in a political environment controlled by newly elected President Ronald Reagan. Elected on a platform that highlighted and targeted the "moral deficiencies" of the "undeserving poor" and "welfare queens," Dr. Curran reminds us that President Reagan and his officials were unwilling to devote needed resources to an issue defined largely by gay men and injection drug users:

> There was really no funding to speak of before the mid-eighties. So it isn't like anybody got much money. There was some money for surveillance—a very small amount. And during the early eighties there was relatively little. I mean public health organizations were getting cut back when Reagan first came in. So there were cutbacks in public health organizations, major cutbacks in the CDC while AIDS was just starting to occur.[31]

Curran comments further that it was not just funding that was affected by Reagan's election, but also the general understanding of which issues could be promoted. He noted that with William Bennett serving as drug czar, issues or policies that focused on drug use were very "high profile" in the administration. However, solutions to such issues were generally conservative or reactionary in nature, focusing on eliminating drug use ("Just Say No!"), instead of prevention or rehabilitation strategies. As Curran says,

> You know this was a highly political era in the Reagan administration. That is when Bill Bennett became the drug czar, and they were coming from a very, very conservative point of view. Drug use issues were high profile, I mean they were as high profile in that administration as they are low in [the Clinton administration]. . . . Bill Bennett has come from a conservative background, he was related to Gary Bauer, he was high profile and so [drug and HIV prevention] wasn't something that we were likely to break into.[32]

Even those Reagan appointees who seemed to be reasonable in their approach to AIDS still operated in a conservative and restricted political environment. For example, former Surgeon General C. Everett Koop told me of a visit by Reagan White House officials who asked him to curtail the use of certain words when talking and writing about AIDS:

> When I wrote the first report [on AIDS] at the request of the president, I was visited by the domestic policy people within three weeks, who asked me if it wasn't time for a second edition. You know there is a protocol about who goes where. Nobody in the White House ever goes any place else unless they really need a favor. And so I knew just instinctively when he made an appointment to come see me in my office that they would be groveling. And when I said, "Why would I want to make a new edition when we still have a million copies left?" they said, "Well, we think maybe you ought to take some words out." And I said, "Such as?" And they said, "Well, penis, vagina, and rectum, and of course condom." I said, "Not negotiable."[33]

Although C. Everett Koop was clearly one of the more respected members of the Reagan administration on the issue of AIDS, he also revealed a contradictory and at times disturbing understanding of HIV and AIDS in communities of color. Specifically, when asked about his office's attention to AIDS among African Americans, Dr. Koop seemed to collapse efforts to deal with AIDS among African Americans with policies targeting Haitian communities. Further, Dr. Koop suggested that the "Spanish" did better because they spoke a different language:

> Very slowly, the IV drug abuse came and although there was talk about the fact that this was a white disease, the Haitians took our mind away from everything. And as I look back on it, my own interpretation may be incorrect, but we paid a lot more attention to Latinos than we did to Afro-Americans because of their separate language. And so by putting out the Surgeon General's Report in Spanish, it made us focus on the Spanish. . . . But when we looked at people who were black, we were looking at Haitians because everybody said Haitians are different. . . . And then the next thing that came up that was particular to Haitians was, "Shouldn't we do some education in Creole?" And I suspect if we had done an educational program in Creole, we would have had even less attention to the Afro-Americans. Now if we had *ebonics* then, then we could have put out a special thing, but I think that the reason Hispanics did better is because we had a focus on them as a language.[34]

While many parts of this statement are troubling, including the idea the Latinos/as are to be thought of as a language, the perception that

"Hispanics did better," or the idea that the way to reach African Americans was to do a special educational program in ebonics, none seem to approach the disrespect of Haitian doctors that Dr. Koop expresses when explaining the spread of AIDS among Haitians:

> It was just men that weren't sterilizing needles, so the doctors were passing AIDS all around. So that however, didn't come out for two years, so for two years the Haitians bore the brunt of that, and one of the things that annoyed me, the government never came out and said we were wrong about the Haitians. We absolve them of everything. Their excuse was we can't undermine the faith of the Haitians in their doctors. Well, you know [I believe] they [Haitian doctors] were already using chicken's blood and cob webs and other things, so I don't know.[35]

We are confronted here not only with the contradictory and troubling comments of Dr. Koop, but with a larger illustration of the inability of Reagan administration officials to create a political environment where every aspect of AIDS and every group dealing with this disease could be provided equal and legitimate status. Thus, when trying to understand the response of the CDC to AIDS in black communities, the hostile political environment of the Reagan administration must be considered as a factor.

Conclusion

Despite the very severe problems listed above, the CDC helped bring AIDS into the focus of most Americans. In the first years of Reagan's reign, the CDC warned that something just as dangerous as Reagan lurked on the horizon. It would therefore be misleading to suggest that the CDC did not provide important and needed information through a very elaborate system of epidemiological study. Undoubtedly, mistakes were made in the first years of the epidemic; however, Dr. Helene Gayle believes that over the years the CDC has learned from its early mistakes and improved the attention they pay to communities of color:

> I think fairly early on the CDC made it clear that this was disproportionately affecting minority communities and [began] a very different response to HIV prevention that [recognized] . . . the need to reach communities of color and . . . to directly fund community-based organizations. . . . This is one of the major breaks in the way we do business because of the

need to make sure the community was more involved. . . . All of the money that goes to state and local health departments for our prevention grants now has to have a community planning group that is representative of the community, that agrees on what happens and how the money is spent—that's been tremendous. . . . In fact, our direct assistance to community-based organizations has components that are specific to minority populations as well as others. There was also another program started, the National Regional Minority Organization . . . again, we saw the need to get organizations involved that might not be AIDS-specific only—some are, some aren't—but nationally represented, you know, [with] a national scope that could be a voice for issues in minority communities.

[All this] has brought new voices to the table and . . . we're empowering a whole generation of people who I think will be community activists beyond just AIDS, who are going to be savvy about things like how you get grants, savvy about how you communicate your needs to a diverse group of people, including Congress and other policy makers.

HIV made us think about a much more multidisciplinary approach. . . . And then I think if we try to reach the communities that we need to reach, then we have to have people who have the same sensitivities and/or similar experiences who can understand the experiences of those communities. I think it makes a big difference beyond HIV; I think it's the right thing to do for public health in general. If we are going to put in place things that are in the best interest of the public, we need to reflect the public. . . . It's also about empowerment. If you don't at some point make changes, then the same people will always be making the decisions for everyone.[36]

However, beyond the lessons learned by the CDC, anyone concerned with the health and, just as important, the representation of marginal groups, should take note of the failures and systemic biases evident in the CDC's response to AIDS. Injection drug users, poor women, and disempowered children, many of whom were African American and Latino/a, found themselves silenced, invisible, and neglected in the early years of this epidemic. Moreover, their absence in an evolving picture of AIDS, I believe, significantly delayed and hindered recognition and response from organizations and individuals in black communities. Again, this is not to suggest that indigenous institutions and elites did not eagerly look the other way and distance themselves from this epidemic. However, information (or the lack thereof) from the CDC made denial, distance, and ignorance that much easier. In the end it may be Dr. Curran who best summarizes the numerous factors contributing to the invisibility of poor injection drug users of color:

> They're poor, they're stoned half the time, they don't have insurance, and some of them don't give a shit, at least part of the time they don't. Now, other than that, they do okay in the sense that I think they're probably at least as smart or smarter than other people. They can survive, so it's not that simple, but I mean it isn't all society's fault that they don't have good health care, but it isn't all their fault either, and so its a combination of things.
>
> So they don't have good doctors; they don't go [to the doctor] at the right time; they go to the emergency room when they get sick. It's not like they've got their family doctor to go to, and so when they get diagnosed with something, it could very well be at the very end. They aren't well liked by providers; they have a hand-and-glove relationship with crime, sometimes, not all the time. And so there are a lot of problems that they have that make them invisible. . . . They also get a lot of pneumonias, so they get treated for something else because the pneumonias are thought to be due to something else.
>
> I have no doubt that there were many cases of pneumocystis missed. The patterns of AIDS in drug users were not quite as well understood early in the epidemic, and it really took the discovery of the virus to start the discovery of the associations. In other words, it was known that other pneumonia deaths, due to bacterial infection and TB, were increasing in drug-using populations. That wasn't appreciated until people could associate it with the virus.
>
> America was to some extent asleep to the TB epidemic, and the reason they were is in part related to the fact that it was in drug-using and homeless populations and in people who had poor access to housing as well as care and also were not good at taking their medications. But also because it was related to HIV, and they were in HIV-infected populations where HIV and TB go together hand in glove. . . . *But initially, the association of this population with AIDS was missed* in part because of other illness patterns, the health care patterns and the general ghettoization of this population [emphasis added].[37]

Again, the CDC's response must be understood within the context of two significant and intersecting factors. The first is the general institutional bias and standard operating procedures of the CDC. The second is the marginal position (while acknowledging differences in magnitude) of those groups thought to be at "high risk" for AIDS. While both gay men and injection drug users are afforded marginal social status, the manifestation of institutional marginalization often took different forms and engaged different discourses for each group. Thus we must recognize differences in the complexity and severity of marginalization with regard to the epidemiology of AIDS if we are to understand the severe exclusion experienced by both gay men and injection drug users, but more cumulatively by the latter.

Finally, we must address the question of intent, because it has become a major part of the discussion of AIDS in communities of color. Repeatedly, when hearing or reading of the CDC's early failures in research on marginal communities, members of African-American communities raise the possibility that the CDC was engaged in some type of conspiracy against people of color. Although it is understandable that community members might see the problems at the CDC as part of a more general pattern of neglect, exclusion, and genocide on the part of dominant institutions, I suggest something a bit more systemic, dangerous, and long-term is happening. Institutional marginalization produces effects that far outlive the sinister actions of individuals. So to those concerned with conspiracy theories at the CDC, I suggest that sometimes the effects of institutional practices of exclusion and ideological narratives of deviance result in a cumulative marginalization more daunting than any conspiracy a few white men in a room could concoct.

CHAPTER FIVE

All the Black People Fit to Print

> Because of the HIV virus that I have obtained I will have to retire from the Lakers today. (Press conference, 7 November 1991)

With these few words, Earvin "Magic" Johnson forever changed, at least in terms of quantity, the coverage focused on AIDS among African Americans. Announcing his seropositive status, Magic Johnson forced both print and television media to cover a story that for so long they had largely ignored. Suddenly, among the over two hundred thousand people classified as having AIDS in the United States through 1991,[1] there was one black man whom reporters, editors, and media institutions could not ignore. Repeatedly, on the nightly news and on the covers of newspapers and magazines there appeared a black face, recognized by all, under the headline of AIDS. This did not mean the media took off with zeal to investigate the manifestations of AIDS in black and African-American communities; instead, a more subtle shift occurred.

Prior to Johnson's announcement, media coverage of AIDS, especially in African-American communities, had been minimal. The number of print and television stories devoted to analyzing the spread of this epidemic in African-American and Latino communities lagged behind those stories in which gay men were central, and drastically lagged behind the number of stories examining the threat of AIDS to "the general population." Further, the substance of this minimal coverage was skewed, with a number of stories promoting black women and children as the "innocent victims" of AIDS in black communities.[2] Unfortunately, Magic Johnson's announcement, along with his accompanying declaration of heterosexuality and the need for abstinence on the part of young people (made in the days following his initial statement), only exacerbated the dominant media's dodging of what some might consider the "seamier" side of AIDS in black communities. In the discussion of Magic Johnson there was no mention of black gay men or black men who sleep with men, only the occasional story written to fan or refute the rumors of Magic's possible bisexuality (Harper 1996). The stories on Magic Johnson did not speak of injection drug users or of programs such as needle exchange, which could curb the rate of transmission among this population. The forbidden topics regarding AIDS in black communities—homosexuality and drug use, those "not so innocent" behaviors—would continue to be ignored, as the press focused on Magic Johnson, smiling sports icon, former "ladies man," and soon-to-be educator of young people about the dangers of HIV and AIDS.

The role of the media in shaping or, at the very least, informing attitudes about AIDS is a subject that has been discussed more than researched. Scholars, activists, and the public have all suggested that during the early years of the epidemic the media played an important role in bringing the epidemic of AIDS to the consciousness of the general public. By mid-1983 most Americans had heard of AIDS, with many stating they received such knowledge from television and newspaper reports. Eleanor Singer, Theresa F. Rogers, and Mary Corcoran (1987), in their article on trends in public opinion and awareness of AIDS, write that "the data also provide evidence that the public credits the media as being an important source of information about AIDS (581–82)." In fact, it is hard to explain the high level of public recognition of AIDS in the early years of the epidemic, before the majority of Americans had any direct contact with individuals living with AIDS, without attributing much of this recognition as coming directly from media reports. Iyengar and Kinder (1987) reinforce this conclusion, suggesting that quite often the media provide information about subjects outside our personal, lived experience. However, before applauding the media for heightening recognition, we should also be aware that while the majority of Americans knew of AIDS by mid-1983, less than a majority had accurate information about routes of transmission, personal risk, and possible preventive strategies (Thomas 1989).

So to what degree did media coverage of AIDS drive public opinion and public awareness, including that among African Americans? This question cannot be answered fully from the data I have available. Certainly the media play a very important role in communicating information and influencing the salience of issues, and AIDS is no exception. The media's impact on public thinking, or at least on public discourse, may be greater than that of any other institution in the United States.

Melissa Shepard, from the CDC, recently commented at a conference sponsored by the Columbia University School of Journalism that "we've been doing tracking since 1985, and still, over 70 percent of Americans get their information about HIV and AIDS from the news."[3] A recently published report from the Kaiser Family Foundation revealed that "46 percent of African Americans cite the media—TV, radio, newspapers, or magazines—as their leading source of information about HIV/AIDS in the month prior to the survey" (Kaiser 1998, 14). Public-opinion and media researchers Page, Shapiro, and Dempsey (1987) comment further that "nearly everyone is exposed either directly or indirectly to what the media broadcasts" (125).

Despite this level of informational penetration into the American populace, there seem to be limits to the media's ability to shape public opinion. For instance, the work of scholars such as Iyengar and Kinder (1987) and McCombs and Shaw (1972) indicates that the media, while pervasive in its ability to reach the American public, is much less successful in changing attitudes already formed. These researchers have found instead that the media possess the ability to alter an individual's concern over, or the priority given to, an issue. This process, called agenda setting, or public agenda setting, works in relation to the time and attention media outlets designate to an issue or event. The more attention given an issue (especially prominent attention at the beginning of an evening news broadcast or on the front page of a newspaper), the more likely the public is to view the issue as having greater importance (Iyengar and Kinder 1987). For example, the increasing attention devoted to AIDS in the early to mid-1980s is believed to have contributed greatly to a process of agenda setting whereby in 1985 AIDS replaced cancer as the health problem a majority of Americans perceived as most threatening (Rogers and Dearing 1988; Thomas 1989).

Again, while the media have a much more difficult time shaping the formal opinions people hold about an issue, they are able to prime or mobilize the evaluative frames or standards individuals use to assess an issue or event (Iyengar 1991; Iyengar and Kinder 1987; Gitlin 1980). In the case of AIDS one can hypothesize that, beyond signaling the salience of this issue, dominant media sources also helped to frame or shape who or what was thought of when thinking about AIDS and those living with it. Iyengar (1991), in his work on political framing, has argued that "the manner in which a problem of choice is 'framed' [the assigning of responsibility in particular] is a contextual cue that may *profoundly* influence decision outcomes" (emphasis added, 11). We can probably conclude, therefore, that given the limited access to alternative information sources (since elected officials demonstrated little interest in or commitment to speaking about this crisis in public) and the emergence of AIDS from what seemed like nowhere (thus absent prior knowledge), individuals based many of their early opinions on AIDS on the information they received from the media. Both dominant and indigenous media institutions were positioned to build an understanding of who suffered from this disease as well as mobilize existing moral judgments of those groups (Fiske and Taylor 1984). Here was a new issue waiting to be framed or, as Allan Brandt (1987) argues, socially constructed, defining who and what to think about when forming opinions about AIDS.

> By assessing the symbols and images which diseases attract, we can come to understand the complex phenomena of illness. The symbols reflect social values—patterns of judgment about what is good or bad that guide perceptions and practice. They tell us how a disease is regarded, how we believe it is caused, who its victims are, and what they are like. Some diseases are viewed as the result of a sinister environment beyond our control; others are blamed on the individual victim and his or her personality and behavior. (5)

During the early years of this epidemic, the media, as a receptor and interpreter of information, largely influenced the social construction of AIDS not only for the general public but also for many elites. Dominant media sources informed policy-makers of the dimensions of this crisis (Hallin 1989; Gitlin 1980). Of course, those responsible for policy do not rely exclusively on the information provided to the general public, but research has shown that at the very least media sources provide "rapid information" and may have agenda-setting capabilities over elite policy-makers (Cook 1989; Cook et al. 1983). In the case of AIDS, elites, claiming no direct knowledge of the behaviors associated with this disease, relied on information they received from government sources (such as the CDC) as well as basic information from the media to map the development of this crisis. Unquestionably, dominant media sources played an important role in the policy process, taking this private and stigmatized issue into the public policy arena.

As we examine the role of the media in shaping attitudes, we need to be aware of a few institutional structures that guide the images and stories produced, independent of AIDS. First, in the area of health issues, scientific and medical journals are important in setting the agenda. Science reporters, in particular, look to journals like the *New England Journal of Medicine,* the *Journal of the American Medical Association* and, in the case of AIDS, the *Morbidity and Mortality Weekly Report* to signify the magnitude of a new issue (Kinsella 1989). For this reason the scientific and medical literature on AIDS in the early years of the epidemic significantly shaped the coverage this new disease received in both print and broadcast media. This reliance of the media on medical sources for information on AIDS was evident in NBC's first network news story on AIDS in June of 1982. Tom Brokaw introduced the segment by saying, "Scientists at the National Centers for Disease Control in Atlanta today received the results of a study that shows that the lifestyle of some male homosexuals has triggered an epidemic of a rare form of cancer."[4]

Second, the media, especially the broadcast media, are generally not very comfortable in following what they consider to be long, drawn-out stories or "old news." Thus, expanded coverage of any story, including AIDS, is driven by new angles and events. Celebrities and "average" people contracting AIDS were seen as new or interesting news, not the increasing numbers of cases in those "same old stigmatized groups."[5] In such an environment AIDS activists worked to find new ways to keep AIDS in front of the media, generating a continued sense of urgency with regard to the epidemic. Except for some major, breaking story such as Magic Johnson's announcement, however, we can expect to find a decline in the number of stories aired or printed on AIDS over the course of the epidemic.

Third, when analyzing the attention paid to any issue by the media, we must be aware of the roles that initiative and personal familiarity play in gaining access to coverage. George Strait, the health reporter at ABC News, states that the focus on white gay men in many of the AIDS stories in the beginning of the epidemic had as much to do with the numbers or "facts" produced by the CDC as with the efforts of gay activists to get their stories on television and into papers. In response to a question on where he received his early information on AIDS, Strait states,

> A lot from the community, and mainly it was the white gay community. My first stories were done there. We took the CDC numbers, but the CDC for a lot of reasons wasn't interested

in helping us actually find victims. Part of it was because of confidentiality, and they shouldn't. But the white gay community saw the problem, saw the need for people like me, and so that is where a lot of my information on the trends, and what worked and what didn't work, and some of the political tensions came from.[6]

In addition to Strait's acknowledgment of the role of media entrepreneurs in the gay community, many media scholars also suggest that a reporter's familiarity with certain groups or communities influences the selection of who will be covered. James Kinsella, in *Covering the Plague* (1989), writes that "news gets covered by a reporter for a thousand and one reasons, many of them personal" (15). And while few reporters, editors and broadcasters across the country were claiming familiarity with primarily white, gay men, fewer still were actively associating themselves with black and Latino/a drug users, gay men, and poor women of color. Understanding some of the institutional biases of the media will, I hope, inform this analysis as we identify and explore patterns of AIDS media coverage.

New York Times

Most of the writing (and complaining) about the *Times*'s coverage of the AIDS epidemic has focused on the lack of coverage by the *Times* in the early years of the epidemic. The *New York Times*, while not known for breaking stories, does have a reputation for accurately and comprehensively following "all the news that's fit to print" (Kinsella 1989).[7] For this reason, those who evaluated the *Times*'s early coverage of the epidemic found such apparent disregard for the subject somewhat surprising. The first *Times* article on the subject of AIDS appeared on 3 July 1981, the day before the CDC made public its second report on this new disease. The article was one column in length and located on page 20 of the first section. This initial article on the possible identification of a new disease would be followed throughout all of 1981 by only two other articles. By the end of 1982, when the number of confirmed cases of AIDS was nearing one thousand, the *Times* had run but five stories on the epidemic, none of which had made it to the front page. The first front-page story on the epidemic appeared in the *Times* on 25 May 1983, when Dr. Edward Brandt, assistant secretary of health, declared AIDS the "number one health priority" of the Public Health Services.

The apparent lack of interest in covering this story at the *Times* becomes even more evident when we examine the type of coverage given to other medical emergencies. For instance, the *Times*'s coverage of an outbreak of Legionnaires' disease in Philadelphia in 1976, involving eighteen cases, consisted of thirteen articles in the first week, with three appearing on the front page. Further, in 1982 during their coverage of the Tylenol scare, which accounted for seven deaths, the *Times* published four front-page articles and ran nearly fifty stories over a three-month period. Although no one can definitely state the reasons for such dismal coverage of AIDS in the early years of the epidemic by the *New York Times,* many have suggested that editors at the *Times* did not perceive issues affecting "the gay community" as noteworthy. Kinsella argues that while reporters at the *New York Times* have generally been accused of showing little interest in reporting on AIDS, part of the lack of interest was created by the costs of covering AIDS. In other words, unless you were willing to give up a chance at getting on the front page or getting in the paper at all, writing a story on AIDS was simply too risky. According to Kinsella,

> Successful reporters work to keep their editors happy, said one *Times* reporter. That is true at any well-run newspaper. But at the *Times,* which employs some of the most ambitious journalists in America, "almost everyone is out to get the story that's going to advance his career," said a current staffer. That is the story that could wind up on the front page, or the series given special play. Under Rosenthal [Abe Rosenthal—former executive editor of the *New York Times* during the beginning of the AIDS epidemic], according to a number of top editors and reporters, homosexuals and the "Gay Plague" stood a poor chance of making it on the front page, or almost anywhere else in the *Times.* (Kinsella 1989, 60)

Over the years, coverage of the epidemic by the *New York Times* improved drastically from its neglectful and biased start, as figure 5.1 shows. Michelangelo Signorile (1992), in an article comparing AIDS coverage by major newspapers between 1990 and 1992, finds that "on AIDS issues alone, the *New York Times* beat out all three other papers, with 20 percent more stories than the *Los Angeles Times,* 50 percent more than the *Washington Post,* and 75 percent more than the *Chicago Tribune.*" Further, a recently released report by the Kaiser Family Foundation's AIDS Media Monitoring Project indicates that in their analysis of designated periods of coverage of AIDS during 1985 and 1996, the

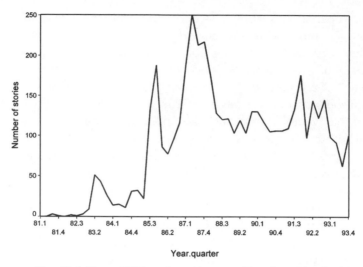

Figure 5.1. *New York Times* **AIDS stories, 1981–1993. (Data from** *New York Times* **index)**

New York Times ran more stories on AIDS than did the *Washington Post* or *USA Today*.[8]

Numerous reasons have been put forth to explain the increasing coverage of AIDS by the *Times*. Some have argued that the mounting devastation of AIDS forced the *Times* to cover the story. Kinsella suggests that personnel changes, such as Rosenthal's retirement, provided a different institutional environment—one conducive to writing stories on AIDS. Others, such as former *Times* reporter Tom Morgan, contend that the realization that favored reporters were living with AIDS also helped get more stories on AIDS into the paper.[9] Still others point to the actions of gay activists as a major catalyst for changes at the *Times*. For example, reporting on AIDS in certain gay newspapers like the *New York Native* is believed to have provided outside pressure and information for reporters at the *Times* eager to write about the emerging medical crisis (Alwood 1996). Just as important in helping *Times* editors reconsider the attention given to AIDS were the protests and less confrontational actions of AIDS activists. In particular, groups such as ACT UP (AIDS Coalition to Unleash Power) and GLAAD (Gay and Lesbian Alliance against Defamation) have been trumpeted as helping to push the *Times* in a better, if not new, direction when covering AIDS. The movement evidenced in the *Times*'s coverage of the AIDS epidemic reminds us of the dialectical relationship between power and resistance highlighted through the framework of marginalization. In spite of recognized changes in the quantity of stories, however, many—perhaps most—AIDS activists, still have major criticisms of the *Times's* coverage of AIDS, with activist and writer Larry Kramer registering some of the most stinging and eloquent critiques (Kramer 1989).

White AIDS activists such as Larry Kramer are not the only ones unhappy with the coverage of AIDS printed by the *Times* and other dominant media outlets. Throughout the epidemic, AIDS activists of color, in particular black AIDS activists and service providers, have repeatedly contested the images put forth by both dominant and indigenous press sources. Although most AIDS agencies in communities of color tend to be preoccupied with securing even basic services for their clients, they have on occasion found time to write editorials and letters to the editors denouncing what they claimed was clearly racist reporting. Most recently, a group of AIDS activists and service providers of color have been meeting through the auspices of the Audre Lorde Project (Brooklyn, New York) in response to what they perceived as the racist coverage of the Nushawn Williams case in Chautauqua County, New York. Mr. Williams allegedly, knowing he was HIV positive, had unprotected sex with up to seventy-five young women and girls in Chautauqua County. This makeshift group of activists, while in no way condoning or excusing Mr. Williams's actions, focused a substantial part of their attention on the bias and racism inherent in the coverage of this event, and the need for greater AIDS education in communities of color. Specifically, on the topic of racism, these activists and others across the country publicly questioned whether the fact that Mr. Williams was black and his alleged victims were white motivated and shaped the coverage this crisis received. A section of the Housing Works newsletter articulates this concern quite effectively, highlighting the role of marginalizing myths of black men's sexuality in framing this story:

> Finally, the attention the case has drawn is clearly motivated by racism. The public's outrage seems focused as much on the number of sexual encounters an African-American man had as on the risk of HIV infection associated with those encounters. And news photographs and television coverage emphasize that many of the young women he knew where white. The outrage evoked by this story reflects deeply embedded cultural archetypes in many white communities of sexually voracious Black men who "prey" on vulnerable white girls.

Media discussion of the unusually high percentage of women infected through contact with this man described him as a "super-secretor," further evoking racist stereotypes of super-potency. The articulation of racism through metaphors of contagion is common throughout modern Western history. In this case, where an actual infectious agent—overtly the virus, in the popular imagination the Black man himself—has been identified, the expression of those racist fears is allowed to rage unconstrained. (31 October 1997, 5)

Tracie M. Gardner, one of the initiators of the makeshift group responding to the Williams case and the policy director for the Harlem Directors Group, also questions the media's motivation in a letter to the editor of the *New York Blade,* a recently established gay newspaper in New York:

There is something fundamentally racist in the media response to this incident. Where have the voices of outrage been when special interest groups put a stranglehold on any provisions for aggressive AIDS education in the schools? Where have the voices been as the epidemic continues to ravage African-American and Latina women in the prime of their young lives? Where have the voices been when not one dime of federal Centers for Disease Control and Prevention dollars set aside for directly funded HIV prevention resources can make its way to hard-hit communities like Central Harlem, and Bedford-Stuyvesant, and Brownsville?

Where is the outrage? Where is the horror? (14 November 1997)

Interestingly, the Black Leadership Commission on AIDS (BLCA), a mainstream black AIDS organization that works to involve *established* black leadership and institutions in the fight against AIDS in black communities, ignored the perceived racism of dominant media sources. Instead, this body of traditional leaders, at their press conference in response to this case, first called on "Black clergy to publicly denounce the actions of Nushawn Williams. . . . The press conference was also used to announce a public health intervention through BLCA's extensive black church network, and to aid public health officials in identifying, testing, and supporting victims of Mr. Williams. Plans designed to educate and help black parents talk to their children about AIDS at next Sunday's church mass were also revealed" (BLCA press release, 3 November 1997).

The Nushawn Williams case is but one example of black AIDS activists, organizations, and service providers condemning and challenging dominant media coverage of AIDS. For example, the media coverage of Magic Johnson's announcement of his HIV-positive status was also condemned, in particular in black newspapers, for the absence of black experts, black AIDS workers, and references to black communities. More explicitly political groups of color responding to AIDS, such as BAM! and VOCAL, also sporadically engaged in challenges to the both dominant and indigenous media. However, with so many issues impacting and shaping the development of AIDS in communities of color, these groups often found it difficult to mount and sustain a campaign targeting media sources. Instead, the response among all those involved in the fight against AIDS in black communities tended to be more piecemeal, with individuals, organizations, and activists reacting to the more outlandish presentations of African Americans with AIDS. Thus, to assess the impact of such actions on the decisions of editors and reporters would be difficult. The evidence presented here, however, suggests that there was, at the very least, periodic contestation of the marginalizing narratives of AIDS found in dominant papers and magazines, on television, and even in indigenous black newspapers and magazines.[10]

In light of the patterns of early neglect evident in the *New York Times* as well as the response from activists across communities, we are left with the question of how to understand the absence of coverage in the early years of the epidemic. Scholars such as Kinsella argue that it was a combination of the institutional hierarchy of power (which allowed one editor the discretion to neglect one of the most important stories of our time) and the personal ideology of Rosenthal (who saw lesbians and gay men and the issues that affected their lives as undeserving of serious attention) which produced such a dearth of coverage. This combination of institutional and personal marginalization provided the framework through which this world-renowned paper would ignore what would soon be a worldwide, devastating disease. While this proposition makes intuitive sense, it seems to ignore the fact that other people, not only gay men, and in particular white gay men, were implicated in the early years of this epidemic. Left unexplored by Kinsella is the quantity and quality of coverage received by other groups, in particular people of color, during the early years of the epidemic.

Using the *New York Times Index,* a group of magnificent students assisted me in identifying all the stories indexed under AIDS from 1981 to 1993, coding each story for its group focus.[11] Figure 5.1 outlines the

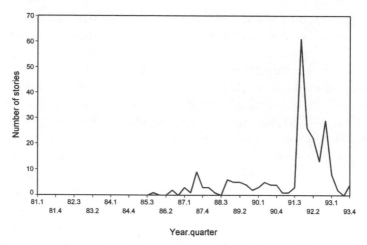

Figure 5.2. *New York Times* stories on AIDS and African Americans, 1981–1993. (Data from *New York Times* index)

general trend in the number of stories printed by the *Times* between 1981 and 1993 by quarter. As discussed above, the *Times*, while clearly negligent in the first years of the epidemic, eventually changed, printing a greater number of stories over the course of the epidemic. As is also evident from the data, coverage of AIDS at the *Times* peaked and waned at different times. For example, the third quarter of 1985 shows a large peak due to the volume of stories written about Rock Hudson, his AIDS diagnosis, and his revealed homosexuality. A similar celebrity-driven peak is evident at the end of 1991, resulting from Magic Johnson's announcement of his seropositive status. The largest peak came in 1987 as a significant number of stories dealt with the topic of HIV antibody testing.

This data can also be used to examine trends in the coverage of stories that focused on AIDS in African-American communities. If we begin by asking how many stories on AIDS actually focused on the manifestation of this epidemic in black communities, we find a very disturbing answer. Over the course of the thirteen years of this analysis, from 1981 to 1993, the *Times* printed 4,671 stories on the AIDS epidemic. Unbelievably, only 231, or five percent, of those 4,671 stories had African Americans as their focus. Even this number is misleading, since the distribution of stories on African Americans is quite skewed, as figure 5.2 shows. Furthermore, when we exclude stories on African

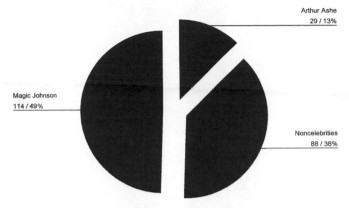

Figure 5.3.   Breakdown of *New York Times* stories on AIDS and African Americans, 1981–1983. (Data from *New York Times* index)

Americans that are about black celebrities with AIDS, coverage of AIDS among African Americans looks even more grim.

Specifically, stories on Earvin "Magic" Johnson accounted for 114, or about 49 percent, of the 231 stories we categorized as focusing on African Americans. Additionally, 29 stories, or about 13 percent of the 231 stories, center on Arthur Ashe. Thus 62 percent of the stories printed by the *Times* which highlighted or made central AIDS among African Americans were about either Earvin "Magic" Johnson or Arthur Ashe, as indicated in figure 5.3. In fact, the *Times* printed nearly as many stories on Magic Johnson (53) in the fourth quarter of 1991 when he announced that he was HIV positive as it had printed on AIDS in African-American communities over the previous ten years of the epidemic (66). From another perspective, we can say that over 70 percent of the stories on AIDS among African Americans printed by the *Times* between 1981 and 1993 were published in the two years following Magic Johnson's announcement.

Regardless of the number of stories on Magic Johnson, however, we are left with the question of whether 231 stories is an adequate number to fully represent the affect of AIDS in African-American communities. The problem with answering this question is of course finding the appropriate comparative framework. For example, should we compare the coverage that focused on the gay community to that which focused on the African-American community, even though these two communities clearly overlap? Between the years 1981 and 1993 the *Times*

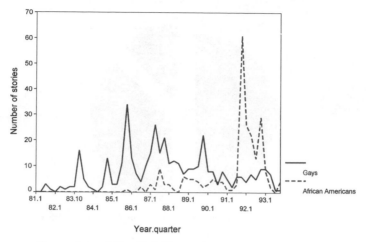

Figure 5.4.   Comparison of *New York Times* AIDS stories on African Americans and Gays, 1981–1993. (Data from *New York Times* index)

printed 369 stories that focused on gay men. And while figure 5.4 tells us something about when coverage occurred and peaked for each community, it does not answer the question of whether the quantity of stories for each group was appropriate.

Most would agree, however, that the levels of coverage indicated in figure 5.4 seem hardly adequate for either group. Again, the comparative framework shapes our understanding of this data. For example, the 231 stories on AIDS among African Americans—actually 88 stories on African Americans and AIDS, since most of the stories on Magic Johnson and Arthur Ashe make no mention of black communities—seem almost excessive when compared to the 64 stories, or 1.4 percent of *New York Times* stories, in which AIDS among Latinos/as was the central focus. Figure 5.5 indicates that in comparison to stories on Haitians, Latinos, Africans, and gays, stories on African Americans were second only to stories on gays in this very restricted analysis. However, if we remove the stories on Earvin "Magic" Johnson and Arthur Ashe, as shown in figure 5.6, African Americans fall into third place behind both gays and Africans.

Whatever the comparative frame, it seems clear, at least intuitively, that when only 5 percent of the stories on AIDS in the *Times* between 1981 and 1993 focus on AIDS in African-American communities, while cumulatively through 1993 blacks constitute 32 percent of all AIDS cases, something systemic and marginalizing is occurring. The inade-

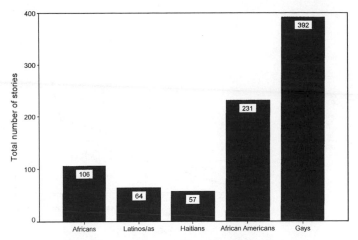

Figure 5.5. *New York Times* cumulative AIDS stories by group, 1981–1993. (Data from *New York Times* index)

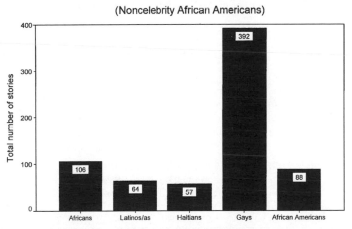

Figure 5.6. *New York Times* cumulative AIDS stories by group, 1981–1993. (Sample comprises noncelebrity African Americans; data is from *New York Times* Index)

quacy of this coverage is especially evident when we examine the *Times* coverage in comparison to the trends in the number of AIDS cases among African Americans. As indicated in figure 5.7, blacks have experienced a consistent and rapid increase in the number of AIDS cases reported to the CDC. The dramatic rise in AIDS cases among blacks is especially apparent in 1993, due largely to the implementation of a revised case definition, which, as can be seen in table 5.1, expanded

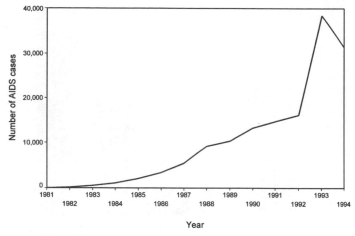

Figure 5.7.   AIDS cases among African Americans, 1981–1994. (Data from CDC *HIV/AIDS Surveillance Reports*)

Table 5.1   Changes in number of AIDS cases reported, 1991–1994 (case definition adjusted in 1993)

	1991	1992	1993	1994
Men				
White	20,716	20,743 (1)[a]	43,987 (2.12)	29,910 (0.67)
Black	11,059	12,035 (1.09)	28,792 (2.39)	22,838 (0.79)
Latino	6,850	6,782 (0.99)	15,301 (2.26)	12,016 (0.78)
Other	468	520 (1.12)	1,085 (2.09)	827 (0.77)
Total	39,093	40,080 (1.03)	89,165 (2.22)	65,591 (0.74)
Women				
White	1,358	1,458 (1.07)	4,103 (2.8)	3,148 (0.76)
Black	3,102	3,394 (1.09)	9,220 (2.72)	8,016 (0.87)
Latina	1,213	1,337 (1.10)	3,324 (2.49)	2,814 (0.85)
Other	57	66	177	103
Total	5,730	6,255 (1.09)	16,824 (2.69)	14,081 (0.84)

Sources: Data from Centers for Disease Control and Prevention, *HIV/AIDS Surveillance Report*, 1991–1994.

[a]Numbers in parentheses are the ratios to the previous year.

the list of diseases, conditions, and tests used to classify someone as having AIDS.[12]

This picture stands in contrast to the amount of coverage dedicated to AIDS among blacks in the *Times*. In fact, a close comparison of figures 5.1 and 5.7 shows that overall coverage of AIDS in the *Times* declines just as the number of cases among blacks is increasing. Further, while 1993 was clearly the most dramatic year in terms of the number of new AIDS cases among blacks as reported by the CDC, there was no corresponding increase in *Times*'s stories on AIDS in African-American communities. Instead, as figure 5.2 demonstrates, 1993 shows a decline in stories on African Americans from the high years of 1991 and 1992 when coverage focused on Magic Johnson and Arthur Ashe.

Some will argue that I have exaggerated the disparity in coverage by not applying the correct comparative standard. In response, I ask, What is the appropriate framework, or how do we determine the appropriate level of coverage, for a disease that is disproportionately wreaking havoc and devastation in black communities unlike any other in modern history? Five percent of stories on African Americans and 1 percent focusing on Latinos/as cannot begin to tell the story of AIDS in these communities. This coverage must be understood as at best neglectful; at worst, as yet another example of the institutional and ideological marginalization of these groups.

Finally, and perhaps most importantly, we must address the question of content. What did the few stories that were printed about AIDS in African-American communities describe? What frames were mobilized, and which segments of African-American communities were again silenced and made invisible? The first story dealing with AIDS in African-American communities did not appear in the *Times* until October 1985, over four years into the epidemic. In the article, an epidemiologist highlighted the overrepresentation of black Americans among those classified with AIDS, and called for educational programs in these communities. While this first article focusing on African Americans did not appear until the end of 1985, there were other glimpses of people of color in the coverage of the *Times*. In fact, numerous stories on AIDS appeared that would attract the attention, anger, and suspicion of many African Americans. For example, throughout 1983 and 1985 the *Times* printed twenty-one stories on AIDS among Haitians in the United States, following the CDC's lead in designating all Haitians as a risk group. These were accompanied by a set of stories in 1985 and 1986, attempting to link African swine fever to the development of AIDS. Knowing the feeling of distrust embraced by African Americans toward dominant institutions, we can only imagine that these articles were perceived by many black Americans as part of a long tradition within the "white press" of naming Africa as the origin of nearly every disease—this time AIDS.

It was not until 1987 that at least one story on AIDS among African

Americans appeared quarterly. In fact, in 1987 the *Times* printed sixteen stories about AIDS among African Americans. These stories were largely in response to two conferences held on the topic of AIDS in black communities. Generally, these early stories focused on the increasing numbers of those with AIDS in black and Latino communities, as well as the calls by public officials for more educational programs and money targeted to fighting AIDS in minority communities. Often these stories were framed as pitting white gay men and their demands against the increasing numbers of blacks and Latinos living with AIDS. Rarely were the intersections of these identities considered.

Articles in the *Times* tended instead to focus on the established institutions of the black community, highlighting their discomfort with this disease and the "immoral" behavior that leads to its transmission. These articles also discussed the limited and constrained efforts of indigenous institutions to serve those with AIDS in black communities. For example, the efforts of black churches or civil rights organizations like the Southern Christian Leadership Conference (SCLC) to counsel and provide services for those with AIDS received a significant amount of coverage, relatively. The complaints of black officials concerning the distribution of resources or the "genocidal" nature of programs such as needle exchange generated a number of stories. As was noted earlier, the framing of AIDS in black communities as a battle over limited resources, with poor blacks and Latinos/as pitted against wealthy white gay men, allowed black public officials to appear to be doing something on this very visible issue without identifying too closely with the stigmatized and secondary segments of the community most at risk.

Missing from much of the *Times*'s coverage of AIDS among African Americans was attention to those segments most at risk in black communities. For example, only three articles focusing on black gay men and AIDS were published between 1981 and 1993. Although male-to-male sexual transmission was recorded by the CDC as the leading route of transmission of HIV among black men through mid-year 1997, those black men engaging in sex with other men, whether they identified as gay or not, did not merit the attention of the *Times*'s reporters and editors (CDC, *HIV/AIDS* 1996). And while drug users received more ink than black gay men, they too were generally neglected in *Times* coverage, in favor of black public officials debating drug policy. In what might be considered a contrast, there were at least nine stories about women of color with AIDS. Again, representation of all of these groups was inadequate, but the ability to portray women, especially through the telling of their personal stories, as the "innocent victims" of the epidemic provided a sort of *moral* cleansing which facilitated their inclusion in this more restricted discourse about AIDS.

Finally, stories on Earvin "Magic" Johnson and Arthur Ashe brought more attention to the question of AIDS in black communities. However, even this approach was limited, since most of the stories on these two celebrity athletes made no mention of black communities and the epidemic of AIDS. In many ways, it was Johnson's appeal to white America, as the ambassador of basketball with the unforgettable smile, that generated much of the media attention around his announcement of his seropositive status as well as his resulting decisions about how to manage his career. And as noted earlier, Johnson's and Ashe's non-traditional routes of transmission gave the media a chance to cover AIDS without full discussions of homosexuality and drug use. In part, it was their declared heterosexual, drug-free, family-oriented (especially in the case of Ashe), celebrity personas that propelled the media to label these two black Americans, in particular Johnson, one of the most important AIDS stories of the epidemic.

However, the question of when and how "the black community" is deployed in these stories differs for each athlete, and is particularly interesting in the case of Arthur Ashe. Articles on Ashe repeatedly told the story of how he was the first black player to integrate and at one point dominate the tennis circuit, winning Wimbeldon, the Australian Open, and the U.S. Open. We are told in these articles of his research and writing on black athletes. We are told of his political commitment to fighting racism, displayed most dramatically in his efforts to end apartheid in South Africa. However, it seems that when AIDS entered the picture, race, or specifically "the black community," dropped out. In none of the stories on Ashe in the *Times* is he reported as expressing any special interest in dealing with AIDS in black communities. Instead, his comments, as reported in the *Times*, center on educating the general population about AIDS, while his fund-raising efforts were directed at children with AIDS. Even when Ashe reluctantly announced that he had AIDS, there was no reported mention of AIDS in black communities, in spite of the fact that David Dinkins, a personal friend of Ashe and at the time mayor of New York City—the city with the largest number of AIDS cases among black Americans—stood with Ashe at his press conference.

None of these comments are meant in any way to tarnish or dispute the importance of the work pursued by both Mr. Ashe and Mr. Johnson after announcing their seropositive status to the world. They are intended to help us question what components or images are necessary to designate a story as focusing on AIDS in black communities. Is a black body on the front page enough? Is a black body necessary at all? Must the individuals involved designate as the target of their work members of black communities? While all of these are questions yet to be resolved, it does seem clear that coverage of celebrated black Americans with HIV or AIDS is not an adequate media response to the continued progress of this epidemic in black communities.

So what do we make of all of this? In light of this data, how do we evaluate Kinsella's claim that the lack of coverage at the *Times* in the early years of the epidemic was largely determined by a hierarchy which centralized control in the hands of an editor who was homophobic? In part I think Kinsella is correct. It seems clear that Rosenthal was homophobic and thus neglectful of a disease understood as located centrally in the gay community. What Kinsella and others who study media coverage of the AIDS epidemic seem to miss or possibly discount is the importance of the marginal position of those drug users, gay men, lesbians, and heterosexual women, men, and children living with AIDS who are people of color. The marginal position of these other groups living with AIDS (some heterosexual) also allowed the *Times* to look the other way on the issue of AIDS. I believe that if this disease had primarily affected gay men and white middle-class heterosexuals, the *Times* and other dominant institutions would have had a different response. Thus, the concentration of AIDS among numerous marginal populations, all of which were generally outside the social world of Abe Rosenthal and many other editors at the *Times*, in large part motivated and allowed his and others' disregard for this story. One fact that many white AIDS activists are still unwilling to admit, however, is that many of the people of color living and struggling with AIDS—even those self-identified heterosexuals—are farther removed from the world of Abe Rosenthal than some white gay men with AIDS. Therefore, to discount racism, in many instances as it interacts and works with homophobia and heterosexism (among other systems of oppression), as a significant determinant of the amount of coverage this story received at the *Times* is to be at best misguided and naive, and at worst, racist.

Television Network Evening News

The coverage of the AIDS epidemic by the television broadcast media, although reaching a larger and less informed audience, displayed generally the same patterns as that of the print media. In much the same fashion as the *Times*, the national nightly news programs, which take their cues from the *Times*, also ignored the AIDS crisis in its early years. There was no coverage of AIDS in 1981 on any national nightly news programs. Only six stories appeared in 1982: three on NBC, two on ABC, and one on CBS. NBC ran the first story on AIDS. As noted earlier, Tom Brokaw began this segment by stating that "scientists at the National Centers for Disease Control in Atlanta today received the results of a study that *shows* that the *lifestyle* of some male homosexuals has triggered an epidemic of a rare form of cancer" (emphasis added; NBC 17 June 1982). The report by Robert Bazell continues, focusing on the experiences of two white gay men with AIDS. And while the segment mentions that "the disease" has also been discovered in heterosexual men and women, the focus is clearly on AIDS as it was experienced by white gay men. Eventually, each network would run at least one story introducing the disease in 1982. These stories, appearing two to four months after NBC's initial broadcast, still emphasized the association between gay men and AIDS, but also included a small segment on the spread of this disease beyond the gay community.

Cook and Colby (1992), in their article "The Mass-Mediated Epidemic: The Politics of AIDS on the Nightly Network News," suggest that during the first five years of the epidemic one can decipher five phases of AIDS coverage. They call the first cycle "The Mysterious Disease." Here the authors argue that reporters presented AIDS as something located almost exclusively in the gay community and linked to the "abnormal" behavior of gay men. This phase also included an early introduction to other groups, such as Haitian refugees and injection drug users, thought to be at risk for AIDS. The second phase, "The Threat to the Innocent," moved beyond gay and other marginal communities to focus on people thought to have acquired HIV because of someone else's indiscretionary behavior. As we would expect, this phase featured stories on hemophiliacs and the possible contamination of the blood supply. "The Epidemic of Fear" described the third phase of coverage. Cook and Colby suggest that many of the reports during this stage highlighted the fear of AIDS that was gripping the country. During this phase, they find journalists trying to report the "facts" of the disease, while trying at the same time to calm fears in the general public. The fourth phase, "The Search for the Breakthrough," centers on scientists and their promising discoveries. During this stage reporters emphasized developments in treatments and the hopeful march toward a cure. The final phase Cook and Colby label "Rock Hudson and the Legitimation of AIDS." The authors suggest that in reporting about Rock Hudson, AIDS as a topic gained some legitimacy, as indicated by longer and special segments, the use of more gay experts in stories, and reports appearing earlier in broadcasts.

Much as Kinsella argued that homophobia at the *New York Times* shaped early coverage of AIDS, Cook and Colby argue that initial television news coverage of AIDS was influenced by the population affected by the disease, namely, gay men, and by the perceived distastefulness of the details of the story. The authors comment that television producers, especially sensitive to what might offend their viewers, were reluctant to feature stories on such an "unworthy" population (1992, 87). By Cook and Colby's account, AIDS did not garner a substantial spot on the nightly news until "worthy" heterosexuals could be entangled in its destruction. Robert Bazell of NBC news supports this assessment, noting at a forum organized by the Scientists Institute for Public Information that "it would be dishonest not to say we couldn't sell the AIDS story early on because it was about gays" (Altman 1986, 16). Bazell is quoted in Edward Alwood's book, *Straight News* (1996), as saying that when he proposed stories on AIDS early in the epidemic, he was told, "Look, it ain't us. We don't want to hear stories about homosexuals . . . [and] drug addicts" (219). Again, we are presented with an explanation, this time of television evening news coverage of AIDS, that focuses on heteronormative assumptions, contending that the seemingly almost exclusive manifestation of AIDS in gay male communities diverted coverage. But this model ignores the role played by poverty, race, and drug phobia in defining worthy subjects and levels of coverage.

To explore the coverage of AIDS among African Americans and the degree to which Cook and Colby's findings apply to that reporting, I enlisted a group of research assistants to help me examine a sample of television news stories on AIDS.[13] Between 1981 and 1993 1,729 stories on AIDS, totaling 3,354.2 minutes, were run by NBC, ABC, and CBS. Viewing each of these stories would have been both financially draining and time-consuming, so I settled for viewing a subset of them. To accomplish this goal, I generated a random sample of AIDS coverage

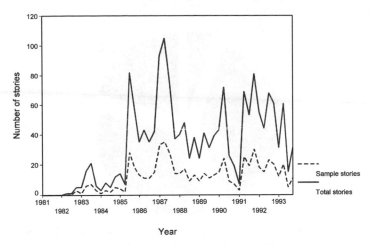

Year

Figure 5.8.   Network evening news AIDS stories, 1981–1993. (Data from Vanderbilt University Television News Archive)

from the stories indexed by the Vanderbilt Television Archives. My objectives in designing this sample were to ensure representation of the different stories aired throughout the entire time period of 1981–1993, as well as to include as many stories as possible in the sample. The final sample includes approximately one-third of all the stories aired on AIDS between 1982 and 1993.[14] There are 598 stories in the sample, totaling approximately 1,220 minutes. Figure 5.8 maps the trend in overall coverage as well as that represented by my sample of stories.

I begin with a general description of stories on AIDS among African Americans. Of the 598 stories coded in my sample, only 38, or 6.4 percent, focused on AIDS among African Americans. As was the case with the *New York Times*, this number is somewhat misleading since the coverage was again extremely skewed. Figure 5.9 details a partial breakdown in story topics. Obviously, much of the coverage I classify as centering on AIDS in African-American communities is really focused on AIDS among African-American celebrities. Twenty-five (66 percent) of the stories on African Americans detailed the experiences of Magic Johnson, Arthur Ashe, or Max Robinson. Only 13 (2.2 percent) of reports on AIDS aired between 1981 and 1993 focused more generally on the manifestation of the epidemic among "ordinary" African Americans.

Again, we need to put the number of stories on African Americans in a larger context, comparing it to the number of stories on other

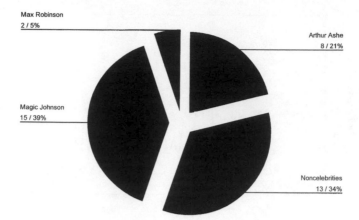

Max Robinson
2 / 5%

Arthur Ashe
8 / 21%

Magic Johnson
15 / 39%

Noncelebrities
13 / 34%

Figure 5.9.   Breakdown of network evening news AIDS stories on African Americans, 1981–1993. (Data from Vanderbilt University Television News Archive)

Table 5.2   Comparison of television evening news coverage of AIDS among Racial, Ethnic and National Groups, 1981–1993

Group	Number of stories	Percent of coverage
African Americans	38	6.4
Africans	18	3.0
Haitians	8	1.3
Latinos/as	14	2.3
African Americans (noncelebrity)	13	2.2

Source: Data from Vanderbilt University Television News Archive.

groups. Table 5.2 indicates that in comparison to other communities of color, African Americans received poor but slightly better amounts of coverage than their counterparts. In the sample 18 (3 percent) of the stories focused on the devastation of AIDS in Africa; 8 (1.3 percent) of the stories detailed the impact of AIDS on Haiti and Haitian refugees; and 14 (2.3 percent) centered on AIDS in Latino communities. Only when we broaden the framework of this analysis can we identify other groups who garnered significantly more coverage on the network evening news. For example, table 5.3 indicates that while stories focused on women numbered only 24 (4 percent) and stories on drug users totaled 22 (3.7 percent), stories on children totaled 49 (8.2 percent). This number is driven in part by the numerous stories focusing on Ryan White, the Ray Brothers, and other young people who gained notoriety

Table 5.3   Expanded comparison of television evening news coverage of AIDS among specific groups, 1981–1993

Group	Number of stories	Percent of coverage
African Americans	38	6.4
Women	24	4.0
Hemophiliacs	12	2.0
Children	49	8.2
Gay men	51	8.5
Drug users	22	3.7
African Americans (noncelebrity)	13	2.2

Source: Data from Vanderbilt University Television News Archive.

because of the discrimination they faced due to their seropositive status.

Throughout this epidemic media sources have shown the most interest in covering AIDS when the "general population" or "innocent victims" could be pulled into the epidemic. However, we should be clear that even "innocent victims" are not treated equally. So while black and Latino children comprise over 80 percent of all pediatric AIDS cases, Ryan White, the Ray brothers, and Kimberly Bergalis are still the most well-known cases of young people with AIDS (CDC, *HIV* 1996).[15] It seems that even among "innocent victims," patterns of marginalization that stratify along characteristics such as race, gender, class, and in this case, route of transmission, are actively at work. Finally, the group garnishing the largest number of stories (only two stories more than those focused on children) in this very constrained analysis was gay men. Stories in which gay men were central totaled 51 (8.5 percent) of all reports on AIDS in my sample between 1981 and 1993. Not surprisingly, nearly 75 percent (74.4 percent) of these stories appeared before the end of 1987, when the media began to redirect the minimal attention given *any marginal group* away from gay men and toward other communities dealing with AIDS.

Much like Cook and Colby, I too was able to identify five phases in the coverage centered on AIDS, not among African Americans exclusively, but more broadly among communities of African descent. Unlike Cook and Colby, my phases were not confined to the first five years of the epidemic, but ran the span of my sample from 1981 to 1993. Actually, the span of this coverage ran from 1983 to 1993 because the first story focusing on AIDS among people of color did not appear until 19 June 1983. This story, on CBS, discussed the difficulties prisoners with AIDS faced, highlighting the personal experiences of two Latino prisoners. In spite of this initial story, the first phase of what I call racialized AIDS coverage focused on the impact of AIDS in Haitian communities and is defined by two stories in 1983. One story described the plight of a young Haitian baby with AIDS, who needed adoption. The other story, broadcast on 21 June 1983 by NBC, discussed "the mysterious connection" between AIDS in Haiti and AIDS in the United States. During one segment of this story, reporters used a hidden camera to film activity at a tourist bar in Haiti catering to "homosexuals mostly from the United States." The owner of the bar explained to the reporter that very poor young men often worked as sex workers for gay male tourists in order to acquire money for food. The report indirectly suggests that AIDS may have entered the United States through the infection of a white gay male tourist who unwittingly had sex with an HIV-positive male prostitute in Haiti. Of course, science reporter Robert Bazell made sure to mention that there was no evidence to support the idea that AIDS had come from Haiti to the United States. However, such reporting, which deployed the marginalizing myth that people and nations of color are the origins of disease, may have resulted in people of color not only being less knowledgeable of the AIDS epidemic, but also more suspicious of the reports coming from the television evening news.

The second phase I identified ran from 1985 to 1987 and had as its core stories on the impact of AIDS in Africa. Many of these reports included segments on the devastation of AIDS in Africa, as estimated by the World Health Organization (WHO). These accounts also emphasized the spread of AIDS through heterosexual sex, including, of course, comments on the perceived "abnormal and promiscuous" sexual habits of Africans. Some reports discussed the discriminatory treatment of Africans in other countries such as Belgium and China, where the governments had ordered the testing of all foreign, primarily African, students. However, the most disturbing and recurring theme found in this phase was the attempt to identify Africa as the origin of AIDS. Repeatedly, these stories hypothesized about the link between the African green monkey or African swine fever and AIDS.

For example, on 15 August 1985, NBC broadcast a report stating that "scientists now believe they know the source of AIDS—Central Africa." The picture suddenly switches to Zaire, and the viewer is told by voice-over that "the AIDS virus almost certainly started to spread from here in equatorial Africa." Reporter Keith Miller goes on to state that "scientists here believe AIDS reached the United States from Central Africa by way of Haiti." The segment proceeds, changing its focus to the African green monkey as the source of the virus. This time the image of a monkey on a street corner eating a banana comes into view. Although we are never informed as much, I assume that the viewer is to believe that the monkey on the screen is an African green monkey. Similarly, I assume the viewer is to believe that monkeys run free in African cities, since this monkey is shown sitting on a corner with pedestrians and cars going by. The voice-over for this segment states, "From monkey to man, that is how some experts believe the virus is spread. The African green monkey carries a virus similar to AIDS. It may have been passed to man through a bite." The report again switches its focus, this time to the change in AIDS from a rural to an urban epidemic in Africa. This part of the story begins with the image of Africans dancing in a club. The reporter informs the viewer that "unlike the United States there are no risk groups. Here everyone is threatened. Here AIDS is a heterosexual disease. Men and women are infected in equal numbers. Scientists don't know why. Unsanitary living conditions and sexual promiscuity could help to spread the disease. The use of a single needle in multiple medical injections could pass the virus to the general population. But no one is certain and everyone is afraid." The report ends on a pseudo-conspiratorial note, with the reporter standing in front of a large building and commenting that "inside this medical compound American, Belgian, and Zairian researchers are conducting a top secret study of the virus. No one is allowed to talk about it."

Clearly, as reporter Keith Miller suggests at the end of the segment, discovering the source of this virus is without question important, if it can assist in developing a cure or at the very least containing its spread. It is, however, the manner in which speculation about Africa, Africans, and disease is conducted that is the general problem of reporting in this phase of coverage. George Strait of ABC news, commenting on such stories, states that

> there is a legitimate and interesting investigation as to how AIDS started. People would like to know what is killing all of these people. People would like to know. And from a scientist's point of view they would like to know because maybe that can

help them figure out how to stop it. But it became politicized. And it again was used as a way to say, "Well we don't have to worry about this because it's them [Africans]. It started over there [Africa]. It started with them. So it also was a way of letting us off the hook. . . . they started it, they are different."[16]

Unfortunately, the reporting in the story detailed above is not very different from many of the stories broadcast during this period. The mobilization of these all-too-familiar narratives about Africa and Africans distracts attention from needed and more accurate information about this unique and devastating disease. Specifically, such framings, in which Africans and by association African Americans were blamed for the spread of AIDS, were reported to have aroused the ire of black Americans following these reports. Researchers Thomas and Quinn (1993) make just such an argument, suggesting that the framing of reports on AIDS among people of color significantly impacts how African Americans view these stories. The authors state that "several reports in the popular black media and numerous anecdotal reports from community-based organizations document that black Americans mistrust government reports of AIDS, believe that HIV is a man-made virus, *have a negative response toward people who say AIDS originated in Africa,* and believe AIDS is a form of genocide" (emphasis added, 328).

The third phase of coverage spans between 1987 and the third quarter of 1991. During this period we find an "upsurge" in the number of stories (nine) dealing with AIDS among African Americans. For the most part these stories were uneventful, yet important. They tended to focus on the rise in AIDS cases among African Americans and Latinos/ as—or as the reporters like to call it, "the changing face of AIDS." Segments usually included some mention of the accelerating statistics on AIDS in minority communities. Some stories then proceeded to discuss the failure of AIDS education and prevention programs aimed at these communities. Other accounts described new initiatives to increase access to educational programs, drug clinical trials, or treatments such as AZT among minorities and women. The segments of African-American and Latino communities highlighted most often in these reports included women and children, with some minor discussion of drug users, those in prison, and sex workers.

One familiar dynamic found in some of these stories is the use of polar and monolithic narratives to define African-American women with AIDS. For instance, one report by ABC on 20 June 1990, examining AIDS among intravenous drug users, included a segment in which a group of primarily black women are *warned* by a black female AIDS educator, who was infected by her drug-using husband, that many *unsuspecting* (read innocent) women are becoming infected by their partners. She states in the report that "a lot of our men are infecting us. They're not telling us that they are bisexual. A lot of our men have been in prisons. They're coming out back into the community, and they're making love to us, and they're making these goo-goo eyes at us, and we are falling for it because of a lot of the voids in our own life."

In another report, however, black women are indicted as the transmitters of AIDS. In this ABC segment on the rates of infection among newborns in New York, no U.S. infecting mother is actually seen on camera or given the opportunity to speak. I specifically say "U.S. infecting mothers," since reference is also made to the rates of infection of babies in Zaire. And while no woman thought to have infected her baby in the U.S. is shown on camera, the picture of a room full of Zairian mothers and their children is displayed on screen. During the story, science reporter George Strait tells us that the small (read innocent) children we see on camera were infected by their mothers, "primarily women who either use drugs or are the sex partners of those who use drugs" (ABC, 13 January 1988). In this story the seropositive status of the mother is an issue not because it threatens the life of a woman, but because it threatens the life of her child.

These two stories represent the familiar tropes of innocent victim or infecting mother used to frame and superficially explore the lives of women with AIDS, in particular black women with AIDS. The experiences of women with AIDS, independent of children and infecting men, are never truly explored in and of themselves (Hammonds 1997). It seems that the complicated struggles of women, such as the different and largely unstudied manifestations of AIDS in women, do not merit the attention of dominant institutions built on the simplicity of singular patriarchal narratives of "good" women and loving relationships between mothers and their children. Institutional rules or norms similar to those which lead the broadcast media to highlight only monolithic and familiar frames of black women, also determine that the stories of black gay men are never aired on the nightly news. Thus it is not surprising that none of the nine stories comprising this phase of coverage or the thirteen stories focusing on AIDS among African Americans aired between 1983 and 1993 discussed the experiences or even the numbers of black gay men with AIDS. I remind the reader that this absence, or nonevent, occurred as male-to-male sexual transmission remained the number one route of transmission for those classified with AIDS in black communities as well as nationally, as documented by the CDC (CDC, *HIV/AIDS* 1997).

The fourth phase of coverage dealing with AIDS among people of color ran from the fourth quarter of 1991 to 1993. The twenty-three stories that comprise this period centered on the HIV-positive status of both Magic Johnson and Arthur Ashe. The coverage of these two celebrities produced more tangential than actual coverage of AIDS among African Americans. In many of the early stories, following closely on the heels of their announcements, the press was eager to explore not only the impact their HIV status would have in black communities, but also the "larger society." So for example, in the case of Magic Johnson, a number of the stories following his announcement highlighted not the effect of his announcement on black community members, but its effect on children. Again, it was the ability of Magic Johnson, in particular, but also Arthur Ashe, to have standing, recognition, and even admiration outside black communities that in some ways made their announcement so newsworthy. As one reporter stated at the end of his report on Magic Johnson, "now everyone knows someone with AIDS."

When thinking about the appeal of stories on Magic Johnson and Arthur Ashe to television news reporters, we should remember that with both Magic Johnson and Arthur Ashe the press not only had black celebrities who were highly regarded outside of black communities, they also had individuals who did not carry "the mark" of other stigmatized risk groups. Johnson and Ashe were respectable "victims." They were respectable not only because they professed to being infected by the more acceptable routes of heterosexual sex and blood transfusion, but also because they conformed to normative ideas of manhood, in contrast to what had been represented for most men with AIDS. Due to their history in sports, the very visible presence of their wives and children, and in the case of Magic Johnson, due to the reported magnitude of his sexual prowess, these two men signified a pseudo-normative maleness not often seen in AIDS stories.[17] Through these stories reporters and viewers alike were presented with worthy tragic figures. The national grief, sympathy, and empathy that the American public felt around AIDS, but held back out of fear that such emotion might somehow be construed as condoning the "immoral" behavior that leads to AIDS, could now be released and directed toward these two national figures. Just such a national catharsis began with Rock Hudson, but was cut short when the public found out he was gay.

However, in spite of the national standing of Magic Johnson and the networks' willingness to cover both Johnson and Ashe, changes in the type of coverage they received are evident as their stories extended over the years. For example, while most AIDS stories are typically presented by the network's science reporter, a number of stories on Magic Johnson were presented by one of the network's sports reporters. As one can imagine, stories developed by sports reporters tended to focus on Johnson and Ashe as sports figures, paying little attention to the other identities and communities that determine their social location. So while Dan Rather introduced the first story on Magic Johnson's HIV infection, Pat O'Brien of CBS sports was the lead reporter on the story and provided most of the commentary (CBS 7 November 1991). In this story, young men playing basketball were the critical audience used to assess the real impact of Johnson's announcement.

The placement of stories on Johnson and Ashe was also different compared to the placement of general stories on AIDS among African Americans, which were evenly placed in the first ten minutes of the broadcast and the second ten minutes of a thirty-minute program. Thus six of the thirteen stories on AIDS and African Americans were broadcast during the first ten minutes of the evening news, while the remaining seven were shown during the second ten-minute segment of a thirty-minute program. The stories on Magic Johnson and Arthur Ashe indicate a different pattern, with the first few stories on Johnson or Ashe broadcast in the early time slot (or first ten-minute span), while later stories were relegated to the second or third ten-minute period of a thirty-minute program. This pattern is especially stark in the case of Arthur Ashe. When Ashe announced that he had AIDS on 8 April 1992, it was the lead story on the evening news, but after the initial coverage of his announcement, every other story aired on Ashe in my sample appeared in the last ten-minute segment of the program, signaling much less importance. It was not until his death that this pattern changed, with one report of his death falling in the second ten-minute span of the broadcast. Media scholars would probably not be surprised by this pattern, since it is generally understood that the longevity of a story increases the probability that there will be less new news to report, dictating the placement of additional stories in the later part of an evening news broadcast.

The fifth and final phase I identified brings us full circle back to the Haitian community. This time five stories were run in 1993 on the detainment and eventual forced release of HIV-positive Haitian refugees and their families at Guantanamo Bay. These stories tended to be very straightforward. They began with some discussion of the horrible conditions under which these individuals were being held. The reports then proceeded beyond the deplorable living conditions to center on the visits of notable figures to Guantanamo Bay (such as Jesse Jackson), or to the judicial decision ordering the United States government to release those detained. After the last story on the release of Haitian refugees from Guantanamo Bay was broadcast on 14 June 1993, no other stories exploring the impact of AIDS in communities of color were identified in 1993.

Again, we are left with the question of whether the coverage provided African-American communities was adequate with regard to quantity and quality. In terms of sheer numbers, 2 percent of television news stories on AIDS devoted to the epidemic among noncelebrated African Americans was not acceptable or sufficient by any standard. The fact that the number of stories aired on Magic Johnson's HIV-positive status surpassed the total number of stories devoted to AIDS among "average" African Americans, a group disproportionately represented among those with AIDS, also signals severe problems in the amount of coverage afforded this community. On the issue of the substantive nature of this coverage, we need only look at the absence of any serious discussion or representation of male-to-male sexual transmission in black communities, the leading route of transmission among black men classified as having AIDS by the CDC over the course of the epidemic (mid-year 1996), to recognize failure in this area. The lack of coverage of black gay men and black men who have sex with men can be viewed as an indicator of the disparity between the reality of AIDS in black communities and the presentation of AIDS in black communities as seen on the nightly news. But the more fundamental question may be: To what or whom do we attribute such troubling coverage? That is, were there so few stories with only superficial content on AIDS in African-American communities because of the personal prejudices of reporters and editors, or did institutional biases shape this coverage?

Cook and Colby (1992) conclude that they "cannot agree that 'media response to AIDS has generally been irrational.' The ebb and flow of AIDS reporting reflects considerable rationality, *but by the standards of 'media logic'"* (111). What Cook and Colby view as the rationality of the media is better understood as the institutional biases of the television evening news, which marginalize and make invisible, in this case, the manifestation of AIDS in black communities. A strict media analysis of AIDS coverage would confirm that, on average, reporters, editors, and producers did what they normally do when covering a story. They used personal stories as their hook; they used authoritative sources such as the government for easy and cheap information; and they examined AIDS from different angles as the epidemic progressed. However, even in following the guidelines for "good" journalism, certain biases lead to the exclusion of marginal groups. For example, those who take care of the health of black communities are rarely the experts tapped as authoritative sources on the evening news. Thus, even in the established rules of the profession, we must recognize the biases that inherently skew or distort what the public sees.

Adding the variable of race to the analysis of television coverage of AIDS provides a very different picture of the evening news coverage than that identified by Cook and Colby. This is not to suggest that the five phases Cook and Colby describe do not exist in this sample. However, if African-Americans viewers watched the same news broadcasts that Cook and Colby examined in the first five years of the epidemic, they might identify additional themes that escaped the gaze or consciousness of Cook and Colby. Such viewers, while also identifying the epidemic of fear in the broadcasts during this five-year period, might see the absence of stories on African Americans as a phase or a phenomenon worth mention in itself. The more troubling scenario, however, would be if these same African-American viewers, seeing few stories or visible images about people of color and AIDS, interpreted this absence as a signal that the AIDS epidemic was not about them or their community. According to George Bellinger, Jr., former education coordinator at the Minority Task Force on AIDS, this is exactly what happened. He states, "The media told us it was a white gay disease. I mean people are about denial that it happens in our [black] community."[18] This same sentiment is shared by Greg Broyles, formerly a staff member at the Black Leadership Commission on AIDS. He explains, "Black people didn't see AIDS as a disease that concerned them because we were always told that it was a gay disease and if it was a white gay disease, why should we be concerned? From the beginning the media called it GRID (Gay-Related Immune Deficiency).

Why should we be concerned with it? We have other problems."[19] The denial that both Bellinger and Broyles refer to is of course only available to those African Americans who have not yet been affected by this epidemic. To many other members of black communities, exclusion and invisibility, not denial, have been the defining characteristics of their experience with AIDS.

Conclusion

During the early years of the epidemic, through the actions of media sources such as the *New York Times* and the television evening news, the social construction of AIDS began to take shape. Of course, decisions about how this emerging crisis would be framed did not take place in a vacuum: activists, lobbyists, and even the readers of the *New York Times* and the viewers of the evening news influenced the coverage. However, the majority of those in the United States passively received their information about AIDS from dominant media sources. The labeling of AIDS as a gay disease in the early years of the epidemic, while instilling great stigma, discrimination, and bias, also resulted in the mobilization of the gay community, where AIDS was perceived as an issue that threatened their survival. Conversely, the absence of African Americans from images and discussions of AIDS undoubtedly supported the denial of black community leaders, who viewed AIDS as a disease they did not need to own. Recognition of the potential impact of AIDS on black communities may not have drastically increased if the CDC had pursued research dealing with injection drug users, women, and children in the early years of the epidemic. Media coverage calling attention to the increasing numbers of African Americans losing their lives to this disease may not have changed the pattern of response evident in black communities. However, an expanded focus in either case may have given those trying to increase awareness of AIDS in African-American communities a powerful weapon to challenge the comfort of black leaders and organizations intent on denying the consequences of this disease for group members.

The response to AIDS by the CDC and the media as outlined in these last two chapters clearly revolves around at least two factors: (1) the institutional practices, rules, and procedures of those organizations involved in the early response to this disease; and (2) the history of ideological, institutional, and social marginalization of those groups thought to be most at risk for AIDS. Institutional structures, independent of the intent of those who work within them, had a significant impact on the ability of individuals to gather the information they needed to be fully informed. When the CDC established procedures which depended on traditional providers for surveillance information about disease, they effectively made invisible many poor people and injection drug users—significant numbers of whom were people of color—who have limited access to adequate health care. When newspapers relied on medical journals for information about this new disease, they inherited and reproduced all the biases of these sources. Thus, regardless of the individual motivations of epidemiologists, doctors, reporters, editors, or television anchors, the structures and procedures of these institutions were set up to pay attention to those with access, largely ignoring those without it.

Beyond structural access, the second factor that significantly explains much of the response to AIDS by dominant institutions is the ideological marginalization of the groups disproportionately affected by AIDS. Throughout the last two chapters we have seen the repeated deployment of ideologies that conceptualized injection drug users and gay men as groups easily disregarded and unworthy of full treatment. Whether such ideas originated from doctors, editors at major newspapers, or television producers, they had the same effect of justifying inaction and negligence. The ideological discourse attached specifically to AIDS not only reinforced those marginalizing strategies that already existed, it also created an additional barrier between these individuals and the resources they needed to survive. In other words, not only were gay men deemed undeserving of full recognition in the society—because of the perceived abnormality of their sexual relationships—but those same relationships were now being deemed the cause of a disease afflicting this community. Similarly, drug users, who had always been constructed as a threat to black communities, were additionally identified as being sick and contagious.

Finally, while this chapter has focused on the construction of AIDS in the early years of the epidemic, similar concerns over treatment decisions and the representation of different groups with AIDS still exist. Most recently, ideologies of marginalization have begun to frame the discussion of new drug therapies for AIDS. Many of us have been encouraged by the progress made by scientists in trying to move AIDS from a fatal disease to a chronic illness. The use of protease inhibitors, in particular, has proven significant, even dramatic, in sustaining the lives of some with AIDS. This medical development has been touted as bringing "The End of AIDS," as one *Newsweek* cover proclaimed (2 December 1996). It has even allowed Andrew Sullivan in the *New York Times Magazine* to write of a time "When Plagues End" (10 November 1996). While the development of new therapies should be applauded, we must also be careful to examine how the full discussion of such progress unfolds.

In the case of reports on protease inhibitors, a troubling discourse has already developed. It seems that protease inhibitor therapies require great discipline, since a patient's medication must be taken, in some cases, every eight hours on an empty stomach. Further, without strict adherence to the defined regimen with regard to the medication, it is possible that a virus resistant to these drugs might develop and spread. Thus the question of which patients or people with AIDS have "enough discipline" to receive these new therapies is now a central part of a new generation of AIDS reporting. Journalists are openly discussing and writing about who should be allowed such treatment. These decisions move us disturbingly close to the rationing of life-saving treatments, based not only on limited financial resources, but also on the marginalizing myths attached to ascribed group traits and behaviors that have nothing to do with individual behavior. Should drug users, who are described as having little regard for their own lives, be given access to treatments that, if used incorrectly, could threaten the longevity of treatment benefits for other more "disciplined" groups of people with AIDS? Should those who are homeless with AIDS, without access to water or food, be given treatments that demand strict adherence to medication requirements? How reporters frame and construct drug users, poor women, gay men, and all groups demanding access to treatment undoubtedly will influence who receives such treatment. Thus, patterns of institutional marginalization or internal biases that "naturally" exclude or limit the access of marginal groups to dominant institutions—whether those institutions be the *New York Times*, ABC, NBC, CBS, or the CDC—have life-and-death consequences.

Confronted by an environment where dominant institutional and ideological strategies served to deny substantial numbers of African Americans with AIDS the access to the services and resources they needed, many looked toward indigenous organizations for support. In this context, where dominant resources were largely out of the control of marginal group members with AIDS, the indigenous actions and attitudes of other marginal group members took on added significance. If community organizations were unwilling either to demand greater resources for group members or to develop resources inside the community that could fill some needs, then who or what entity would work to demand a place for these groups on the agenda? I take up the question of the indigenous response to AIDS in the next few chapters.

CHAPTER SIX

Conspiracies and Controversies

In November of 1990, almost ten years into the AIDS epidemic, *Emerge,* a news magazine aimed at the black middle-class, published one of the first cover stories on AIDS in the black popular press. Many black AIDS activists and service providers considered this story to be one of the most complete and accessible articles published on the topic to date. However, one glaring fact about the story seemed out of place in 1990: the title, "We Are Not Immune." Almost ten years into the epidemic, with over 52,329 black men, women, and children dead from or living with AIDS—New York City alone accounting for over 10,000 of those individuals—the publishing staff at *Emerge* magazine still believed there was a need to tell members of black communities, especially middle-class blacks, that they were not immune from AIDS (CDC, *HIV/AIDS Surveillance Report,* July 1991).

The perception of editors at *Emerge* magazine that the black community, even as late as 1990, had not yet reckoned with its connection to the AIDS crisis was supported in many of my interviews with those doing work on AIDS in black communities. Almost every person reiterated the idea that too many black people still did not see AIDS as a disease that threatened them. I repeatedly heard the refrain that "the white media" told the black community that AIDS was not happening to them and was therefore not their concern. This is not to deny the shouts of activists and the whispers of more traditional leaders acknowledging that some in the community—black gay men, injection drug users, their partners, and children—were "coming down" with AIDS. However, the appearance of AIDS among these clearly defined and bounded segments of black communities was quickly attributed to misguided individuals with lifestyles, such as homosexuality, that were not inherently among the behaviors and norms of black communities. Underlying such explanations was the assumption that "moral" or "good" black people need not worry or talk about this disease.

These patterns of silence and invisibility, supported and justified by dominant ideologies of marginalization, allowed the deadly impact of AIDS among black Americans to go largely unrecognized. More and more members of black communities were left to die in the midst of insignificant sustained political action on their behalf, little public recognition of their loss, and underfunded and constrained efforts to prevent others from following this same path. In the next two chapters I examine what role the black press played in reinforcing or challenging the denial of black communities concerning AIDS. Specifically, I am interested in how internal standards and norms provided the framework for the black press's reporting on AIDS.

Ideas, discourse, and debate are fundamental components of any functioning democracy. Without the provision of information from multiple perspectives and multiple sources, people are left without the tools or materials necessary to carefully evaluate issues, to reformulate their political positions, and to identify those standards thought to advance the society. Traditionally, political scientists have focused on the role that dominant institutions play in providing such information, imparting meaning to our actions and attitudes (Smith 1997; Conover, Crewe, and Searing 1996; Zaller 1992). This inquiry builds on that literature by considering how indigenous institutions—in this case the black press—replicate, challenge and reconstruct the categories and definitions used to motivate and inhibit behavior. A fundamental part of this analysis, therefore, involves a careful look at those indigenous institutions and cultural symbols that confer meaning on the actions, behaviors, and choices of other group members. As discussed in chapter 2, marginalizing narratives and ideological strategies work to constrain not only the way individuals interpret events, but also the way institutions frame and respond to everything from daily developments to worldwide pandemics.

One mechanism for evaluating the indigenous responses to AIDS in black communities is to examine the representation of AIDS in the black press.[1] As scholars have discovered, often the trusted, culturally sensitive, indigenously constructed sources of information are those most effective in educating and changing behavior with regard to AIDS (Herek and Capitanio 1994; Stevenson and Davis 1994). Further, academic studies—for example, Freire's (1972) discussion of a "pedagogy of the oppressed," McAdam's (1982) recognition of group consciousness in social movement participation, and Scott's (1990) focus on the "hidden transcript" as a basis of resistance—all emphasize the importance of indigenous sources of information in creating alternative or oppositional understanding and action.

Furthermore, in the absence of media attention from dominant institutions, indigenous sources of information become one of the only ways for marginal group members to assess the impact of an issue on themselves and their communities. For example, the gay press, another indigenous information source, was instrumental in helping to focus the concern of gay and lesbian community members on the issue of AIDS when few mainstream sources wanted to deal with the subject (Alwood 1996; Kinsella 1989). Because significant parts of the dominant media largely ignored the impact of AIDS on black communities, as shown in chapter 5, any consistent knowledge about AIDS among African Americans had to be communicated to black people through the efforts of black indigenous institutions and activists.

My concern, of course, is not just with the number of stories published on AIDS in the black press, but also with the actual content of these stories. The black press, as an indigenous media source, is well positioned to reconstruct or redefine the way AIDS has been characterized by the dominant media and is consequently understood by African Americans. Therefore, we might hope to find in the black press oppositional framing of this issue that highlights not only the health threat posed by AIDS, but also the political threat intrinsic to this crisis. At the very least, we might expect the black press to paint a picture that highlights the struggles of all in black communities affected by this epidemic more accurately than that found in the mainstream press. In the absence of such oppositional or alternative framing, we will need to identify those sources of power and constraint dictating the replication of dominant portrayals of this disease.

Finally, and perhaps most importantly, I begin this examination of the response to AIDS by indigenous institutions with the black press because, historically, this institution has been integral in providing information that helped shape the political agenda for black Americans. Whether it be the *North Star* in the 1850s, or the *Crisis* in the 1920s, or *Emerge* in the 1990s, the black press provides a semi-autonomous vehicle by which traditional black leaders and journalists can impart to community members the relative importance of different issues. Most traditional black leaders, such as elected officials, directors of national civil rights organizations, and ministers of large black churches, read and utilize the black press to reach community members. Because of the resources these leaders control, they are afforded significant access to most black media sources. For example, letters or guest columns from traditional black leaders regularly appear in the pages of their local black papers. This practice of providing a vehicle for black elites to speak to the masses of black people not only shapes discussion of issues within black communities, it also signals the relative importance attributed to different topics. Moreover, the localized focus, in particular, of black newspapers means that they have the added ability to influence local debates, speaking to the conditions of communities within a specified geographical area. Thus these publications tell us what is significant, who is important, and how or if we should move politically.

Undoubtedly, not every black person, not even the majority of black community members, reads these newspapers and magazines, but the dissemination and impact of the ideas presented through the black press generally extends far beyond the numbers registered through circulation surveys. As Wolseley (1990) notes, "There is much pass-along circulation in the black press market" (12). Few in the black community have walked into a barber or beauty shop that did not have at least one copy of *Jet, Ebony,* or *Essence* being passed around. Or how many black Americans have never been in a friend's or relative's house where there were no copies of black magazines stacked neatly on the coffee table? The importance of these indigenous information sources should not be underestimated, especially when they report on issues perceived as dismissed or misrepresented by dominant media sources. Stephanie Sears (1997) discusses the importance of the black press in mobilizing black communities around the Million Man March:

> The Million Man March/Day of Absence [MMM/DOA] was reported and promoted primarily through the Black media agents such as radio, BET, and the Black press. Only in the late stages did it receive attention from the general interest media (WPOST 10/15/95). For example, while all Black press used [in this research] have articles prior to August 1, 1995 [on the MMM/DOA], the first article to appear on the MMM/DOA in the NYT [*New York Times*] was found on October 2, 1995. A survey of participants at the march supports this observation. Only 33% of the respondents identified major daily news as the most important source of information about the March. [Sixty-five] 65% of the respondents relied on word of mouth, 44% on radio and 44% on black newspapers.

Historically, the black press has been thought to present a more fair and accurate (usually meaning positive) representation of black Americans. As noted above, African Americans who were skeptical of "white reporting" turned to the black press for crucial information about the political issues, actions, and agenda of the black community. The black press was also thought to provide an accounting of what was happening in black communities that could not be found in dominant media outlets. Thus, the black press has functioned as a source of information formulated from the perspective of black Americans as distinct from white Americans. It has also served as a source of perseverance and resistance used to build self-esteem, a sense of community, and a common historical narrative of struggle—all necessary components of collective political action. Jannette L. Dates (1990) writes that

> in print journalism black responses to white influence and control this time meant that the black press needed to become— and, in fact, became—an established alternative for expressing African American views. Thus the war over who would provide images of the African American, so important in molding both self-esteem and opinion and setting the public agenda, became the catalyst for instituting a black press. (345)

Early black newspapers focused primarily on opposing slavery, within a larger framework of attempting to provide a more factual/ positive representation of the black community. The pursuit of this larger goal was explicitly highlighted in the first editorial of the first black newspaper, *Freedom's Journal* (1827). John Russwurm, cofounder of the paper with Samuel Cornish, wrote,

> We wish to plead our own cause. Too long have others spoken for us. Too long has the public been deceived by misrepresentations in things which concern us dearly, though in the estimation of some mere trifles; for though there are many in society who exercise toward us benevolent feelings; still (with sorrow we confess it) there are others who make it their business to enlarge upon the least trifle, which tends to the discredit of any person of colour; and pronounce anathemas and denounce our whole body for the misconduct of the guilty one. (Dates 1990, 347)

It is important to remember that the goal of the accurate representation of black people by the black press has always been accompanied by the equally important proactive function of crusading for the rights of black Americans. And while other media outlets have commented on and sometimes championed these same struggles, members of the black press have most often pursued these issues beyond superficial examinations. For example, although Abolitionist papers called for the end of slavery, it was in the pages of black publications like Frederick Douglass's *North Star* that calls for full citizenship for black Americans were heard (Dates 1990, 348).

With the abolition of slavery, the focus of black newspapers shifted from one dominated by campaigns to end this "peculiar institution" to one defined by broader campaigns intent on securing equal rights for black Americans. Despite changes in the specific political struggles of African Americans, resentment toward white representations of black communities remained constant, fueling the further development of the black press. Roland E. Wolseley (1990) citing the work of Roi Ottley, historian for the black newspaper the *Chicago Daily Defender*, reinforces the ideas of Russwurm and Cornish written almost two hundred years ago. He notes, in particular, the history of suspicion and mistrust that black Americans felt toward the mainstream press as one of the major reasons, *past* and *present*, for the survival of the black press:

> Also for many years the black people have mistrusted the white press. As Roi Ottley explained, the white press services earned the suspicion of black citizens in the first half of this century because they could not be trusted to tell the truth about blacks. These white agencies were accused of favoring whites against blacks, i.e., tailoring the news to fit the publication's prejudice or at least those of their owners. Both northern and southern papers followed the practice of race identification of blacks only and ignoring entirely anything but unfavorable black news. (10)

Over the years competition from other communication mediums, namely, television and radio, as well as constraints imposed by business and professional standards, have led the black press to make changes in content and appearance. This is especially true with the advent of black popular magazines like *Ebony, Essence, Jet*, and *Black Enterprise*. Black magazines, while dating back to the 1850s gained special currency in the 1940s with the arrival of publications such as *Negro Digest* and *Ebony*. These more popular black information sources have come to emphasize entertainment, family issues or professional interests over strict news coverage, locking down a consumer market geared toward the black middle class. They have attempted to blend the presentation of black culture for mass consumption with the goals of fairly representing African Americans and providing news about black communities often left out of dominant newspapers and magazines. This combination is most often manifested in the repeated presentation of legitimate, mainstream, middle-class black subjects:

> The black press includes popular consumer magazines, aimed primarily at the black middle class and designed to serve African American communications needs and interests that lie beyond what is offered in mainstream publications. Over the years, most black press magazines have addressed and presented African Americans as cultured, urbane, sensible, contributing middle-class citizens. By implication, these publications thus refute the notion, often implicit in general market press coverage of activities involving blacks, that somehow the group almost always represents a social problem. (Dates 1990, 372)

Dates once again highlights a dominant characteristic of the black press: the general tendency to emphasize what are thought to be the positive, or more specifically, respectable and legitimate attributes of the community and its leaders. Again, many black newspapers and magazines see their job as presenting images and stories that *prove* to both whites and blacks that African Americans *share* the goals, dreams, and behaviors of white Americans and thus deserve equality and respect. So while important news stories that might be judged uncomplimentary to the community will undoubtedly find their way into the pages of black newspapers and magazines, there is generally a concerted effort to highlight the more affirmative and mainstream characteristics of the community. This tendency is especially evident in reporting on black leaders, where the pattern is to praise and defend black elites and celebrities. Linda Villarosa, a senior editor at *Essence* magazine, discusses the tensions this practice may bring to reporting:[2]

> Even beyond black elites, we see it more in our celebrities. We could never do a *Vanity Fair*–like story of a black celebrity because we don't say anything bad about black people. We've gotten better about asking harder questions. . . . Even sometimes when I'm reading something in the black press and I read something negative, maybe it's a knee jerk reaction, but I think, what is this doing in here? I think it's a function of the past, where there was nothing positive about us, so then the

black press came along to say in part, oh, here are some positive stories. So now that history has changed, it will be interesting to see if the black press changes.[3]

The degree to which the black press has improved at asking the
tough questions separates what some call the old black press from the
new. Specifically, the degree to which the black press is willing to turn
its lens internally, to examine differences and failings within black
communities, seems to define a new generation of reporting among
black journalists. Tom Morgan, formerly a reporter at the *New York
Times* and president of the National Association of Black Journalists
(NABJ), elaborates on this idea of a new generation of black journalists,
offering *Ebony* and *Emerge* as two distinct examples:

> I think there is a new generation of the black press. Not the
> *Ebony* magazines of the world, but *Emerge* for example, run by
> George Curry. They are the new black press. And they have
> a different kind of ideal. The new black press tries to reach
> a black audience on a different intellectual level that is not
> simply holding up the standard for the race.... I think the
> newer generation has more training in the journalistic tradi-
> tion. We have people examining their lives and society in ways
> that were never written before. That has led the push for the
> black media to be more critical of what's happening within our
> own environment.[4]

Morgan's comments seem to suggest that the new "intellectual level"
being pursued by the new black press is one centered on critical analysis. A new generation of journalists no longer sees advocacy as the
primary or sometimes exclusive purpose for their writing. Now, the
need to advocate in a society still dominated by racism is comple-
mented by a need to hold accountable, both outside and inside black
communities, those who help to determine the opportunities and barriers African Americans encounter daily. This more complicated mission of the new black press, attentive to the power located in both
dominant and indigenous institutions and leaders, holds promise for
reporting on AIDS. But in spite of the possibility of a less advocacy-
centered journalism among the new black press, structural constraints
still exist which can inhibit a rigorous gaze into black communities by
reporters at black newspapers. Morgan suggests, for example, that the
financial imperative to make a profit may impair the judgment of editors at black newspapers and magazines, especially as it concerns what

is written about African-American leaders and celebrities, since many of these well-known individuals are friends of these same editors and owners:

> If you are trained as a businessman, you are concerned about financial interests, whether or not the magazine is going to make money. If you are trained as a journalist, you understand that the magazine has to make money in order for you to keep publishing, but your goal is not to make money; it is to tell and to write good stories. Two totally different orientations. That is why in most magazines and newspapers you have the business staff and the editorial staff. They are very deliberately separate. . . .
> Most of the black press is run by business managers who worry first about survival, as is understandable. But that fear for survival dictates editorial policy. They will be less likely to criticize a friend who's in a social circle if it might affect the business—even if that friend is doing something harmful to the whole black community.[5]

Financial constraints are but one set of explanations for the social and editorial conservatism found in some parts of the black press. For example, the central role played by the black church in reifying more conservative middle-class social norms can also be understood as a limiting factor in the reporting found in black newspapers and magazines. Wolseley (1990), while shying away from detailing the reasons for such social conservatism, acknowledges its impact on the reporting found in major black newspapers. Moreover, he suggests that major black publications leave the more progressive reporting for smaller or political weeklies:

> For the most part, on national issues aside from race, the bigger publications are socially and politically conservative or moderate, but not reactionary. Liberal viewpoints are to be found in the small community weeklies, the publications of militants, and some of the purely opinion publications more often than in the big-circulation newspapers and periodicals. (20)

Despite the socially conservative tendencies of major black newspapers and magazines, Wolseley argues that they can be moved politically. He offers as an example the impact of the social movements and progressive political campaigns of the 1960s on the reporting found in

Ebony magazine: "With the rise in black militancy and the impressions upon the black society made by groups such as the Black Nationalists and the Black Panther party, *Ebony* became more outspoken in behalf of more rapid improvements in the living conditions, educational opportunities, and vocational acceptance of blacks" (143–44). Thus, while the black press may start out presenting a conservative understanding of an issue, pressure from groups within black communities can effect some change in reporting.

Recognition of the economic constraints under which many black publications operate leads to the identification of a third distinct component of news coverage in black media, namely, the absence of news coverage. Due in part to small staffs and limited resources dictated by the financial constraints that many black newspapers face, the pages of these publications are often filled with as much commentary and editorial opinions as with news stories. Lewis Martin (1984), in his article on the role of the black press in shaping attitudes on Africa and African foreign policy, remarks, "Historically, the black press—over 200 newspapers with an estimated 12 million readers—has been much longer on commentary than on ongoing news coverage" (51). Wolseley (1990) also comments on the decreasing space in black newspapers devoted to news stories: "The contention is that it takes too much staff, and hence too much money, to cover the black community" (383).

Despite conditions of social conservatism, extensive commentary, financial constraints, and a reported decrease in circulation, these papers remain an indigenous source of information that gives black writers the opportunity to present an oppositional understanding of issues threatening black communities. The black press can serve as a vehicle for elites and organizations seeking to challenge dominant images and representations of issues. Thus, it is a "trusted," although limited, source of information that has the potential to influence opinions as well as political agendas. In the case of AIDS, we know that dominant media sources paid little attention to the resulting devastation in black communities. We can now explore to what degree the black press unleashed its resources, raising the consciousness of its readers by detailing the importance of this issue for black communities. With this understanding of the black press as a locally oriented, socially conservative, generationally divided, and often struggling advocate, we begin to examine its role in the response to AIDS in black communities.

The New York *Amsterdam News*

To explore the type of coverage AIDS received in major black newspapers, I used the *Black Newspaper Index* as my central means of tracking numbers and trends over time.[6] I focused specifically on the coverage printed by the *Amsterdam News*, a well-established, Harlem-based weekly newspaper in part because it is the black paper with the largest circulation in New York, in part because of its national reputation, but also because it is the only New York–based black newspaper that is indexed.[7] The New York *Amsterdam News*, like many now-defunct black newspapers, was founded in the early part of the twentieth century (1909) by James H. Anderson. Over the years the paper changed owners as well as its reputation. During World War II, when the paper was run by Dr. C. B. Powell, it was known nationally for its advocacy concerning the treatment and rights of black soldiers. Since the 1970s, however, scholars have pointed to a decline in the quality of reporting as the paper increasingly sensationalized its coverage. Wolseley (1990) comments that recently "more space than earlier was given to gossip and political promotion" (102). He goes on to note that the changes at the paper have also affected its layout. "Until 1979 the *Amsterdam* had been a standard- or broadsheet-size weekly. That year it became a tabloid; new editors promised to print more interpretive copy similar in type to that found in the nation's newsmagazines, a policy now followed in cities of heavy competition by other black papers or the regular white press" (103). Despite such changes the *Amsterdam News* still remains one "of the mostly widely known and oldest of the major black newspapers," and undoubtedly *the* black newspaper of New York. Currently, the *Amsterdam News* has a readership of about sixty thousand (Ethnic Newswatch).[8] As noted earlier, we can assume that these circulation numbers underestimate the true distribution of the ideas and positions presented in the paper.

The first stories on AIDS by any black newspaper, as documented through the *Black Newspaper Index*, did not appear until the end of 1983. The *Amsterdam News* ran only two stories on AIDS in the last quarter of 1983. The first story, which ran on 17 December 1983 highlighted the award of a $5,000 grant to a Haitian group to fight AIDS (12). The other story, printed in the 24 December issue, detailed the work of a Newark, New Jersey, Alderman to block the relocation of prisoners with AIDS into a neighborhood hospital. Alderman Ronald Rice argued that there was no way to secure the hospital and, just as important, that such a plan might derail efforts to "improve and upgrade the environment" (9). The announcement by Newark City Council President Ralph T. Grant that Alderman Rice's efforts had been successful and the New Jersey Department of Corrections would not transfer inmates with AIDS to the city hospital was the only story published on AIDS in 1984 by the *Amsterdam News* (14 January 1984).

This late start in reporting on AIDS, over two years after the epidemic had been identified by researchers, might be explained by the fact that it was not until 1983 that the Centers for Disease Control (CDC) began reporting the racial breakdown of AIDS cases in any regular fashion. While such an explanation seems plausible, the initial stories on AIDS printed in black newspapers had nothing to do with the racial categorization of AIDS cases. Very few of these early stories attempted to detail who was getting AIDS in black communities, especially those segments most at risk—black gay men, black men who have sex with men, and black injection drug users. Instead, significant attention was paid to the actions of black elites and the accomplishments of black organizations regarding AIDS. Thus, holding true to the tradition of the old black press, positive reporting emphasizing the awarding of grants, the holding of public hearings and community forums, and other generally symbolic events sponsored most often by black public officials were the mainstay of early reporting on AIDS in the *News*. Complementing these topics were other acceptable subjects, such as black and Latino/a children with AIDS, alternative drug therapies for AIDS, and conspiracy theories about the development of AIDS.

FRAMES OF REPORTING, 1985 AND 1986

As early as 1985 and 1986, a clear and identifiable pattern of stories that would come to form the base or boundaries of AIDS reporting in black newspapers and magazines over the next ten years was evident. Specifically, my examination of AIDS stories published in the *Amsterdam News* revealed that by 1986 almost all the major themes or frames (about seven) used to cover the epidemic had been mobilized. Guiding the reporting on each of these topics were at least three fundamental aspects of reporting in black newspapers identified in the introduction. First is the historically learned mistrust of white leaders and dominant institutions. Second is an extreme effort to portray the positive or mainstream characteristics of black communities. Third, and closely related to the second, is a social and conservative moralism with regard to behaviors seen as bringing shame or negating legitimate claims for equality and respect by most African Americans.

The presentation of general information on AIDS as it was shaped for black communities, confronting an entrenched denial of the impact of this disease on African Americans, was one such frame or pattern identified. These stories use black experts, most often black doctors, to communicate information on AIDS. The image of the black doctor serves at least two purposes. First, she signals that the information being provided is probably accurate, which the reader might not expect or accept from a white AIDS expert. Second, black doctors also serve as examples of the success, perseverance, and inherent ability of African Americans. In August of 1985 the *Amsterdam News* published the first of many stories that would fit into this category. In J. Zamgba Browne's article, two Harlem physicians refute the idea that blacks are immune from AIDS, calling additionally for a massive educational program on AIDS in black communities (17 August 1985, 3). In a similar article published in the issue for 2 November, entitled "Black AIDS Rate Higher," Henry Duvall reports on the efforts of doctors from Howard University Hospital, including Dr. Wayne Greaves, formerly of the CDC, to bring attention to the high incidence of AIDS among blacks.

While doctors based in black communities were often used as experts on the incidence of AIDS among African Americans, other individuals professing expertise regarding AIDS were also highlighted in the pages of black newspapers. Controversial claims by numerous "specialists" that the use of alternative treatments could cure or significantly improve the condition of those with AIDS was a second theme that would help define much indigenous AIDS coverage. In the first cover story ever run on AIDS in the *Amsterdam News*, the headline read, "Scientist Says Proper Diet Can Cure AIDS" (14 September 1985). In the article, also written by J. Zamgba Browne, diet specialist Angelo P. John outlined his belief that dietary changes could bolster the immune system and strengthen resistance to AIDS. Stories of this sort were enmeshed in a tradition of reporting that tapped into an ever-present suspicion in black communities toward dominant institutions and in this case "Western medicine." The *Amsterdam News* marshaled and replenished this line of thinking by publishing numerous articles on alternative and holistic treatments, such as herbal remedies and the controversial drug Kemron.

The nearly complete absence of stories on black gay men and their experiences with AIDS epitomizes a third pattern of reporting. This category is distinguished more by what is not there than by what is there. Specifically, the lack of stories about black gay men and injection drug users as well as the hostile tone of many of the stories written on those most at risk and most stigmatized by AIDS defines this frame. Unlike dominant media sources that almost exclusively, early in the epidemic, defined AIDS as a disease of gay men, the *Amsterdam News* gave little attention to this segment of black communities. Articles or letters published during the early part of the epidemic were often contradictory or even hostile when discussing AIDS among gay men and injection drug users. For example, the first article to deal with AIDS among black gay men was published in 1985 in the 12 October issue of the *News*. While the article calls attention to the plight of black gay men with AIDS, in particular their faster rate of death after diagnosis than that among white gay men, it also presents a very hostile depiction of gay men's role in the spread of the epidemic. In fact, at one point in the article the author, Abiola Sinclair, writes, "Gays are seen as selfish people who *irresponsibly* and perhaps *deliberately* spread AIDS to the hospital blood supply because they feel that a cure would be found faster if everybody had AIDS!" (emphasis added, 26).

This marginalizing narrative, in which gay men, this time because of AIDS, are constructed as threats to society, was even more stridently argued in a letter to the editor printed in the 19 October issue. The author, Jerry Weiss, suggests that those who test positive twice through a mandatory testing process should be made to wear "a lavender star on their clothing. . . . Then our youth would no longer be at risk of corruption by those loathsome creatures." Mr. Weiss goes on to say that "walls should be built around such places as Greenwich Village and the entire City of San Francisco. Those who can prove they have never had a homosexual experience or that there has been no incidence of homosexuality for three generations in their families, will be allowed to emigrate from these ghettoes" (12).

While I recognize that the media are thought to have a responsibility to print all rational sides of a debate, I can only wonder who at the *News* thought such homophobic ranting about "a final solution capable of ending this matter once and for all" was rational. I cannot imagine that a similarly racist letter would have found its way into print. Further, while objectivity is said to be a basic principle of good journalism, much of the distinctiveness of the black press has been built on the premise of challenging the purported objectivity of dominant media institutions. In fact, one can identify a pattern of advocacy in the reporting of black newspapers and magazines which suggests that not all viewpoints have a right to publication. I believe the views expressed above fall into this category.

In the absence of mass mobilization in African-American communities around AIDS, (and stories on black gay men), the gestures of black elites, traditional organizations like the black church, and mainstream social service agencies toward the crisis define a fourth framing of this epidemic in black newspapers. Historically, black newspapers have presented in a positive light the work and activities of local and national black leaders and elected officials. *Amsterdam News* coverage of AIDS in 1985 continued that tradition by consistently reporting on the primarily costless and often symbolic activities of black officials and organizations addressing the AIDS epidemic in black communities. For example, on 2 November the *Amsterdam News* reported on the plans of two black City Council members, Enoch Williams and Archie Spigner, to introduce a bill "to have the city hold hearings on whether teachers, students, and all school personnel should be tested for AIDS, whether the city should shut down gay bathhouses, and whether the city should build special medical centers to treat AIDS patients" (9). Council member Williams stated that the information gathered from the hearing would be the basis of a public education campaign. In a similar manner, on 30 November, Simon Anekwe wrote in the *News* on a public hearing held by Congressman Charles Rangel to examine "the problems of drug trafficking and abuse and the relationship of IV drug abuse to AIDS" (12). As we might expect, parts of Congressman Rangel's opening statement were reprinted in the article, as was a listing of other public officials who attended the hearing in Harlem. Finally, in a 2 November story, the establishment of an AIDS memorial by a local church rounded out this genre of reporting (37).

The process of gathering information and hearing directly from people with AIDS, through such vehicles as public hearings and community forums, is not only important but necessary to any plan aimed at dealing with this crisis. My concern is that the act of sponsoring a hearing becomes conflated with "real" political activity on the issue of AIDS in black communities. Rarely are officials who sponsor such hearings involved in more proactive political action. The pages of the *News* contained very little detailing legislation that elected officials were sponsoring or calls for mass political mobilization in response to AIDS. Instead, the action or demand of choice, when there was one, centered almost exclusively on the safe call for more AIDS education. This approach was universal in its appeal and effective in conflating or even ignoring differences in the risk, need, suffering, and social position of individuals in black communities. Demands for AIDS education, an important need in black communities, was an "act" that did not cost officials much, but paid well in the pages of the *Amsterdam News*.

The airing of public stories leads us to the fifth pattern of reporting, namely, a focus on the innocent victims of the epidemic—women and children. This theme took hold in 1986 and only grew stronger. Attention to the impact of AIDS on children and the provision of information on AIDS for teen-agers was an especially strong theme in reporting on AIDS at the *Amsterdam News*. For example, a 22 February 1986 article highlighted attempts by Hale House, a Harlem social institution providing services and living arrangements for drug-addicted babies, to acquire funds to provide care for babies with AIDS. Another story on 30 August detailed arguments over whether children with AIDS should be anonymously let into public schools (31).

Similar to the construction of children as innocent victims was the representation of black women as the victims of AIDS for whom we should feel most sorry. Often the stories of black women with AIDS came in the form of personal testimonies at public forums or in the pages of the *News*. While such coverage often gave women who previously went unnoticed in discussions of AIDS voice and presence, the presentation of and response to such stories became almost scripted. These women were being asked to tell their stories not as an empowering act in their struggles against AIDS, but instead so they might become worthy victims for the attention and concern of both black officials and readers. Their stories were often used as a respectable way to bring along "the black community" in the fight against AIDS. Thus, stories in the *Amsterdam News* which detailed the personal experiences of women with AIDS do not contradict the work of other scholars, who have noted the processes silencing black women in the epidemic (Hammonds 1992). In this case, the narrow and routinized presentation of personal narratives is, in fact, consistent with an understanding of the multiple processes of marginalization and silence encountered by black women. So, while black officials were willing to listen to and deploy the personal stories of individual women affected by AIDS, there was a silencing of, and silence among, those who wanted to step out of the model of innocent victim to challenge their secondary position in black communities as well as the inactivity of black elected officials in response to AIDS. Black women were allowed to speak as long as what they said did not threaten the respectability of community members, in particular black male elites. Highlighting stories on black women and children instead of, for example, black gay men is facilitated by myths that construct black women and black children as community members who need and "deserve" protection and are not fully capable of independent group membership. This is an interesting contrast to many dominant narratives of black communities structured around the strong, black matriarch protecting or destroying, depending on your perspective, her family, and black men in particular. This is a form of reporting and response to which I will return later.

A sixth pattern of reporting evident in 1985 and 1986 centers on the possible involvement of government agencies in the development of AIDS. Again, this type of coverage gained legitimacy not because of the individuals making such claims, but because of the previous actions of the government. Whether the controversy be over the Tuskegee Syphilis Experiment, or the perceived influx of drugs brought into black neighborhoods by government operatives, or the targeting of black officials and militant black organizations for destruction and defamation by government programs like Cointelpro, there exists a deserved mistrust of the government among African Americans. Having acknowledged just some of the devious actions of the government, we must also be wary of the manner in which such suspicions are manipulated by both blacks and whites. Often these issues are raised in ways that make activist intervention difficult to imagine, beyond the scope of black people's power. Rarely do these stories of conspiracy call for the mobilization of black communities around the issue. Instead, readers are encouraged to be personally outraged and satisfied with uncovering another deadly plot on the part of government conspirators.

Two stories and one letter to the editor promoting and exploring conspiracy theories of CIA involvement in the creation and spread of AIDS constituted this coverage in 1985. In "Did the CIA Create AIDS," Abiola Sinclair initially discounts the idea that the CIA created AIDS, but later offers research by Dr. E. Danquah Tyler suggesting that AIDS emerged among Haitians through the "cruel and illegal experiments [on Haitian boat people] during their imprisonment at detention centers in [1983–84]" (9 November, 30). The author quotes Dr. Danquah as saying, "Haitians who have contracted (AIDS) are by and large victims or subjects of medical experimentation" (30).

The second article on the CIA's possible link to AIDS was published in the 30 November issue. In this story Dr. Nathaniel S. Lehrman accused the CIA of engaging in bacteriological and chemical experiments against "homosexuals, drug addicts, and African Americans" (12). He also suggested that the CDC participated in bacteriological experiments. This article was followed by the final discussion in 1985 of the CIA's link to AIDS, in the form of another letter from Dr. Lehrman. This letter, appearing under the heading "Some Minor Inaccuracies," reiterated his suspicion of CIA involvement in the spread of AIDS, while denying the claim made in the original story that he included the CDC as a participant in biological warfare.

A seventh and final pattern of reporting is actually a nonfinding in the *Amsterdam News* coverage of AIDS: the absence of comment on stories which filled the pages of dominant media sources. For example, in 1985 when mainstream print and broadcast media sources were filled with discussions of Rock Hudson's AIDS diagnosis, his revealed homosexuality, and his eventual death, not one story in the *Amsterdam News* (at least among those stories indexed) had Rock Hudson and AIDS as its major focus. Further, very few stories appeared on white gay political groups like ACT UP that challenged dominant constructions of people with AIDS, while also offering an example of the type of activism that might be mounted against this disease. This nearly exclusive attention to events in black communities effectively points out the unique construction of AIDS by indigenous media sources. Such absences undoubtedly skew the reporting on AIDS found in black newspapers, but they also signify the possible impact of black media in providing an alternative or even oppositional understanding of the AIDS crisis in black communities.

Between 1985 and 1986 the *Amsterdam News* printed twenty-one stories and two letters to the editor on AIDS. These reports laid the groundwork for future stories on AIDS. Repeatedly, articles that high lighted the work of black officials and local leaders filled the pages of the *Amsterdam News*. Stories on children and women with AIDS, reports on government involvement in the development and spread of AIDS, as well as articles highlighting alternative therapies also appeared. There were even a few stories that discussed efforts to engage in collective political action around AIDS, but they centered almost exclusively on the political actions of Haitian communities protesting the CDC's on-again, off-again designation of Haitians as a high-risk group.[9] Of course as new events came to light, such as Magic Johnson's announcement that he had tested positive for HIV, coverage evolved to include these new topics. Nevertheless, in the twenty-one stories printed between 1985 and 1986 we find the roots of AIDS coverage as it would develop in black communities and in black newspapers.

NEEDLE EXCHANGE

Over the years, coverage of AIDS in the *Amsterdam News* would expand, driven at times by the development of recurring stories or the work of activists challenging the lack of stories in the paper. But most often it was controversy that drove the expansion of coverage of AIDS in the *News*. The role that controversy played in generating news stories is seen most explicitly in the coverage of AIDS provided by the *News* in 1988. In that year, the number of stories printed on AIDS jumped from sixteen in 1987 to fifty in 1988, over a 200 percent increase (see table 6.1). In part this boost was spurred by the increase in the number of blacks diagnosed with AIDS, generating more political, legal, and medical activity around the epidemic. However, fourteen, or nearly one-third (28 percent), of the fifty articles were written in re-

Table 6.1   AIDS stories in the *Amsterdam News* (year/quarterly)

Year	Yearly totals	Quarterly Totals			
		1st	2nd	3rd	4th
1981	0	0	0	0	0
1982	0	0	0	0	0
1983	2	0	0	0	2
1984	1	1	0	0	0
1985	11	0	0	2	9
1986	10	3	0	4	3
1987	16	0	7	4	5
1988	50	5	3	23	19
1989	17	5	2	4	6
1990	28	6	4	13	5
1991	20	4	2	1	13
1992	56	8	22	14	12
1993	9	2	3	2	2
Total	220	34	43	67	76

Source: *Black Newspapers Index*, 1981–1993.

sponse to plans by city and state health officials to initiate a needle-exchange program.

The controversy over needle exchange emerged in 1986 when New York state officials proposed an intervention program for injection drug users. According to the plan, a small number of injection drug users would be allowed to turn in their used hypodermic needles, or dirty works, for clean ones. The program was designed as an experiment to see if the provision of clean needles might decrease the rates of HIV transmission among this population. On 15 November 1986 the *Amsterdam News* printed its first article in response to this proposal. The article, entitled "Addicts Needles Supply Idea Bad," actually focused not on the specifics of the pilot study, but on the objections to this experiment by the directors of two drug rehabilitation programs in Harlem. In the story the directors "blasted state health officials for studying the possibility of giving some drug addicts free needles to halt the spread of AIDS" (3). The directors claimed that health officials were offering a Band-Aid approach to a systemic problem. Sydney Moshette, director of Reality House, argued further that "providing needles would encourage individuals to think that drug abuse is condoned in some form or fashion."

Condemnation of needle-exchange proposals by black indigenous leaders would be a constant theme in the pages of the *Amsterdam News*, with comments ranging from a mere rejection of the plan as unfeasible or poorly planned to the labeling of such programs as genocidal. The most intense period of this controversy came in 1988 when the state, ready to implement the project, encountered public objections and outcries from almost every black public official and traditional leader in New York City. As we might expect, articles in the *Amsterdam News* presented the objections and legal efforts of black public officials to stop the implementation of the program. The position of the *News* on this issue was made clear on 5 November, when Wilbert A. Tatum, chairman of the board and editor-in-chief of the *Amsterdam News*, wrote and published a front-page editorial with the headline "Koch Must Resign: Koch's Needle Exchange Program":

> The utter arrogance of Edward I. Koch and his Commissioner of Health, Stephen Joseph, who have the audacity to impose their flawed wisdom in a situation so fraught with danger that anyone but a fool can see it. These two less than brilliant men have decided to go ahead with what they refer to as a Needle Exchange Program. . . . They say that this will prevent, or help

to prevent the spread of AIDS. Thus in the name of AIDS ther-
apy, and on the backs of the Black and Latino communities,
these two "hopelessly white" men have unilaterally decided
what is best for these communities. . . .

What Koch is saying is: Your clergy doesn't matter. Your politicians don't matter. Your medical community sucks wind.
Your community leaders are cowards, and you Blacks and Latinos are dumb as hell. I will do precisely what I want, 'cause
I am the mayor'. (1, 14)

In trying to understand the response to needle exchange mounted
by black leaders such as Tatum, it is important to remember at least
three characteristics that generally defined the reply. First, drug use
per se was not really the issue; instead much of their rage was in response to what they perceived to be the "inappropriate" actions of
white elites. Attention to the link between drug use and AIDS generally occurred only when pushed by the actions of white government
officials. Prior to the proposed needle-exchange program, for instance,
little was said and even less was written, except by a few experts such
as Charles Rangel, on the danger of AIDS to the black drug-using population. Again, discussion of any subject should not be equated with
action on the issue.

Second, these discussions were often centered around assertions of,
and contests over, the authority of black elites to speak on behalf of
black communities. Repeatedly, black leaders, in legitimating their opposition to needle exchange, reminded white officials that they more
directly experienced the imploding drug crisis in black communities.
They, more than any white official, were positioned to take the lead
in defining, or at least approving of, the appropriate solutions to this
problem. Hence, in Tatum's response we see not the defense of the
black drug-using population, but the defense of local black leaders'
ability to decide authoritatively what is best for black communities.

Third, when discussions of drug use and AIDS were forced onto the
front pages of black newspapers, these discussions contained normative judgments as well as the designation of blame. Thus, while some
black leaders in challenging the needle-exchange program seemed to
embrace the needs of the black drug-using population by demanding
more resources for drug treatment or drug treatment on demand, they
often reverted to an "us versus them" framework in which the survival
of black drug users was portrayed as a threat to the survival of the
"larger" black community. Few leaders, for example, sought to frame
the fight over needle exchange as a fight for the individual rights of

drug users to be empowered to define and mobilize around their needs. Instead, most arguments were structured around how best to protect "the community" from more drug use and more drug users. During many phases of the needle-exchange debate, black leaders would offer unproven arguments suggesting that the provision of clean needles to injection drug users was a threat to other, presumably more important segments of black communities, such as children who might more easily start to use and become addicted to drugs with free needles "floating" through black communities. The "us versus them" model, in this case, was not whites versus blacks, but a dichotomy among African Americans themselves. Much of the discussion surrounding the needle-exchange controversy mirrored in important ways the process of secondary marginalization discussed in chapter 2. Remember that the process of secondary marginalization is built on differences in behavior, attitudes, and socioeconomic status that exist in black communities. However, secondary marginalization has the greatest impact when moral judgments are used to explain and justify differences between segments of black communities. Through the imprinting of moral judgment, certain segments of marginal groups are depicted as less valued by black communities than those thought to be morally superior.

Some may argue that moral judgment is not only appropriate or right, but necessary for maintaining social order in any society or community. Clearly, communities must decide how to constitute the boundaries of acceptable behavior. It is, however, the power invested in some and not in others to make such decisions that requires careful analysis, even within marginal groups. Moreover, it seems necessary to conceptualize decisions, especially moral judgments, as areas necessitating persistent and intense debate. Thus the bonds of community, the institutions of information, and the infrastructure for mobilization must constantly be reevaluated with an eye toward their effectiveness not only in promoting unity, but in allowing for debate and movement.

The amount of attention paid to needle exchange and peripherally to black and Latino drug-using populations did not carry over to other at-risk populations in the black community, in particular black gay men and black men who sleep with men. Once again we find that the experiences of black gay men, as they struggled against AIDS, remained largely cloaked. While fourteen of the fifty AIDS stories printed in the *Amsterdam News* in 1988 dealt with needle exchange, only one of them focused on AIDS among black gay men. The nearly complete invisibility of discussions of sexuality, in particular that of gay sexuality, in comparison to the prominent and more numerous discussions of drugs in black communities, should not be confused as a move toward embracing drug addiction and drug users as a defining issue of black communities. Instead, such discussion was forced in part by the actions of white officials. It has also been suggested that black leaders were more willing to talk about issues of drug use because drug addiction is recognized as a debilitating behavior visible in certain segments of black communities. Black gay and lesbian sexuality, on the other hand, is still perceived as a behavior or lifestyle largely located outside of black communities.

The *Amsterdam News*'s treatment of both black gay men and black injection drug users serves as an empirical example of the process of secondary marginalization in black communities. In particular, the absence of stories on these groups seems to reflect the belief of editors at the *News* that these segments of black communities were unimportant to their readers and thus unworthy of coverage. This point was made clear in 1988 when William Egyir, managing editor of the *News*, was asked why the paper had not run more stories on AIDS. Mr. Egyir was quoted as saying, "We have a family newspaper here. . . . These people [black gay men and drug users?] don't read the paper" (Kinsella 1989, 243).[10]

KEMRON

While the controversy surrounding needle exchange helped to generate the large number of stories found in 1988, similar spurts in articles on AIDS, also generated by controversy, are evident at other times. As with needle exchange, these moments often involved not a need to communicate more information to community members about the threat of AIDS, but what or who dominant institutions such as "the white press" had ignored or misrepresented. For example, table 6.1 shows a general decrease in the number of stories on AIDS between 1988 and 1992 from the high of fifty stories in 1988. In 1990, however, there was a small increase in articles printed; the *Amsterdam News* published nearly 50 percent more stories than it did in 1989. As we might expect, this increase in AIDS stories is directly connected to the development of a new controversy concerning AIDS in black communities. This time the discussion concerned Kemron, a controversial drug treatment for AIDS. Over one-third (eleven) of the twenty-eight stories published in 1990 focused on Kemron, with four of them located on the front page of the *News*.

The drug Kemron, which was developed in Kenya by researchers at the Kenyan Medical Research Institute in Nairobi, was touted in the *News* and by a number of black leaders as being a possible cure for AIDS. The first story on Kemron printed in the *News* landed on the cover of the 28 July issue and followed the headline "High Hope for Reported Cure for AIDS in Kenya." The newsworthiness of this story for the *News* was underscored or perhaps made primary because of the generation of this drug in an African country. This treatment was portrayed by many, in particular Afrocentric, black leaders as yet another example of the *positive* contributions of Africans and those of African descent to the world. Reporter Vinette K. Pryce wrote that "African historian Dr. John Henrik Clarke said, [at a forum discussing the drug] 'I'm not at all surprised, this is old hat, we've [people of African descent] been doing this for a few thousand years.'" The reporter notes that "Clarke, who received a standing ovation from the crowd, is a longtime believer in the wonders of Africa. . . . His message brought hope and inspiration to everyone who felt a part of this amazing discovery" (1).

The controversy around Kemron, as it played itself out in the pages of the *Amsterdam News*, centered less on the effectiveness of the drug, and more on the absence of attention and legitimation from, in particular, dominant white media sources. The second story printed on Kemron in the *News*, also written by Vinette K. Pryce in the same issue, led with the headline "Racist Media Silent on Miracle Cure for AIDS." Pryce begins the article by writing, "World racism is being cited as the reason for an international news blackout on a miracle drug breakthrough in Kenya which reportedly reverses the HIV-negative virus in six months." While I attribute the exaggerated claims about the drug to the reporter and not the medical researchers, what stands out in this article is the perceived institutional racism and dismissiveness of stories concerned with Africa, Africans, or more generally blacks on the part of "national white media." For example, Gary Byrd, a local black radio talk show host on black-owned WLIB, and one of the people most involved in bringing information on Kemron to black communities in New York, states, "If this happened in London, Paris, or Rome, the news would cause near pandemonium. But the fact a cure is coming from the very place blamed for bringing the disease, skeptics say, 'Africa is too primitive to come up with this (10).'" [11]

As noted earlier, one of the primary goals of black newspapers has been to report the positive accomplishments of blacks. The importance of such reports varies from correcting the inaccurate and often racist portrayals found in nonblack publications to highlighting the achievements of blacks as a means of proving our worthiness as workers, neighbors, and citizens. Thus, we should interpret the patterns of reporting on Kemron to be driven largely by institutional norms of the old black press committed to highlighting the positive achievements of black people thought to be ignored by dominant media. While this story was clearly fueled by the pattern in dominant white media sources of ignoring or distorting those stories that originate in or focus on Africa, we must also acknowledge the institutional pull at the *Amsterdam News* toward AIDS stories thought to be unencumbered with the details of "distasteful" and "immoral" behavior. In much the same way that Magic Johnson provided dominant media sources with a new way to cover AIDS that was not "marred" by discussions of sexuality and drug use, Kemron presented editors at the *News* with a way to report on AIDS which highlighted everything that was thought to be positive, creative, and innovative about people of African descent. This story was about a possible miracle cure for AIDS, not about the "sinful" behaviors that lead to this condition. There was no need to highlight those characteristics or behaviors that point to the fractured status and lived experience of black people. Instead, the story could focus on our unifying pride in the discoveries and creations of African people, wrapped in an Afrocentric vision of history that, while glorifying people of African descent, makes invisible power and hierarchy within black communities. Unfortunately, instead of fully discussing the limits and benefits of Kemron, the *News* found itself, too often, in the position of defending or even exaggerating the effectiveness of a treatment about which little was known.

EVOLVING COVERAGE AND CLASS

It would be unfair to leave the reader with the impression that black newspapers like the *Amsterdam News* never changed or improved their coverage of AIDS. In fact there are examples of such movement in the reporting on AIDS found in the *News* later in the epidemic. Again, change came not only as a story developed, but also through the demands and urging of AIDS activists. While most white AIDS action groups paid little attention to the reporting in black media sources, black AIDS activists groups like BAM! would periodically write letters to the editor as well as push to have essays penned by their members—articles that would be more inclusive and proactive in their analysis—published in the paper. However, even in the absence of sustained political action or attack, black newspapers like the *Amsterdam News* evolved in their reporting on this crisis. For example, coverage of AIDS in 1991 began in January with another story on Kemron. However, this story did not flaunt the capabilities of this drug. Instead, it highlighted the call by New York State Assemblywoman Geraldine Daniels for clarity on the effectiveness and status of Kemron in the United States. Specifically, Assemblywoman Daniels requested that Surgeon General Novello and CDC Director Roper provide information on the effectiveness, availability, and price of Kemron.

Needle exchange also reappeared briefly in 1991. In an article published in the 16 November issue of the *Amsterdam News,* Lynn Zimmerman and John P. Morgan revisit, but from a different position, the issue of needle exchange, marshaling both international and domestic evidence to demonstrate the effectiveness of this intervention. The authors also note that "a number of public officials in New York have recently reversed longstanding opposition to a needle exchange program." They focus, in particular, on Representative Charles Rangel, writing that "even Rep. Charles Rangel (D–NY), one of the staunchest opponents of needle exchange, has announced his willingness to 'explore' the idea" (14).

It was also Rep. Charles Rangel who in 1991 presented one of the clearest class-based analyses of the AIDS epidemic in black communities. Repeatedly throughout this chapter I have hinted at the importance of class (as well as gender, sexuality, and drug use) in shaping perceptions of the personal and community threat posed by AIDS, the worth and "membership" of those segments of black communities thought to be at greater risk, and the appropriate responses to this disease in black communities. Nowhere in the coverage of AIDS in the *Amsterdam News* is the role of class so prominently showcased than in an essay written by Representative Rangel entitled "An Appeal to African American Professionals: Show Outrage at AIDS." In the essay Rangel called on middle-class blacks to give back to their communities by "speaking out against and educating the minority community against the deadly threat of AIDS (16 November, 3)." Congressman Rangel seemed to assume that this class segment of the black community was not suffering directly from the disease. Moreover, Rangel located male-to-male sexual transmission as a problem of white communities, while transmission caused through drug use is described as the defining character of AIDS in black communities. He writes, "This silent killer in recent years has gone from being largely a gay white man's disease caused by homosexual contact to one that is casting its largest shadow over the country's African American and Hispanic communities." He describes the link between AIDS and drug use: "It is a one-two knockout punch for African Americans, killing more young African Americans than did the Vietnam War. . . . Did I hear young African American professionals say that they were looking for a way to give something back to their communities? This is it. We need help right here. . . . This is a *moral* plea for you to take a close look at what AIDS is doing to our community and help us come up with a strategy" (emphasis added, 3).

Rangel's "moral plea" for help is very reminiscent of numerous historical moments, in particular during the years of the northern migration of southern blacks, when middle-class blacks were asked to help those less fortunate, less educated, and less "cultured" segments of black communities. Repeatedly in church newsletters, black newspapers, and in the speeches of black leaders, middle-class blacks were called on to guide, educate, and socialize newly arrived "southern Negroes" to the proper ways of Northern industrial life (Grossman 1989). As suggested in chapter 2, it has often been perceived the "duty" of middle-class blacks to act as a buffer, regulator, or socializer of working-class and poor blacks. This duty is performed not only because of a shared racial identity that promotes the idea that each member has a commitment to the other, but also because of a shared racial identity in which the misstep or misbehavior of poor and working-class blacks is perceived as threatening the material and social capital acquired by more privileged members of black communities. While the motives underlying Rangel's call for help from African-American professionals are not known, we need to recognize such appeals as part of a larger historical pattern in marginal communities. Finally, while it is important to hold all segments of black communities responsible for fighting this disease, it is alarming when individuals are presumed to have expertise as well as distance from the direct impact of AIDS based on their class and occupational status. Does Congressman Rangel really believe that there are no middle-class black gay men or injection drug users?

Earvin "Magic" Johnson

Despite the return of old stories to the pages of the *Amsterdam News* and the more obvious than usual class analysis provided AIDS in 1991, what was probably the most surprising development in reporting that year was the lack of stories on "Magic" Johnson's announcement that he had tested positive for HIV. Most people even vaguely familiar with the history of AIDS remember 1991 as the year Johnson announced his seropositive status. This one event shaped AIDS coverage by dominant media sources at the end of 1991 and for the next couple of years. Surprisingly, this was not the case at the *Amsterdam News*. In contrast to the attention dominant media sources like the *New York Times* devoted to Johnson's announcement, the *News* printed only two stories on this event. The first appeared on the cover of the 16 November issue, with the headline "Magic Sparks New AIDS Awareness Among Blacks." The other story, found in the same issue, contemplated the financial implications of Johnson's announcement. Unlike dominant white media sources that focused much of their early discussion of Johnson on his contribution as a sports superstar, the coverage in the *News* suggested that Magic's announcement would enhance black communities' relationship to this crisis by moving it from the grip of white gay men. In the cover story, reporter Vinette K. Pryce wrote, "Johnson's announcement raised the level of consciousness on AIDS for many Blacks who easily stigmatized the disease as a homosexual problem."

Earlier themes found in stories on AIDS among blacks, such as appropriate treatments, genocidal theories, and discrimination, were all featured in these two stories on Magic Johnson. In one section of the cover story Johnson is urged by a local black physician to avoid using AZT or DDI since they were "considered toxic by many who have suffered through their side-effects." The reporter continues on this theme, mentioning the work of Peter Duesberg, "a scientist [who] blamed the drugs for ultimately causing the disease." She continues, "Duesberg believes the developers of the drug are profiteers who are guilty of genocide. He called the drug 'poison' and charged a conspiracy with the FDA and developers" (34). The same story expressed concern over the discrimination that might be inflicted against black women in the wake of Magic's assertion that he received the virus through sex with a woman. Reporter Vinette K. Pryce writes, "Black women, already scarred by mass media as promiscuous, believe Johnson's statement that he had many casual affairs may further stigmatize them and are concerned that the mass media must remedy the problem by presenting Black female role models who will explain the color-blind, nondiscriminatory disease" (34). This attention to the consequences of Johnson's announcement for black women was a distinctive frame found in the *News* and a few other sources. It does, however, fit within a model of reporting in the paper where women with AIDS were represented as subjects in need of protection.

A final theme embedded in the Johnson story was again the failure or racism of the white press to accurately report the story. Pryce discusses the charges of discriminatory coverage by major news organizations made by Debra Frazier-Howze, director of the Black Leadership Commission on AIDS. The focal point of Frazier-Howze's concern was the omission of black experts from white media reports on Johnson's announcement and especially the absence of comment by black women. Pryce writes,

> In a letter to the board of commissioners of the Black Leadership Commission on AIDS, Debra Frazier-Howze, executive director, asked the group to send telegrams to the networks in reprimand of the "white out" of Black experts in the coverage of the Johnson story. . . .
> "Every television show has solicited comments from Black youth on basketball courts and then panned right over to White AIDS activists for expert comments," she explained.
> She is also outraged that no Black woman had been asked speak to the issue in light of the fact Johnson admitted sleeping with so many women he was unable to determine which could have infected him. (34)

While stories specifically on Magic Johnson were published only twice in 1991, his announcement apparently had some impact on the amount of AIDS coverage generally. The cover story on Magic was the first AIDS story to be printed in the fourth quarter of 1991 and was followed by twelve more stories on AIDS that same quarter. As table 6.1 shows, this was a marked increase from the one story published in the previous quarter. Thus, while the *Amsterdam News* did not cover Magic Johnson's announcement in the same proportion or from the same frames that dominant white media did, it seems that this story refocused attention on the subject of AIDS at the *News*.

The coverage of AIDS at the *News* varied over 1992 and 1993 as it had throughout the epidemic. The number of stories published on AIDS ballooned from twenty in 1991 to fifty-six in 1992 and then dropped to nine in 1993. Again, we might expect part of the escalation witnessed in 1992 to be a direct result of Magic Johnson's announcement. And while coverage of Johnson by the mainstream media may have helped to legitimize this topic, stories specifically on Johnson were not the reason for the increase at the *News*. In fact the *Amsterdam News* published only two stories on Magic Johnson and three stories on Arthur Ashe during 1992. Instead, the increase in stories was generated in part by an increase in the number of small stories documenting fundraising efforts, community forums and conferences, and numerous attempts to mobilize and educate community members regarding the AIDS crisis. The other major factor fueling the increased number of stories was the development of new controversies around AIDS in black communities. These disputes ranged from questions about the effectiveness of AZT for black Americans to discussions of whether HIV was really the cause of AIDS to concerns raised by the alleged statements of black City Council member and new chair of the City Council's Health Committee, Enoch Williams.

ENOCH WILLIAMS

In this particular conflict Councilman Williams was alleged to have made disparaging comments on homosexuals and homosexuality to a *New York Post* reporter. On the front page of the 25 April edition of the *Amsterdam News*, reporter Karen Carrillo writes, "The [*New York Post*] article quotes the Bedford-Stuyvesant council member [Enoch Williams] as saying that the Black community believes that condoning homosexuality promotes the spread of AIDS and that he had voted against a 1986 law to outlaw anti-gay discrimination because he thought its passage would encourage sexual activity among closeted homosexuals." Williams in responding to these allegations claimed the statements were either not made or taken out of context. His second line of defense was to refocus the debate from his statements to the more sinister motives of others, suggesting subtly that the controversy really arose because certain individuals did not like the fact that he was investigating inequities in funding between primarily white gay organizations and those providing services in communities of color. Carrillo continues, "In a prepared statement Williams pointed out that his interview with the *Post* reporter took place after an oversight hearing on AIDS in communities of color. The focus of the hearing was to address whether minority communities receive a fair share of scarce AIDS funding."

Councilman Williams found himself faced with detractors not only from white gay-oriented AIDS groups, but also from some black AIDS political groups and service providers. As noted in chapter 3, black AIDS political groups, black lesbian and gay organizations, as well as some black service providers mobilized in response to this controversy. Certain groups released individual press statements, others worked collectively to pool their resources and strength, while others chose to meet privately with Williams where they could express their concern and hear his side of the story. As we might imagine, the most active groups pursued some or all of these strategies, and many more. However, as numerous groups from multiple communities called for his resignation as chair of the City Council's Heath Committee and demanded that Mayor David Dinkins not appoint him to the HIV Health and Human Services Planning Council, Enoch Williams mobilized a strategy previously used by many black politicians perceived to be in public relations trouble: he used the local black newspapers and other public forums to rally the support of black community members. Few were surprised on 16 May when the *Amsterdam News* published an article by Williams entitled "The Changing Face of AIDS." In the essay, Williams again voices his concern that communities of color are not receiving the funding they need to fight this disease. "Now, 10 years after AIDS hit our shores, we face another dilemma of public opinion. The problem is that the demographics of the disease have changed, but the treatment, prevention, and education services aimed at eradicating the disease are still concentrated where the problem was most severe" (13).

Thus, in attempting to mobilize the support of black communities, Williams accurately points out that funding streams had yet to adjust their giving to the changing demographics of this crisis. However, in describing the harm to come from the neglect of black communities in funding decisions, Williams retreats to yet another familiar stance of highlighting those who are perceived to be the "innocent victims" of this scourge in black communities—women and children:

> The saddest part of the AIDS epidemic (if indeed there is any part of this tragedy that is not sad) is the drastic increase in infected children. Here too, it is the minority communities that are hardest hit. Not only is the number of pediatric AIDS cases growing by leaps and bounds, but nearly 90 percent of the

cases among children are in the Black and Latino communities. . . .

It is clear that the resources available to battle this epidemic must be shifted to where the problem is worst. And here in New York City that means that Black and Latino community agencies must begin to get more of the limited resources that are being distributed. The future of our community is at stake. For instance, AIDS is now the number-one killer of Black and Latino women between the ages of 15 and 44 years, *the prime child-bearing years.* (emphasis added, 21)

Williams' article does not discuss the impact of AIDS on black gay men or black injection drug users, those groups comprising nearly 90 percent of all black men with AIDS in New York City through 1992 (NYC Dept. of Health, *AIDS Surveillance Update,* second quarter, 1992). Instead, Williams chooses to focus attention on the impact of AIDS on black children and black women in their "child-bearing years," two groups deemed more respectable by many of the black middle and working-class voters Williams would need in future elections. However, as we will see repeatedly in the words of black leaders, Williams emphasizes not just the impact of AIDS on women, but specifically women in their child-bearing years. Thus, it is the reproductive capabilities of black women as "producers" for the black nation, not black women in their totality per se, that Williams seems to be most concerned about. As he states, "the future of our community is at stake." Throughout all of this ordeal, Williams repeatedly sounded a familiar and largely accurate refrain among black politicians—that whites receive funds disproportionate to all those in need. This time, however, the target was the white gay community, portrayed as hoarding resources needed in black and Latino communities.

Conclusion

As I suggested earlier, many of the patterns of reporting on AIDS in the *Amsterdam News* were in place by 1985, and while the frames of analysis used by reporters evolved over time, the major players and themes remained intact. Articles highlighting the words and actions of black leaders became a staple of coverage throughout the epidemic. Controversies surrounding possible interventions, alternative treatments, and the possible involvement of government agencies in the development of HIV and AIDS also drove reporting on this disease. Largely missing from the printed stories were the words and experiences of members of black communities most commonly stricken by AIDS: black gay men and black drug users. Of crucial importance is the distinction, for example, between general discussions of drug use and honest inclusion of the particular stories of those who use drugs in black communities.

In conclusion, it seems that the *Amsterdam News* devoted relatively more print to the story of AIDS in black communities than did its white counterparts. It also replicated many of the inaccuracies and oversights of the mainstream media. However, we are left again with the question, Was there "enough" coverage in the *News*. For example, some black AIDS activists have suggested that a story of this magnitude should find its way into the paper every week. They point to gay papers that not only ran stories every week about AIDS, but established weekly sections that did nothing but report on developments and political activities around HIV and AIDS. Some of these papers, it should be noted, were among the most successful in gay communities. Critics of this proposal argue that no black newspaper can run a story every week about AIDS and survive. They point out that black communities are so inundated with numerous issues and ills that threaten the survival of the community that such a unidimensional approach is less feasible. Yet the pressing nature of AIDS—now the number one killer of black women aged 14–44 and black men aged 25–44 in New York City—makes this an issue that deserves disproportionate attention. The debate over how much coverage is appropriate will undoubtedly rage until the end of this crisis.

Beyond the question of the amount of coverage given AIDS in black newspapers, there is also the equally important concern over the quality of the coverage provided. It seems clear that while AIDS made it into the pages of the *Amsterdam News*, such exposure entailed considerable constraints. The experiences of black gay men and black drug users struggling with HIV and living with AIDS were largely made invisible. Instead, reporting tended to take three directions. The first highlighted and glorified the positive efforts and sometimes symbolic acts of, in particular, black social service agencies, churches, and public leaders that offered assistance to those with AIDS. The second followed and generated controversies around AIDS in black communities. The third focused on the actions or inactions of white or dominant institutions. Of course these three patterns of reporting cannot account for all the coverage observed in the *Amsterdam News* and other major black newspapers. Sprinkled through these categories were stories highlighting those with AIDS, especially children and women, as well as the occasional article aimed at communicating the enormity of this crisis in black communities, using CDC and other "official" statistics and reports. However, while the *Amsterdam News* was able to mobilize new and different frames than those tapped by dominant media sources, it did little to present an oppositional understanding of AIDS, one that would challenge the marginalizing normative power defining AIDS both inside and outside black communities and would help mobilize resistance to this crisis.

CHAPTER SEVEN

Unsuspecting Women and the Dreaded Bisexual

Black newspapers like the *Amsterdam News* are not the only indigenous sources of information for black community members. In fact there are a number of black magazines that comprise a significant portion of what has been labeled the black popular press. National monthly and weekly magazines such as *Jet, Ebony,* and *Essence* can tout a much larger readership than most local and national black newspapers, reaching between one and two million readers monthly.[1] These media vehicles are also national in focus, and thus should be less beholden to local black elites. This chapter explores the coverage of AIDS in some of the national magazines as well as alternative media sources originating in black communities. In particular, I am interested in the degree to which reporting patterns identified in black newspapers were replicated among other segments of the black press. Were the stories and lives of black gay men and black drug users again ignored in the reporting on this epidemic? Did the words and actions of black leaders receive disproportionate attention from black magazines? More generally, who and what black subjects were deemed worthy enough to cover?

Black Popular Magazines

Table 7.1 combines data from the *Index of Black Periodicals* and the *Reader's Guide to Periodical Literature* to characterize AIDS coverage in four popular black magazines: *Ebony, Essence, Jet,* and *Black Enterprise.*[2] I choose these four publications because they are among the most well known and well read in black communities and because they represent a range in terms of reporting style, subject matter, and targeted audience. The first articles to be published about AIDS in a popular black magazine came, as with the *Amsterdam News,* in 1983 when both *Essence* and *Black Enterprise* each published one article. A cursory review of table 7.1 indicates that since 1983 there has been a consis-

Table 7.1   Number of AIDS stories in black consumer magazines

Year	Ebony (monthly)	Essence (monthly)	Jet (weekly)	Black Enterprise (monthly)
1981	0	0	0	0
1982	0	0	0	0
1983	0	1	0	1
1984	0	0	4	0
1985	1	2	15	0
1986	0	1	17	0
1987	3	2	25	1
1988	3	2	4	1
1989	2	2	9	0
1990	1	5	4	2
1991	2	2	16	0
1992	5	5	21	2
1993	0	3	6	3
Total	17	25	121	10

Sources: *Index to Black Periodicals*, 1981–1993, and *Reader's Guide to Periodical Literature*, 1981–1993.

tent, yet minuscule, number of articles written about AIDS in the popular black magazines I examine. *Essence, Ebony, Black Enterprise,* and now *Emerge,* all monthly magazines, seem to publish one or two articles a year. However, an examination of the numbers tells us little about the subtleties of the coverage found in each magazine. Only through a brief review of the stories published can we assess the degree to which these magazines replicated or deviated from reporting patterns evidenced in both the *Amsterdam News* and dominant media sources.

JET

No discussion of the black popular press would be complete without paying some attention to the weekly magazine *Jet,* so we begin there. *Jet* has been a staple in the black community network of information since its inception in 1951. Often described as a black *People* magazine, *Jet* is known for its sensationalist stories of black Hollywood as well as for its dedication to providing news of the black community overlooked by the white press.[3] As indexed in the *Reader's Guide to Periodical Literature,* this pocket-sized magazine has demonstrated a better pattern of reporting on the subject of AIDS, as measured in sheer numbers of articles, than other popular black magazines. In considering the numbers in table 7.1, we must note that *Jet* is published weekly, while other magazines under review are published monthly. In many ways the more accurate comparison for *Jet* is with the *Amsterdam News*. Such a comparison reveals that coverage by the *Amsterdam News* has outpaced that of *Jet*, especially in the later years of the epidemic. But even if we take into account the frequency of publication, *Jet* generally printed on average more articles on AIDS than the other popular black magazines.[4]

The first article on AIDS in *Jet* appeared in 1984, in the 19 January issue. That initial story focused on an "AIDS baby" who reportedly had been abandoned by her Haitian mother in Miami, Florida. And while this first story centered on the "most innocent of victims," a baby with AIDS, the content of future articles on AIDS ranged from the presentation of scientific information to discussion of the changing dating patterns of heterosexuals in the era of AIDS. Beyond the range of stories, the reader should also note that while *Jet*, at its peak, published twenty-five articles on AIDS (1987), the articles were often less than a page in length and focused on more sensationalized aspects of the disease. For example, the impact of AIDS on the kissing habits of Americans, in particular celebrities, was one theme that received repeated coverage in the early years of the epidemic. The issue for 9 September 1985 ran an article under the headline "Should Actors Take AIDS Test Before Filming Kiss?" In the 9 December issue of the same year the article "AIDS Fear May Cause Less Kissing Under the Mistletoe" appeared. Yet another article on kissing was published in the 28 September 1987 issue with the headline "AIDS Scare Changes Way Stars Make Love on TV."

None of this is written to discount or trivialize *Jet's* reporting on the AIDS epidemic; I offer these headlines as an example of some of the sensationalist tendencies to be found in the early reporting on AIDS in *Jet* magazine. Despite this more dramatic start, much of the reporting in *Jet* can be said to have matured in its approach. Increasingly, many of the medical developments reported by government agencies such as the CDC found their way into the health section of the magazine. Further, many of the black medical and AIDS experts quoted in the *Amsterdam News*, *Ebony*, and *Essence*, such as Dr. Wayne Greaves or Dr. Benny Primm, also appeared as experts in *Jet*.

Although coverage of medical advancements expanded the type of reporting on AIDS to be found in *Jet*, the behavior of black celebrities remained a defining characteristic of the magazine generally, and reporting on AIDS specifically. Whether it be stories on the "charity" work of Dionne Warwick and the eventual scandal such questionable efforts would cause, the homophobic statements of Donna Summer— that AIDS was God's punishment to homosexuals—and her eventual apology for making such statements, or rumors that celebrities such as comedian Richard Pryor had AIDS, these celebrity-driven articles were the backbone of *Jet* magazine. As we might expect from such a star-centered publication, Magic Johnson's HIV status and Arthur Ashe's AIDS diagnosis came to dominate AIDS coverage at *Jet* after 1991. Of the twenty-one AIDS stories printed in *Jet* in 1992, fifteen, or nearly 75 percent, of these articles centered on either Magic Johnson or Arthur Ashe. In 1993, four of the six AIDS stories published focused on Magic Johnson.

Like the *Amsterdam News*, which focused much of its AIDS coverage on the efforts (symbolic or real) of black elites, much of the coverage at *Jet* was also defined by the actions (real or rumored) of black elites, in this case celebrated black personalities. However, unlike the *Amsterdam News*, *Jet* did not include the more controversial and racialized stories about AIDS. For example, *Jet* ran only one story explicitly dealing with the topic of needle exchange. Further, only after 1990 did the reporters at *Jet* devote any extended coverage to the AIDS epidemic in Africa or among Haitians. Again, the reporting on AIDS at *Jet* largely reflected the reporting more generally in the magazine. While not serving an exclusively middle-class readership, editors at *Jet* seemed intent on confining their coverage to those individuals in black communities who had already arrived at some level of legitimacy, be it through their celebrity status or their economic, social, or political accomplishments.

As we might expect, then, the coverage of AIDS at *Jet*, like that of most black media outlets, did not include stories on black gay men and injection drug users. Questioning the sexual practices of, in particular, noted black male celebrities was a part of *Jet's* coverage, but reporting on the lives of black men who openly identified as gay or bisexual was not. Even more hidden from the readers of *Jet* were the black men and women who were at risk from AIDS through injecting drugs. So while some may characterize *Jet* as a magazine for working-class black people, it seems to operate as an indigenous media outlet with middle-class aspirations, at least as those norms constrain and limit subject matter and reporting patterns to be found in the pages of this magazine.

BLACK ENTERPRISE

AIDS coverage at *Black Enterprise* began one month prior to that at *Jet*, in the December 1983 issue. The first article, written by David J. Dent, detailed the discrimination experienced by Haitians across the country after the CDC designated Haitians an official high-risk group. This article was followed by a few stories every other year or so on subjects similar to those covered in the *Amsterdam News*. Articles highlighting individuals such as Dr. Helene Gayle, then a leading black epidemiologist at the CDC and now the head of the HIV/AIDS Division of the CDC; stories debating the effectiveness of the drug Kemron; reports describing Haitian political activity; and discussions of the courage exhibited by both Magic Johnson and Arthur Ashe were representative of AIDS coverage at *Black Enterprise*.

Given the focus of *Black Enterprise* on black business and economic advancements, possibly the most surprising stories to be published on AIDS in the magazine were two articles in which the activity, or specifically the inactivity, of black elected leaders was raised as an issue of concern. In both articles—"It Doesn't Stop with Magic," published in the February 1992 issue, and "Do Black Reps fight AIDS?" published in the February 1993 issue—the authors pose the question of whether black leaders have done enough in the fight against AIDS. While the answer is never forcefully pursued in either article, just the posing of the question is a departure from the uncritical praise of black leadership evident in the *Amsterdam News*. This points again to the variation, as modest as it may be, to be found in more centrist or conservative media sources in black communities. However, the unwillingness of editors at *Black Enterprise* to conclusively pursue an answer to this question, presenting instead quotations from members of the Congressional Black Caucus who then pointed their fingers, and rightly so, at the inactivity from the federal government, also underscores the discomfort such sources feel in holding black leaders accountable for their action, or lack thereof.

ESSENCE

Coverage of AIDS at *Essence* was very different from that exhibited by *Black Enterprise*. Anyone familiar with *Essence* will not be surprised to learn that personal narratives largely defined the articles printed in *Essence*. Repeatedly the magazine ran stories in which middle-class, heterosexual black women told their tales of family members and friends living with and dying from AIDS. The first story of this genre, "AIDS in the Family," by Marie Blackwell, was published in the August 1985 issue. This article told the story of a young black woman whose gay brother was dying from AIDS. In the mode of a number of stories that were printed in *Essence* in those early years of the epidemic, the focus of the narrative is not on the brother, but the impact of his suffering on his sister. The *indirect* impact of AIDS as a threat to the family members and heterosexual black women was theme of much of the early reporting on AIDS at *Essence*.

Complementing stories highlighting the indirect effects of AIDS were a few articles in which the provision of very basic information on AIDS was the primary goal. The first article published by *Essence* on AIDS, entitled "What (and Why) You Should Know About AIDS," had this as its mission. The article, written by Eric Copage and run in the July 1983 issue, provided some very brief and introductory information on the disease. And while *Essence* continued throughout the epidemic to publish articles aimed at providing direct and factual information, stories appeared with more alarmist messages regarding the threat that AIDS posed to heterosexual women. Such stories, while trying to provide general information on the epidemic, were often centered around the exaggerated threat to middle-class heterosexual women in particular. Linda Villarosa, a senior editor at *Essence*, talked about the frames she used when writing one of the first pieces on AIDS for *Essence*.

> I remember the first story I wrote, and it was one of the first stories ever. We really had to convince [the editors at *Essence*] there was a problem. Being gay, I had read a lot about AIDS. We didn't really go at [the story] from a black standpoint. We just wrote a general piece like a lot of the [mainstream] press was doing. I'm so embarrassed now; the title was something like "Nobody's Safe." It was totally alarmist. It talked about how everybody can get AIDS, but it wasn't specifically targeted to the black community. There was no knowledge that it should be; it was more just at a time when everybody was starting to write those pieces that heterosexuals were going to get AIDS.[5]

As the epidemic progressed and more black women were counted among those with AIDS, the coverage at *Essence* shifted, with articles beginning to detail women's own personal struggles with being HIV positive or having AIDS. In fact the first cover story on AIDS to be published at *Essence* appeared in 1994 and detailed the story of Rae Lewis-Thorton. In the article, Ms. Lewis-Thorton, a black, professional, heterosexual woman, discusses how she became infected through un-protected sex. In addition to detailing her route of infection Ms. Lewis-Thorton takes great pain to describe how she has lead a life that would not typically lead to AIDS, distancing herself from those women most often portrayed as at risk for AIDS. She writes, "I am the quintessential Buppie: I'm young—32. Well educated. Professional. Attractive. Smart. I've been drug- and alcohol-free all my life. I'm a Christian. I've never been promiscuous. Never had a one-night stand. And I am dying of AIDS" (63). Later in the article, she says, "I made a way out of no way. Stayed off the welfare rolls and managed never to get pregnant. I grad-uated magna cum laude from college. I've worked with and dated the best and the brightest. It's scary that eventually I will have to surrender my independence and my vibrancy to this disease."

According to the increase in calls by black women registered by na-tional AIDS hotlines across the country after the article was published, her story of success and unexpected vulnerability resonated with many of the magazine's readers. While Lewis-Thorton's narrative is compelling and important, these stories often included a tacit message about the exceptional nature of their infection. These articles seemed to suggest that women such as Lewis-Thorton should be absolved from any blame for their infection. They have played by the rules and done nothing "wrong," making instead a success of their lives. Thus, either because of their sexual identity or their class status, these women should not have to deal with problems like AIDS. Less success-ful black women, those who were perceived as having brought AIDS upon themselves through bad behavior—namely, injection drug users, sex workers and "promiscuous" black women—rarely found their way into the pages of *Essence*. Instead, they remained the voiceless compar-ative framework from which women like Lewis-Thorton could tell their distinguished story of victimization.

Interestingly, it was most often through these personal narratives that discussions of sexuality, and in particular black gay men, were introduced into the coverage of AIDS. Giving weight to the commonly held belief that many black women have black gay men as their best friends, a number of the personal stories published in *Essence* were written by middle-class black women whose best friends or brothers were dying from AIDS. Unfortunately, this was most often the only vehicle for talking about gay sexuality and AIDS. Very few stories gave black gay men the opportunity to tell their own stories or to speak for themselves concerning AIDS. There were even fewer stories on the impact of AIDS on black lesbians. Instead, the core of AIDS coverage, as with the magazine more generally, was on AIDS as it impacted black, middle-class, heterosexual women. Again, I am describing the general trends or themes found in these articles. There were, of course, articles in which the storyteller or the subject of discussion was a working-class or poor woman, or black lesbian, but these instances were the exception and not the rule.

One of the more interesting articles published by *Essence* during the 1981–1993 time period began by focusing on the numerous genocidal theories about AIDS and concluded with yet another plea to the middle class for help. In a September 1990 article entitled "Is It Genocide?" Karen Grigsby Bates outlined several conspiracy theories, citing black leaders such as Minister Louis Farrakhan, Dr. Barbara Justice, and Dr. Frances C. Welsing as proponents of such theories. What Bates does that is so unique is to offer "the opposing view," including quotations from black researchers such as Dr. Wayne Greaves, chief of infectious diseases at Howard University, and Dr. Alvin F. Poussaint, associate professor of psychiatry at Harvard Medical School, who both contest such theories. Bates concludes this section of her article by stating that "however AIDS managed to invade our community, we bear the primary responsibility for halting its spread." She continues by urging black communities to "put aside our personal prejudices about homosexuality" and to "own up to the drug problems in our communities" (116).

After such a heroic beginning the article takes an unexpected turn as the author imposes her class-analysis of the black community. Specifically, Bates makes a final plea similar to that made by Rep. Charlie Rangel in the *Amsterdam News:* she appeals to the leadership of middle- and upper-class blacks, writing, "Better-off Blacks must begin to take some responsibility for AIDS and drugs—which they perceive to be a grass-roots problem" (116). She follows this up with a quotation from Stephen Thomas, formerly codirector of the Minority Health Research Laboratory at the University of Maryland, who states that "because most of the people who are suffering from AIDS are in the so-called underclass, the middle-class won't get involved in a political agenda until it's too late" (116).

The importance of class in defining and shaping not only *Essence's* coverage of AIDS, but more generally the political response to AIDS in black communities is a theme that has been raised before. But it is the subtle and constant appeal to middle-class black women in most of the articles on AIDS published by *Essence* and the explicit appeal to "better-off blacks" in the Bates article that expose the significant role class played in defining AIDS in black communities. The presumed leadership and responsibility of middle-class black women is a constant theme not only in the pages of *Essence,* but also in the speeches of its editor-in-chief, Susan Taylor. For example, Taylor is quoted as saying in one of her lectures, "The continuation of the pain in black America is dependent on what we do today. Blacks in this nation, *the underclass,* are counting on you . . . to do what you are supposed to do no matter how *professional* you may become" (emphasis added; Wolseley 1990, 263). Nonetheless, it becomes clear as we review the reporting on AIDS in *Essence* that analyzing AIDS through a singular framework such as race, class, sexuality, or gender is unproductive and misleading. Instead, it is the intersection of multiple identities that determines how black Americans will experience this disease. In the case of *Essence* the experiences of black, middle-class, heterosexual women took precedence when it came to the "selling" of AIDS in this popular black magazine.

EBONY

Between 1981 and 1993 *Ebony* published fifteen stories on AIDS, the first story coming in the October 1985 issue. As with *Essence,* a number of these stories were meant to provide basic information on the disease. Thus, the facts and figures of AIDS would again be delineated, most often using black medical experts to certify the information. In addition to the basic information on AIDS, other familiar themes, such as the impact of AIDS on heterosexuals, also appeared as the central focus of articles published in the magazine. The centrality of Magic Johnson to AIDS coverage after his 1991 announcement was also evident in *Ebony.* In fact, three of the five stories printed on AIDS in *Ebony* in 1992 centered on Johnson.

The discussion of sexuality that developed in the pages of *Ebony* through articles published on AIDS is also familiar, but includes a few twists. As in other major black magazines, nearly all of the stories dealing with sexuality or relationships in the age of AIDS focused on the threat AIDS posed to heterosexuals. Only one of the fifteen stories in

Ebony between 1981 and 1993 focused explicitly on a black gay man with AIDS. In comparison, seven of these fifteen stories explicitly described the new patterns in dating that emerged among heterosexuals because of the threat of AIDS. Again, the concern over heterosexual transmission, while valid, is clearly disproportionate to the actual threat posed in black communities.[6] However, a focus on heterosexuals, in particular middle-class, professional heterosexuals, is not surprising for the socially conservative *Ebony*.

While the lives of gay men were not the focus of full-length articles in the magazine, there was some mention of the marginalized position of gay men in black communities. Thus, one twist to the AIDS coverage at *Ebony* was the surprising reference not only to homosexuality, but to the stigmatized nature of homosexuality in black communities, and thus the impulse of many blacks to deny association with a disease seen as a gay disease. In the first article ever published on AIDS in *Ebony*, entitled "AIDS: Is It a Major Threat to Blacks?" Thad Martin begins by briefly describing the aspirations and struggles of a black gay man with AIDS (October 1985). He goes on to write, "Another view suggests that because of what some perceive as an uncompromising intolerance toward homosexuality within the Black community and the stigma placed on AIDS as a 'gay White disease,' many Blacks who have contracted the disease have been reluctant to seek treatment, choosing instead to suffer in silence while keeping their affliction secret" (92). The exploration of the stigmatized nature of homosexuality in black communities generally goes no further than the quotation above; however, the mere mention of the marginalized position of many black gay men is more than many other media sources offered.

AIDS coverage at *Ebony* not only raised the marginal position of black lesbians and gay men, it also stepped past the traditional dichotomy of gay and straight. Unfortunately, it was the demonization of bisexuals that was the second twist in this coverage. Several stories on the threat AIDS posed to heterosexuals invoked the image of the "dreaded bisexual," specifically those black men who "pretend" to be heterosexual while having sex with other men, unbeknownst to the women with whom they are involved. This framing was made explicit in a January 1988 article entitled "The Hidden Fear: Black Women, Bisexuals, and the AIDS Risk." The author, Laura B. Randolph, offers up the stories of black gay men who "confess" to sleeping with women before they were "completely certain" of their sexual identity. The article begins as follows:

Until his early twenties, Gil Gerald, director of the Minority
Affairs National AIDS Task Force and the former executive director of the National Coalition of Black Lesbians and Gays,
says he regularly dated, and slept with, women. Craig Harris,
chairman of the Lesbian and Gay Caucus of the American Public Health Association, says he too, has dated and had sexual
relationships with women. David Redmond (a fictitious
name), . . . not only dated women but married. Twice. None of
the men told the women about their sexual dalliances with
men. None of the women suspected their lover's secret. And,
say all three men, they are not alone. (120, 122)

Randolph continues, explaining that homosexuality, or the repression of open talk about sexuality, is not the problem. Instead, the threat
these men pose to unsuspecting women is the critical aspect of this
story. She writes,

This poses a problem that has nothing at all to do with gay or
homosexual lifestyles. The problem, put bluntly, is that women
who have unknowingly slept with bisexuals—persons who
date both men and women—could have been exposed to AIDS
and could have unknowingly passed the virus or the disease
on to their sexual partners since then.
    And so the central issue is not homosexuals or homosexual-
ity but the mounting anxiety of an increasingly large number
of Black women who believe they have been exposed to the
virus or the disease by an apparently small group: undercover
bisexuals with a double sex life and high risk factor. (122)

Left unexplored in this and similar articles are the complex environment and history which frame discussions of sexuality in black communities. Randolph seems to ignore the norms and other structures
that repress open discussion of sexuality and experimentation with
sexual partners of different genders. Instead, attention and blame are
focused on "undercover bisexuals or men exposed to AIDS in casual
encounters in prisons or in the armed forces," or those black men who
learned their homosexuality outside the black community (122).[7]
    Black women's concerns about their partner's sexual experiences are
sensible and not to be trivialized, yet the larger context producing such
scenarios is relevant to their anxieties, and is associated with a more
general failing of black communities to accurately assess the impact of
this epidemic on multiple segments of the black community. When
such concerns are constructed as the fault of a "small group of undercover bisexuals," this ignores other systemic power relationships in

black communities that frame how we think about AIDS. For example, how do we assess the significance of a patriarchal structure that largely guides the relationships between men and women in black communities? Although different than the patriarchal privilege many white feminists have attributed to white men, patriarchy as it is manifested in black communities still allows black men, be they gay, bisexual, or straight, to operate in family, economic, and indigenous political relationships where women are relegated to secondary positions and denied full equality and accountability. Further, the conservative social structure of many black communities, in which the morality of black churches sets the normative tone for the community, while strengthening certain aspects of communal interactions, also rigidly censors discussions of sexuality that might provide women with more information from their sexual partners, as well as more sexual choice for themselves.

None of these normative power structures that frame and influence discussions and behavior regarding AIDS are fully explored in the pages of *Ebony*. The editors chose a different path, one in which conservative dating practices were touted as a positive by-product of this epidemic. They chose a path in which bisexuals (and sometimes drug users) were scapegoated in a very uncomplicated analysis of HIV transmission. Undoubtedly, this response has much to do with the presumed interests of the readership of *Ebony*, but is that reason enough? Is the role of the black press, or any indigenous media source, merely to cater to the values and opinions of its readership as they are currently constructed? Or do indigenous sources of information, in this case the black press, have an additional responsibility to engage and move forward the knowledge and consciousness of marginal black communities?

Alternative Press

It seems evident from the data presented so far that popular black newspapers and magazines, while reporting on AIDS in black communities, did not lead efforts to challenge the dominant discourse. This does not rule out the possibility that such battles were fought in the pages of alternative indigenous sources of information. In this section I briefly explore alternative community information networks, evaluating their response to the AIDS crisis. In particular, I am interested in the coverage of AIDS found in black publications defined as left, progressive, or oppositional. To explore this, I consider briefly the *City Sun*, black and Third World publications indexed in the *Alternative Press Index*, and Muslim papers rooted in black communities.

A focus on left or alternative black publications allows exploration of the hypothesis that alternative or progressive segments of the black press, adhering to a more comprehensive or systemic analysis of oppression, are less judgmental on issues such as sexuality and drug use. We might expect this part of the black press to provide an oppositional framing and understanding of AIDS in black communities. Further, we would expect such groups to articulate a more inclusive vision of those affected by the disease, and to be more attentive to the cross-cutting social issues that provide the general framework for the development of AIDS in black communities. Finally, we would expect articles appearing in such media to focus on a political analysis of the epidemic, prescribing ways to include and make primary the issue of AIDS in struggles for justice and liberation.

The *City Sun*

In many larger black communities there is often at least one, usually smaller, black paper that is distinctively more progressive or "radical" than others in its framing and analysis of events in black communities. In New York City the *City Sun* was one of the papers that fulfilled that role. The *City Sun*, first published in June of 1984, was a local New York paper with the expressed goal of "speaking the truth to power." Due to financial considerations, the *City Sun* stopped publishing in October 1996. The *City Sun* traditionally staked out a more progressive stance than its larger counterpart, the *Amsterdam News*. Reporters at the *Sun* followed developments in divestment and liberation struggles in South Africa, monitored continuing debates and mobilization around police brutality, repeatedly examined the living conditions of poor black people in New York City, and detailed the action and inaction of black leaders in ways unfamiliar to many in the black press. However, beyond pursuing a range of left-oriented stories, the *Sun* also demonstrated a continued interest in the development or evolution of a story, sometimes covering the same story for weeks or months. Thus it is important to see if a paper with such an explicit commitment to covering the struggles of more marginalized segments of black communities provided readers with a different or oppositional conception of the AIDS epidemic than that outlined by either dominant media sources or major black magazines and newspapers such as the *Amsterdam News*.

While no index exists that can provide a complete overview of the pattern of AIDS reporting pursued by the *City Sun*, a survey of all its weekly issues between 1984 and 1993 suggests that the coverage of AIDS clearly differs from that found in the *Amsterdam News*. *City Sun* reporters paid closer attention to those most at risk in black communities, and even repeatedly criticized black officials. This less than systematic examination of AIDS coverage in the *Sun*, however, does not allow me to confidently assess whether the amount of coverage provided AIDS in the *Sun* was as extensive as that found in the *Amsterdam News*.

The *Sun* ran its first story on AIDS on 14 August 1985, over a year after the founding of the paper. The story, "AIDS Casts a Deadly Shadow over Prisoners," written by David Egner, focused on the issues and concerns of those "not-so-innocent victims": prisoners with AIDS. This article was followed by an editorial a week later: "Blacks Are Dying from AIDS, Too" (21–27 August 1985, 18). The essay, initiated by a city health report which highlighted the devastation of AIDS in black and Latino communities, did what the *Amsterdam News* had seldom done. It called on the black community and, in particular, black elected officials to organize and battle this epidemic, as gay communities were doing.[8]

The first *City Sun* cover story on AIDS ran on 25 September 1985, focusing on the "innocent victims" of the black community, namely, children with AIDS. The article, however, presented the unusual position (at least in 1985) of not only supporting the inclusion of children with AIDS in public schools, but also framing this issue as one to be owned by black and Latino communities. Specifically, the reporter, Christopher Atwell, argued that since most of the children with AIDS were black and Latino/a, excluding them meant imposing a new form of segregation on minority children. The opening paragraph says, "The mounting hysteria over AIDS in the city's public schools is threatening the rights of children—perhaps primarily minority ones—with a damaging and unwarranted form of segregation, the head of a 250,000-member parent group told the *City Sun*." Atwell frames this issue as one directly affecting black communities, and demands that community leaders and members own this issue and the population being threatened. Undoubtedly, this task was made easier because the subjects of this controversy were children.

Throughout the epidemic, *City Sun* reporters demonstrated a commitment, although sometimes sporadic, to informing their readers about AIDS in black communities. Fundamental to this reporting was the use of methods and angles not commonly evident in the pages of major black papers. This coverage differed, in particular, from that of the *Amsterdam News* in the subject matter it explored. For instance, the *Sun* repeatedly confronted, challenged, and condemned black officials for their lack of response to AIDS. In a July 1986 cover story, "Doc Sees Conspiracy of Silence on AIDS and Blacks," Dr. Benny Primm, a nationally known black medical expert on drug use, accused black leaders of participating in a genocidal silence on the subject of AIDS. He was quoted as saying, "We should speak out about the risks facing our people [because] if we don't, we will be guilty of conspiratorial genocide" (4). Primm goes on to highlight an additional subject rarely discussed in the black press: the existence of black lesbians and gay men. Dr. Primm suggests that black leaders have ignored both black gay men and injection drug users in their discussions of AIDS because of the community's conservatism and embarrassment: "At the same time, we're facing a very serious problem in that the Black community is very conservative when it comes to acknowledging that Blacks are also a part of the gay community (the group that has the highest reported cases) and that Blacks make up the highest percentage of intravenous drug abusers. . . . Most of our elected officials and community leaders are too embarrassed to deal with these facts. They're swept under the rug" (4).

This cover story was followed by an editorial on 30 July 1986, "The AIDS Epidemic: Only the Political Power Structure Seems Immune." Here the editorial staff questioned whether black political leaders were sufficiently concerned with AIDS. They also repeated Dr. Primm's charge of conspiratorial genocide, concluding, "We couldn't agree more" (18). This editorial was followed a month later by another editorial attacking local officials for their "tough talk" on drugs, and an absence of funding for programs designed to address the issues of drugs and AIDS in black communities. The editorial again included criticism of black officials who had done little or nothing about the AIDS crisis in black communities:

> But the silent crisis remains. And no amount of tough talk is going to solve it. While all the tough talk goes on, the AIDS

epidemic continues unabated, showing no signs of letting up. And the segments of the population most at risk are Blacks and Latinos.

We have raised this issue again and again—that the AIDS epidemic, which really has manifested itself in a new generation, will take its harshest toll on Blacks and Latinos.

Our Black elected officials, many of whom have taken their turn at demonstrating for the cameras, have done little, if anything, to pressure Cuomo and Koch into delivering on this urgent need. (17–23 September 1986, 22)

As can be gleaned from the preceding quotation, the *City Sun* was also distinct in its willingness to write about the impact of and response to AIDS among different communities of gay men and lesbians.[9] For example, the topic of gay activism found its way into the pages of the *Sun* on numerous occasions. Unlike other black media that refrained from covering the political action of groups like ACT UP, based in the primarily white gay community, the *Sun* ran stories documenting the activity and mobilization of these organizations. As early as 11 December 1985, the *Sun* reported on an action in which "about 600 gays and their supporters" demonstrated outside the *New York Post* while accusing the paper of "bigoted headlines" and running "anti-gay columns and editorials" (8).

Another example of the coverage gay men and lesbians received in the *City Sun* is an October 1988 article highlighting the struggles of Richard Noble. Reporter Leslie T. Sharpe explains that Noble, a twenty-year veteran teacher in the New York Public School system—and also an Italian gay man—had recently withstood a small and ineffective campaign to remove him from his job. While the details of the case are bizarre and disturbing, the worry was that because Noble was gay, he *might* have AIDS. Sharpe uses this case to discuss the more marginalized or stigmatized experience of gay men who are HIV positive: "Gays are regarded less as victims than as potential victimizers of the rest of us. The view of gays as 'victimizers' plugs into the standard prejudice against gays as teachers. That's what makes Richard's case so tough—and so sensitive. At best, he would be a 'guilty' victim, whereas kids like Ryan White are 'innocent.' Should they [gays] be treated differently?" (21).

A similar sympathetic or even supportive approach to dealing with AIDS among gay men is evident in a March 1992 cover story. This report centered on Tony Glover, an openly black gay man who discussed the loss of family, friends, and lovers to HIV-related illnesses. The article, written in the first person by Mr. Glover, details in an open and honest way the struggles of those with HIV or AIDS who are located in both gay and black communities.

The *City Sun* made great efforts to challenge the idea that gay men and lesbians were inherently positioned outside of black communities. Furthermore, the paper continued its nontraditional coverage, challenging the established leadership of the black community and focusing on those most affected by the epidemic but usually left out of discussions by other segments of the black press. Kimberly Smith, formerly a reporter at the *Sun*, explains why the deployment of different topics and noncustomary frames is observed so often in the *Sun*. She states, "The *City Sun* celebrates the fact that not all black people think alike. Therefore, we don't have to support all black politicians, and we don't have to pretend to be objective. We can be subjective but fair. We provide an analysis; we don't just describe."[10]

One pattern of reporting at the *City Sun* similar to that identified at other black papers was its focus on black women and, in particular, black children with AIDS. However, even in stories on the perceived "innocent victims" of the epidemic in black communities, the *Sun* often pursued these subjects from a different or slightly altered perspective. For example, in "Young Women and Death, New York City's Quiet Crisis" (13 September 1989, 30) James Rempel provided a broader frame for understanding the life and death of young women in New York, in particular black and Latino women. AIDS is a part of this discussion, but so too are the crises of homicide, housing, and substance abuse which confront many young women. While there were the familiar references to the child-bearing potential of these young women, the article moved beyond this liability. At one point Rempel offered what some might label a feminist critique of patriarchal power: "Unfortunately, the deaths and the illness and misery that surround them [young women] get only a very peripheral attention in the political agenda of the men who control most of the religious, economic, and political institutions of New York City" (30). The story concludes by mapping an integrated response to the "seemingly genocidal pattern of disease and death concentrated ethnically, geographically" among these young women (30). He suggests a four-point response: the provision of decent housing; the initiation of a neighborhood-based health-promotion campaign; the development of more drug treatment programs; and the declaration of a state health crisis.

Efforts on the part of the *City Sun* editors to provide nontraditional coverage of conventional AIDS topics were similarly evident in an April 1992 cover story detailing the life of Phyllis Sharpe, a former intravenous drug user now living with AIDS. In the story Sharpe discussed how she and her daughter struggled against and survived the many obstacles presented by HIV and AIDS (April 22–28, 1992). Like the story on Tony Glover, this article not only featured a subpopulation of black communities most often silenced in discussions of AIDS, but again the *Sun* took the unconventional approach of allowing this article to be written in the first person, with Sharpe telling her own story.

This very brief analysis of the *City Sun* does not suggest that this alternative weekly offered perfect coverage of AIDS in black communities. The *Sun* covered many of the same stories on which the *Amsterdam News* reported. The topic of needle exchange, which received so much attention in the *Amsterdam News*, garnered similar criticism from the *City Sun's* editorial board. Stories on alternative treatments for AIDS, especially herbalistic ones, also appeared in the paper, along with the topic of inequalities in the distribution of resources for dealing with AIDS. Interestingly, the *Sun* carried noticeably fewer stories on Kemron, the interferon drug used by Kenyan scientists, and fewer stories exploring varying conspiracy theories of the advent of AIDS. There were, however, a number of stories on the impact of AIDS in Africa and disputes over whether Africa was the origin of AIDS, topics that were a part of dominant media coverage of AIDS.

Finally, while it seems clear that the *City Sun* was more willing to highlight all those in black communities affected by this disease—in particular gay men and injection drug users—the *Sun* showed little interest in detailing or calling for the political activism needed to truly challenge the crisis of AIDS in black communities. To be clear, the *Sun*, more than most other black newspapers reporting on AIDS, put forth a progressive political analysis that located AIDS within the many crises that confront black communities. Further, they repeatedly mobilized a political framing of this epidemic, one that moved beyond its medical or social resolution. However, like other black newspapers, the *Sun* chose to discuss the political dimensions of this disease without also forcefully telling its readers that mobilization on the part of community members would be necessary to secure and guard the rights of those affected by AIDS in black communities. Instead, the *Sun* most often presented black officials as though they were the only political players in this struggle. The paper indirectly suggested, through its commentary, that if only black officials did the "right thing," then black communities would get the resources and attention needed to conquer this crisis.

This analysis demonstrates the variation in voices, hidden transcripts, and sources of information to be found in marginal communities. Looking only at the *City Sun* and the *Amsterdam News*, we notice that each used different methods and story lines to focus attention on the impact of AIDS in black communities. Undoubtedly each paper's coverage was affected by the different political ideologies in which the publishers, editors, and reporters of these papers were rooted. Representing what Tom Morgan calls the differences between the old and the new black press, William Tatum at the *Amsterdam News* seems to hold very deeply the principle that indigenous black media are vehicles for presenting a more positive and often more accurate image of black community members and leaders. On the other hand, Andrew Cooper, the former owner of the *City Sun*, seems to prioritize a political commitment to empowering black community members by holding black community and elected leaders accountable. Jannette L. Davis (1990) notes that

> Kaggwa [faculty member of the Department of Journalism at Howard University] believes that black newspapers need to see their role as one of a responsible, critical watchdog for the black community. The *City Sun* of Brooklyn, New York, took such a role very seriously: in the 1980s it consistently discussed public leaders and the black establishment despite pressures from others to distance itself from such issues. Andrew Cooper, publisher of the *City Sun*, believed . . . that the way to have influence and increase readership in the black community was to cover the community—warts and all. (384–85)

It is clear that the criticism of black leaders in the *City Sun* will never be replicated in the *Amsterdam News*. However, those who believe that the reporting found in the pages of the *Sun* symbolizes the type of oppositional voice needed in marginal communities must recognize that the circulation at the *Sun* never approached that of the *Amsterdam News*. Nor did the *Sun* receive the degree of respect and attention from traditional black and white leaders accorded the *Amsterdam News*. These differences, in particular in readership and revenues, ultimately led to the demise of the *City Sun*. Tom Morgan, commenting on the failing of the *Sun* stated, "Andrew Cooper was not a businessman like

Tatum, but the *City Sun* was far above, in terms of quality, what the *Amsterdam News* was. Two different orientations: one survived, one didn't."[11]

BLACK LEFT PUBLICATIONS

The analysis of the *City Sun* shows that alternative frames communicating the impact of AIDS on black communities were presented, at least sporadically, through this more progressive media outlet. This one example, however, does not begin to explain the degree to which other black progressive or alternative publications replicated such reporting. To pursue an analysis of left publications, I rely on those sources indexed in the *Alternative Press Index*, which was begun in the 1960s and "indexes those publications which report and analyze the practices and theories of progressive culture, economic, political and social change. Areas covered include, but are not limited to: African-American studies, alternative culture, anarchism, ecology, ethnic studies, feminism, gay and lesbian studies, indigenous people's studies, labor studies, Marxism, organizing, socialism, and 'Third World' studies."[12] The *Index* currently comprises "approximately 250 alternative, radical and left periodicals, newspapers and magazines," including race-oriented journals such as *The Black Scholar* or *Race and Class*. Unfortunately, even with such a large listing of indexed publications, the number of black left publications available for examination is relatively small. The paucity of left journals and magazines aimed squarely and somewhat exclusively at the black community makes any extensive examination of black progressive and left reporting difficult. Thus, this section employs an expanded notion of the terms *progressive* and *alternative* in order to approximate the range of possible reporting angles to be found in black communities; I supplement the data from the *Alternative Press Index* with data from the *Index to Black Periodicals*.

Reviewing the data from both the *Index to Black Periodicals* and the *Alternative Press Index* helps to outline trends in AIDS coverage, especially as they relate to the quantity of articles in alternative black publications. Unfortunately, the most evident trend is the neglect of AIDS. Table 7.2 details the number of articles on AIDS appearing in black or Third World journals and the percentage of those articles published in black lesbian and gay publications. The data suggest that magazines and journals promoting a black alternative analysis have generally ig-

Table 7.2   Number of AIDS stories in alternative black press

Year	Stories from black alternative press (N)	Stories from black lesbian/gay publications (N)	AIDS stories published by black lesbian/gay publications (%)
1981	0	0	—
1982	0	0	—
1983	0	0	—
1984	0	0	—
1985	0	0	—
1986	4	3	75
1987	11	0	0
1988	10	5	50
1989	6	0	0
1990	25	20	80
1991	30	26	87

Source: Data from *Alternative Press Index*, 1981–1991.

Note: The percentage of publications indexed that had a black or Third World focus ranges between 3 percent and 5 percent during 1981–1991. Only two black lesbian and gay publications indexed during 1981–1991: *Black/Out* and *BLK*. Percentage of publication indexed that focused on black lesbian and gay issues never reached 1 percent between 1981 and 1991.

nored the impact of AIDS on black communities. In years like 1987 and 1988, when the number of articles on AIDS finally reached the double digits, these spurts were often produced when one publication devoted an entire section or issue to the subject of AIDS. So in 1987, when eleven articles on AIDS appeared in black or Third World journals, the *New Internationalist*, a monthly magazine focused on Third World issues, published eight of the eleven articles indexed. Again, the low numbers reflect, in part, the small number of such journals indexed by the *Alternative Press Index*. These figures, however, also signal a real neglect on the part of these publications. Journals like *Race and Class, Sage, The Black Scholar* and *Africa News*—known for their attention to the struggles of people of color around the world—were noticeably absent from most discussions of AIDS in black communities. Whether because of homophobia or the feeling that discussions of AIDS circumvented those issues of more critical importance to the black community (e.g., class), many progressive members of black communities seemed unwilling, especially early in the epidemic, to turn their attention to this devastating issue.

The data in table 7.2 also reveal a general pattern: much of the writ-

Table 7.3   Alternative press stories on AIDS

Year	Total of AIDS articles	AIDS stories by lesbian/gay publications	Stories on AIDS by lesbian/gay publications (%)	Publications indexed that are lesbian/gay in focus (%)
1981	1	1	100	4
1982	22	16	75	5
1983	173	145	84	4
1984	166	150	90	4
1985	275	240	87	5
1986	366	288	79	5
1987	457	290	63	4
1988	615	381	62	3
1989	451	282	62	3
1990	503	304	60	3
1991	444	303	68	3

Source: Data from *Alternative Press Index*, 1981–1991.

ing about AIDS from left-oriented publications was produced primarily by lesbian and gay publications. Table 7.3, for instance, indicates that lesbian and gay publications led the struggle to force publications on the left to confront this crisis. Although more sporadic in their contribution, in part because only two black lesbian and gay magazines—*Black/Out* and *BLK*—were indexed during the first ten years of the epidemic, black lesbian and gay publications consistently contributed over half the stories written on AIDS by black and Third World alternative publications. When black lesbian and gay publications were in print (and indexed), they generally seemed to lead the coverage of AIDS in black communities among alternative black publications.

As we might expect, the coverage of AIDS found in black and gay alternative media sources was generally more expansive than that found in the mainstream press or more popular and commercial sources in black communities. Magazines, journals, and newspapers such as *Black/Out*, *BLK*, *B&G*, *Ache*, and *ColorLife*, those rooted in black lesbian and gay communities, discussed AIDS as it affected the entire black community, while paying special attention to the struggles of black gay men with the disease. For example, the articles in these publications openly discussed black gay men—their experiences of loss, depression, anger, and rejection—in a manner not found in other media outlets. Publications oriented toward the black gay community, a group that had been made invisible in both the dominant media and the indigenous black press, took it as their mission to detail the experiences of this neglected group as it struggled with HIV and AIDS. Thus, black lesbian and gay magazines, comfortable with their identity and marginal status in the community, sought to challenge the constraints imposed by homophobia, sexism, drug phobia, and class as constituted in dominant and indigenous ideologies. Consequently, the plights of black women, prisoners, sex workers, and gay men were all to be found in the pages of these magazines. As many black gay men and lesbians had done at the beginning of the epidemic, these magazines sought to serve and include all in the community affected by the disease, without compromising their focus on those who identified as black and gay.

However, as much as these magazines sought to present themselves and their subject matter differently from other publications in the black press, some general patterns found their way into these articles. First and foremost was the lack of a call to action around the issue of AIDS. Even among black gays and lesbians few gave explicit encouragement to take to the street or even to write to local representatives. These articles seemed to mirror those in the *City Sun* which advocated for the rights of those associated with AIDS, yet left out of their stories a complementary catalyst for activity to claim the rights denied. A second familiar pattern was the targeting of white lesbian and gay or AIDS activists for sometimes well-deserved criticism. Thus, one unsurprising characteristic of the analysis presented in black lesbian, gay, and queer publications was the inclusion of white lesbians and gays among the groups inhibiting the leadership and progress of those with AIDS in black communities. In one version of the analysis, not only are government officials, the heterosexual population, and some black officials seen as denying the rights of black lesbians and gay men with AIDS, but white lesbians and gay activists who proceeded in their planning and actions without the support, input, and consent of lesbians and gays of color are also seen as domineering and oppressive in their actions.

Finally, the third pattern identified in these articles is a failure to harshly criticize and openly attack the indigenous institutions of black communities. Therefore, while an article might question the lack of activity from the black church or black elected officials, there was little outright hostility or accusation of abandonment or neglect against institutions and leaders. Instead, a strategy of constructive engagement was utilized to deal with the "mainstream" of the black community. Resembling the questioning of black elected officials found in *Black Enterprise*, the articles in these publications sought to raise issues and concerns without destroying the possibility of future cooperation. Gil Gerald, an early black AIDS activist and former executive director of the National Coalition of Black Lesbians and Gays, suggests that the aforementioned compromises were often dictated by "the reality of the various conflicting 'battle fronts' and/or sources of 'support' (alliance) we had to balance—[the] broader (white) gay/lesbian community, the emerging AIDS industry, the Black community, local, regional and national political structures, and the reality that Black lesbian and gay organizing into formalized political, cultural, or advocacy groups was just beginning when HIV came on to the scene."[13] Similarly, some black AIDS activists described such a strategic decision as necessary to involve the entire community in the fight against AIDS. Others, however, viewed this aversion to a more public battle as replicating a system in which black lesbians and gay men were rendered silent and invisible in exchange for community membership.

BLACK MUSLIM PAPERS

This final section explores the coverage of AIDS in papers originating in Black Muslim communities. Coverage of AIDS in Black Muslim communities is especially relevant for two reasons. First, because significant numbers of black Americans hold to Muslim traditions, this institution has great sway in some black communities. Second, since the Black Muslim community has a reputation for responding to and drawing in some of the most marginal members of black communities, we might expect this group to be in direct contact with certain subpopulations of black communities thought to be at greater behavioral risk for AIDS. While the Black Muslim community has a history of embracing the most vulnerable in the community, once individuals have accepted the religion, they are expected to adhere to a strict moral and behavioral code. Homosexuality and drug use, for instance, can be excused, with varying levels of acceptance, as misguided negative behavior pursued prior to acceptance of the Muslim religion. Such "evils" cannot be tolerated, however, once one converts. Further, while the ideology of Black Muslims is thought to be oppositional at its core—advancing the tenets of black self-determination and liberation—some segments of this community, such as the Nation of Islam, also embrace conservative or traditional values such as self-help through the promotion of black capitalism and patriarchal dominance in home and community (Lincoln 1997, 1973). Thus the ability of Black Muslims to offer an oppositional view to dominant constructions of those with AIDS might be limited by these conservative tenets of the faith.

Since 1978 a split has existed among Black Muslims in the United States. One segment follows the teachings of the son of Elijah Muhammad, Wallace Muhammad, or Warith Deen Muhammad. The other segment adheres to the teachings of Minister Louis Farrakhan. Before the separation of the followers of Wallace Muhammad and Louis Farrakhan, the paper of note representing the Black Muslim community was *Muhammad Speaks.* The paper began in the 1960s as a column written by Malcolm X for the *Amsterdam News,* entitled "Mr. Muhammad Speaks to the Black Man" (Dates 1990, 365). By the 1970s, *Muhammad Speaks* reached its peak, with a circulation of nearly six hundred thousand. However, the popularity of this publication, as well as others of this time such as the *Black Panther,* waned as more radical black political movements suffered from external, often state-sponsored, attacks and internal divisions. Because of the split, two distinct papers now serve the Black Muslim community. The *Final Call* is the paper of the followers of the Nation of Islam. This paper, while featuring the teachings of Minister Louis Farrakhan, is also known for commenting on current issues facing black communities. The *American Muslim Journal* is the voice of the followers of Wallace Muhammad. This paper tends to be less strident than the *Final Call* in its racial demarcations. Using data from the *Index to Black Newspapers,* I examine the type of coverage devoted to AIDS in each of these publications.[14]

Analysis of the data from the *Index to Black Newspapers* shows relatively sparse coverage of the AIDS epidemic in the *American Muslim Journal.* Coverage of the AIDS crisis did not begin in the paper until 1985, and since that time (through 1991) the number of articles on AIDS in any one year has reached double digits only once—ten in 1989. The content of these articles suggests that they differ little from that found in other black newspapers. A significant number of the articles were written by guest columnists, such as television host and author Tony Brown. Story topics over the years have ranged from conspiracy theories to elite commentary on AIDS and the Muslim faith (often from Imams) to discussions of AIDS in Africa. Not surprisingly, there has been little call to action. Instead, the political analysis has focused on the evil and genocidal plots of the government, without any serious dialogue about how to address such insidious attacks.

Again, there is evidence that religious norms which sanction the behavior associated with the transmission of HIV as immoral have influenced the coverage devoted to AIDS in this paper. For example, a 10 January 1992 article on Magic Johnson ran under the headline, "Earvin Magic Johnson: A Victim of Negative Influence and Environmental Deceit!" In the article, Habibullah Saleem, who says he has met Johnson and knows his mother, suggests that it was not his parenting, but hanging with the wrong people and straying from the word of God that produced an environment in which Johnson would become infected with HIV. He writes,

> Magic Johnson received quality parenting right up until the time of his signing a contract to play professional basketball with the Los Angeles Lakers. So what went wrong? It is called "Negative Influence and Environmental Deceit"! It is the life of the professional athletes and entertainers that can very easily catch you swimming in those waters that are much deeper than you could ever imagine. Just the environment alone can play a major role in destroying the strongest individual, unless he or she remain God-conscious in thought and in action. . . . Even though we are allowed input, the ultimate protection is God and only God. Depend on Almighty Allah, instead of the dollar and the ego. (21)

Much of the coverage of AIDS in the *Final Call*, like that in the *American Muslim Journal*, invoked the twin themes of a conspiracy and the moral boundaries crossed by those with AIDS. In fact, the first article on AIDS in the *Final Call* that I can identify (there is no index for this paper) was written by an anonymous inmate. The author suggests "that there are more ways than those stated by prison authorities to contract this deadly disease" (vol. 4, no. 1 [1984], 24). The author continues, arguing that only in the *Final Call* can the truth about AIDS be told. He writes, "We also feel that the only way for the truth to be conveyed to the public will be for us to write this to the *Final Call* Newspaper! How else can Black people know the truth about this disease, if we don't tell them." A similar claim, that the *Final Call* is one of the few publications telling black people the truth about AIDS, is made by Dr. Abdul Alim Muhammad, a surgeon who directs the Abundant Life Clinic for the Nation of Islam. He is probably most well known in the area of AIDS for his promotion of alpha interferon (Kemron) as an effective low-dose treatment for symptoms associated with AIDS. In the article, "A.I.D.S.: Widespread Death—Clearing the Deck for a New World Order," Dr. Muhammad puts forth a number of theories about AIDS. First, he suggests that AIDS is divine justice. "From the Divine perspective, AIDS—an altogether new disease—must be viewed as a part of the Judgment of the wicked by Almighty God. The only safety against AIDS is the righteousness of God!" Second, Dr. Muhammad proceeds to argue that public health officials have "tried to keep the 'lid' on the AIDS pandemic," and asks, "'Why the cover-up?'" In response he offers two very general explanations. One is the power of the "Gay Rights Lobby." He complains that "many public health and political officials are sensitive to the 'Gay Rights Lobby' [and] are engaging in dirty sexual practices themselves." The other explanation for the cover-up is that "the AIDS virus is a man-made biological weapon of war," and the government is therefore intent on keeping this quiet. He concludes by suggesting that "AIDS victims and carriers should be quarantined and isolated from the general population. Strong laws must be enforced against homosexuality, and homosexuals should be banned from occupations which bring them into intimate contact with the public" (14 February 1986, 28).

Dr. Muhammad's article, while the most extreme in pressing the idea that AIDS is "divine justice" and the fault of homosexuals, was not the only such essay to be found in the *Final Call*. In fact, a number of stories published after the Muhammad essay referred to his arguments. As in much of the black press, however, marginal improvement occurred even in this reporting as the epidemic progressed. The language attacking homosexuality, while never fully eliminated, was toned down, and on rare occasions such homophobic narratives were even challenged in the *Final Call's* own pages. For example, an article by Sovella X Perry, on a conference on AIDS and black communities sponsored by the National Coalition of Black Lesbians and Gays (NCBLG), quotes Gwendolyn Rogers, chairperson of the political action committee for NCBLG: "[The] time has come, when it is irresponsible not to address homophobia in the black community. The hatred and fear of anything that has to do with homosexuality is allowing our brothers and sisters to die" (30 August 1986, 18).

Throughout the epidemic, stories on AIDS periodically appeared on the cover of the *Final Call*, but calls to action were few and far between. Once again we find that an organization with a reputation for biting criticism, analysis of dominant strategies of marginalization, and an ability to mobilize at least its own followers stopped short of calling for mass action around the politics of AIDS. It seems that Minister Farrakhan and the staff at the *Final Call* attempted to provide what they viewed as an alternative understanding of AIDS for those in black communities—at the same time defining AIDS as Allah's retribution for immoral behavior and demanding that the government recognize alpha interferon as a treatment for AIDS. And while this alternative reporting, in some cases, awakened the consciousness of community members, little attention was paid to generating the type of political mobilization that would seem naturally to accompany such analyses of AIDS. Maybe leaders in the Nation of Islam worried that fighting for the empowerment of members of black communities with AIDS would make them appear to be "sensitive" to the gay and drug-using segments of black communities, those who suffered from secondary marginalization. Or worse yet, maybe these leaders worried that such action on the part of contested members of black communities would suggest that these leaders were engaged in "dirty sexual practices" themselves.

Conclusion

Most people in this country receive their political information through the dominant media. Americans turn to the evening news and national newspapers to find out what issues will affect their lives and those with whom they identify. However, for some segments of the population, specifically marginal groups, the information received from such sources is not only seen as suspect, but more often than not incomplete. The theory of marginalization discussed in chapter 2 suggests that the history of deceit, misrepresentation, and neglect that characterizes much of the coverage from dominant news sources on black Americans, leads members of this marginal group to look to indigenous media sources to supplement their information. Thus historical and current processes of marginalization underscore the importance of the black press as an alternative and possibly oppositional voice in the politics of black communities.

In light of the failure of dominant media sources to communicate consistent information on AIDS in black communities, indigenous sources of information with an established history within black communities had an opportunity to awaken the consciousness of black people about this disease. The problem, however, was that these popular media sources—the *Amsterdam News, Jet, Ebony, Essence* and *Black Enterprise*—avoided extensive coverage of AIDS. Further, when they did choose to provide information, the articles were often structured around the threat AIDS posed to heterosexuals, the largely symbolic acts of black leaders, or the genocidal theories of the advent of AIDS. Missing from many of these stories were the full experiences of black gay men and lesbians, injection drug users, and poor women—the majority of people with AIDS in black communities. In choosing to distance and misrepresent the AIDS epidemic as it developed in black communities, the black press let stand, and in some cases reinforced, processes of secondary marginalization and ideologies of otherness that designated certain segments of the community as not worthy of group resources, activism, or coverage.

Much of the black press is rooted in the indigenous culture and values of the community. The press takes its direction from an internal organizational structure dominated by the black church as well as black public officials who reinforce moral and conservative ideologies of acceptable behavior. Reporters for the black press have complained that the religious and moral judgments of clergy and elites in the community, communicated to publishers and editors, have impeded sufficient attention to AIDS in general and to the impact of AIDS on black gay men and injection drug users specifically. Clearly, the black press was helpful in making sure that people had basic information about AIDS. Whether one agreed with the stories or not, multiple frames were presented, especially with regard to how the disease developed and how it should be treated. Further, the disparities in resources allocated to fight this disease—between black communities and other groups—was also a topic to which the black press gave well-deserved exposure. In spite of such contributions, however, the constrained and morally bounded coverage in much of the black press did little to confront dominant constructions of those thought to be at risk.

The failure of the popular black press to fully engage the politics of this disease was probably most clearly exposed when compared with the coverage AIDS received in the *City Sun* and left or alternative publications coming out of black lesbian and gay organizations. These publications, while not providing perfect coverage, were much more expansive when discussing AIDS in black communities. They were also much more likely to hold accountable not only dominant institutions, but also indigenous institutions and organizations rooted in black communities. These alternative publications engaged in a process of transforming the consciousness of black people, moving AIDS from being purely a health issue to one embedded in politics. Again, much of the more progressive and inclusive coverage of AIDS came from articles written and magazines published by black lesbians and gay men. These articles and publications attempted to force black progressives to engage in an alternative discourse about AIDS—one that was more inclusive and more political. But even with internal pushing, social and political constraints such as homophobia, sexism, and classism seem to have muted any full discussion of the possible political responses of black communities to this epidemic. The popular black press, generally, left intact dominant representations of AIDS. Instead of engaging in battles to transform the consciousness of black people, offering an oppositional understanding of AIDS as a political issue fundamental to the survival of black people, the black press focused on elite declarations, conspiracy theories, celebrity fund-raisers, and the provision of basic information. Hence in 1990 *Emerge* magazine felt compelled to remind black communities, "We Are Not Immune."

CHAPTER EIGHT

Willing to Serve, but Not to Lead

The role of black institutions in helping to formulate and transmit opinions and ideas among black Americans has been documented by numerous scholars (Dawson 1994; Henry 1990; Morris 1984; McAdam 1982). Whether the issue is AIDS, abortion, or "ebonics," black organizations, through the words and actions of their leaders, have shaped, refocused, and significantly influenced how African Americans think about and act upon political issues (Allen, Dawson, and Brown 1989; Zaller 1992; Conover, Crewe, and Searing 1996). Shared group experiences of marginalization, especially as such oppression has been manifested in segregated residential, work, and social environments, have heightened the importance and recognition given by African Americans to indigenous black leaders and organizations. In the absence of valuable information and interventions from dominant institutions and elites, marginal groups are forced to develop their own networks of organizations, leaders, and information to address their needs and advance their struggles.

Community members, believing that indigenous leaders and organizations share a similar desire for justice, equality, and truth in the lives of marginal group members, bestow upon these individuals and organizations the special status of "authentic." Such essentialist notions of leadership emerge from the belief (often learned through actual interactions) that only those who have lived with the multiple systems of marginalization common to most black people can be trusted with the fight to liberate black communities. Thus the power that is invested in indigenous leaders and institutions is based not in fear or coercion, but in the ability or authority of these individuals to mobilize group members by speaking from a common experience of exclusion and oppression (Burns 1978). This is not to say that African Americans indiscriminately embrace all national and local black organizations professing to struggle for black people. Nevertheless, recent scandals challenging the financial efficiency of organizations such as the National

Association for the Advancement of Colored People (NAACP) and the questionable comments of leaders such as Minister Louis Farrakhan of the Nation of Islam seem to suggest that institutions and leaders perceived as having contributed positively to black communities and having been the targets of dominant white institutions intent on destroying black leadership, are given the benefit of the doubt during times of controversy.

As discussed in chapter 2, practices of marginalization are neither uniform nor static. And while the categorical and, to a lesser degree, integrative marginalization of African Americans has rested in large part on the institutional political exclusion of black people, advanced practices of marginalization have evolved to operate with the formal political incorporation of African Americans. Scholars of black politics have studied the second formal incorporation of black voters that occurred during the late 1960s and early 1970s (Preston 1982; Nelson 1982; Allen 1969). Moving from what Bayard Rustin labeled "protest to politics," black leaders and organizations have, over the years, gained more access and influence in the policy-making arena, especially in the realm of racial consensus issues. Robert Smith (1981) writes of this expanding influence:

> The most important consequence of the development assayed in this article is the entrance of black interest organizations into the competitive, pluralist interest-group system characteristic of the "middle level" of power in the United States. This is particularly evident at the federal level. As late as 1968, studies of the process of formulating federal policy found an absence of access by blacks. Very few blacks were found among the policy-making elites, and blacks did not on the whole possess access to centers of decision making in the federal policy process. . . . Since the late 1960s, however, blacks have made significant progress toward the development of a political voice of their own in Washington, that is, political organizations and leaders actively involved in the articulation of black interests. (440–41)

Like Smith, other scholars have commented on the expanding, but in no way equal, role of black organizations and leaders in the policy process. Dianne Pinderhughes (1995), in her examination of the political activity leading to the 1982 extension of the Voting Rights Act, finds that black and Latino organizations established themselves as important players in this policy struggle: "Despite significant economic problems of the populations they serve, black and Latino groups have created sufficient moral resources and have organized in ways that minimize the information costs of mobilizing their constituencies and disseminating information. They have defined a very important role in the policy arena and have played an important role in defining the civil rights coalition and shaping its long-term direction" (219). Huey L. Perry (1995) argues that the expanding access and influence of black organizations can be found both inside and outside the domain of civil rights legislation: "Since acquiring full-scale voting rights with the passage of the 1965 Voting Rights Act, black political and organizational leaders have participated in and influenced the development of several other public policies beneficial to blacks. These include the Equal Employment Opportunity Act of 1972 and the Public Works Employment Act of 1977" (29). He goes on to note that "since 1965 black organizations have also influenced the actions of Congress and presidents in the nonpolicy areas of nominations to the federal judiciary and support for the King national holiday legislation" (31). Finally, Adolph Reed (1994) comments on the incorporation of nongovernmental black organizations that took place during the Carter presidency:

> A fourth and related dimension of incorporation is the integration of non-governmental organizations—private civil rights and uplift organizations of various sorts—into a regime of quasi-corporatist race relations management driven by incrementalist, insider negotiation. The tracings of this process could be seen rather dramatically at the national level during the Carter administration with the inclusion of Jesse Jackson's Operation Push and the National Urban League as line item accounts in Department of Labor budgets (though, in keeping with the current spirit of bipartisan largess, I should note that Nixon and Ford were only less formalistic in their practice in this regard). (5)

As noted in chapter 2, leaders of organizations representing marginal communities are on occasion allowed *conditional* entrance and *limited* power in dominant institutions and decision making, with the unspoken understanding that they are merely there to represent the views (and temper the actions) of marginal group members. Through such a process of incorporation, moving from potential or solidary groups to interest groups, it is assumed that a stable set of civil rights and race-based organizations will emerge to represent the presumed largely homogenous interests of African Americans (Truman 1958;

Gamson 1968). Moreover, it is expected that as dominant elites become familiar with these organizations and the individuals who guide them, they will be able to funnel their interactions with African-American communities through this restricted group of black leaders. While in certain cases the mere participation of different voices at the table can significantly change the tone and direction of institutions and decisions, often the problem with such "participation" is that inclusion in, not transformation of, dominant political institutions becomes the measure by which the progress of marginal groups is judged. Thus, the standards for evaluating the success of black incorporation have centered less on the actual transformation of the conditions or outcomes under which black people exist, and more on the symbolic, categorical representation of formerly excluded group members (Wolfinger 1974; Guinier 1994).

When scholars do focus on the actual progress brought about by the incorporation of black officials at national, state, and local levels during the 1970s and 1980s, there is real debate about the sustained effects of such access on the lives of most black people. In fact, serious questions have arisen over the ability of black officials and organizations, using primarily mainstream political strategies, to improve the everyday existence of African Americans and to challenge political and economic systems which reinforce their marginalization. For example, scholars of urban politics have criticized the corporatist development policies and progrowth regime governing coalitions of many black mayors (Stone 1987; Reed 1988; Nelson 1987; Eisinger 1982). Researchers studying black elected and appointed officials at the national level have also noted the dominance of the traditional party structure in defining the legislative agendas of these officials (Reed 1986; Marable 1985; Barnett 1982). Even the insider interest-group politics of black nongovernmental organizations have received scrutiny (Reed 1994; Pinderhughes 1995). Therefore, we are left with the question of whether black organizations and leaders, after incorporation, can provide the leadership necessary to *transform* dominant political institutions as well as the lived conditions of black Americans.

Clarence Stone (1990), in his paper "Transactional and Transforming Leadership: A Re-examination," builds on Burns's (1978) distinction between transactional and transformative leadership, applying these categorical models of leadership to the civil rights movement. Stone notes that Burns sees transactional leadership as entailing "modal values—means or procedures that enable transactions to occur that otherwise might not take place" (6). He quotes Burns as commenting that in legislative bodies, "the classic seat of transactional leadership" according to Burns, "leadership is necessary for the initiating, monitoring, and assured completing of transactions, for settling disputes, and for storing up political credits and debits for latter settlement" (6). Transformative leadership, on the other hand, is presented as leadership which seeks fundamental change by appealing to a greater moral purpose, transforming both group members and political targets: "Transforming leadership combines profound purpose with situational factors to bring about social change. Neither purpose nor situation alone is sufficient; both are part of the engagement between leader and followers that makes transformation possible" (33).

In applying these models to the civil rights movement, Stone (1990) discovers that not every organization concerned with the advancement of black people provided transformative leadership or engaged in what has been called transformative politics. He finds that it actually was less the entrenched heads of organizations than new leaders who were willing to be confrontational and nontraditional in their demands for equality. According to Stone,

> The experience of the civil rights movement suggests another contextual factor, one concerning who is most likely to constitute the membership in a transformative mobilization. Specifically, the civil rights experience suggests that evocation of a morally purposive identity around which mobilization can be built occurs most readily with those who are still in a formative stage, not among those who have already achieved a stable identity.
>
> The point should not be exaggerated and the many exceptions not overlooked, but it was younger ministers and newly formed organizations, not older and established ministers and organizations that were central. It was students and a younger generation more than an older generation that constituted the footsoldiers of protest and movement activism. In some cases, the struggle was as much within the African-American community as between blacks and whites. (32)

Of course, transformational and transactional politics are not the only dimensions of black leadership that need concern us; other characteristics of leadership speak to an organization's or leader's ability to promote the progressive struggles of black Americans. For example, throughout *Transcending the Talented Tenth* (1997) both Lewis Gordon, who wrote the foreword, and Joy James, the author, define two often gendered types of black leadership:

> One type of activity is *consensus-building*. Its concerns are with matters of speech and agreement, and the heart of its values is a commitment to democracy. Another type is *instrumental*. Its concerns are primarily functional and administrative. . . .
>
> Given our two conceptions of political activity, we can see straightaway how, in the struggle against race, gender, and class oppression, this distinction emerges in the difference between the classical sociological model of the charismatic leader-intellectual and the leader-intellectual who is guided by a sense of vocation and public responsibility.
>
> While W. E. B. Du Bois and Paul Robeson have become well-known as charismatic leaders and consensus builders, Ella Baker's and Claudia Jones's many hours have been rendered nearly invisible. . . . Similarly, political activity and leadership in black churches tend to be sought among the male ministers, in spite of the fact that day-to-day administering and developing of those institutions stand in the rarely seen but essential boards and officers and key congregation members, members who are predominantly women. . . .
>
> The distinction between the charismatic leader and the instrumental question of facilitating responses to community needs comes to the fore on the question of a demonstrated track record. . . . The consensus-building model requires a charitable relationship of presumed membership, whereas the instrumental model requires earning the community's trust and thereby earning membership. (xiv–xv)

Recognizing distinctions in leadership types, whether it be consensus-building and instrumental or transactional and transformative, is critical to our evaluation of the response to AIDS on the part of national black political and religious organizations and leaders. Only through comprehending the different types of political leadership available to the individuals heading our often closely aligned indigenous organizations, can we begin to discern the extent to which their political interventions are geared toward transforming dominant institutions and discourse, making them accessible and responsible to the most marginal in our communities. Further, by appreciating the changing context of personal and group interests that makes certain leaders and organizations more apt to engage in radical or inclusive progressive politics, we are better able to evaluate the leadership capacities of different black organizations.

Consequently, understanding leadership as multifaceted helps to focus our attention not only on whether leaders and organizations responded to AIDS, but also on the nature and impact of that response. While one line of research might focus exclusively on the level of political activity emanating from national black leaders and organizations in the early years of the AIDS epidemic, a broader research project might also explore the form of that activity. Did black organizations and leaders find new ways to talk about AIDS among African Americans? Did these organizations and leaders target the most stigmatized in black communities for prevention and treatment? Did they seek to transform the way dominant and indigenous organizations conceptualized and responded to AIDS, especially as it developed in black communities? Or did traditional black leaders and organizations work within established paradigms, replicating an ineffective framing of this crisis between those we blame for their illness and those we designate as "innocent victims?" Were national black political organizations and leaders content to receive funding from dominant institutions and provide important yet basic education and prevention programs in black communities, when a more political and inclusive response was needed?

The story of the response to AIDS on the part of national black political and religious institutions and leaders is a complex one, as we might expect. Some institutions did all they could do to disassociate themselves and their constituencies from this crisis. Others, primarily black lesbian and gay organizations, such as the now defunct National Coalition of Black Lesbians and Gays (NCBLG), saw AIDS as a defining moment in their organization's development and early in the epidemic committed significant resources to responding to this disease.[1] However, most indigenous black institutions, like the varied sectors of the black press, provided a mixed, limited, and often reluctant response to this epidemic. The AIDS programs initiated by these organizations were designed not only to provide needed services to segments of black communities, but also to fit within a constrained moral and political framework, where anything from a lack of expertise on this issue to the word of God were offered as reasons for doing less.

This chapter considers the complementary and contradictory ways in which a few national political organizations and the black church responded politically to AIDS in African-American communities in the early years of the epidemic. I use a simple typology to characterize the responses of these organizations to the emergence of AIDS. The four categories are (1) service, (2) awareness, (3) distributive claims, and (4) recognition and redefinition. Activity classified as service includes those efforts meant to directly and indirectly address the material and emotional needs of individuals with AIDS, as well as others affected by this epidemic. Awareness strategies include those actions aimed at increasing community understanding of this disease. Dissemination of culturally sensitive information about AIDS is a major activity within this category. And while discourse impacting awareness tends to be rooted in the experiences and perspectives of black communities, there is generally little effort to challenge and expand existing paradigms for understanding and talking about AIDS in black communities. Thus these indigenous sources of culturally sensitive information often provide a different language or images to frame paradigms not that different from dominant messages about the epidemic.

The third category of responses is distributive. Activity in this category most often centers around demands for a more equitable distribution of resources to fight AIDS. The racial demographic breakdown of those who are HIV positive and those who are living with AIDS has been used by black leaders to underscore the disproportionate impact of AIDS in black communities and the inequity in current distributive policies. Thus public contests over such issues as the allotment of AIDS funding or the allocation of slots in clinical trials have been issues attracting the attention of some black leaders. The final category is that of recognition and redefinition. Through such strategies, leaders and other political entrepreneurs use the devastation of AIDS to highlight the secondary position of certain segments of black communities at greater behavioral risk. Redefinition of a problem may also reorient discourse about AIDS, constructing it not only as a medical disease and social crisis, but also as involving a political fight for the improved living status of many black Americans and the empowerment of those suffering from secondary marginalization within black communities.

It is not difficult to detail a picture of the failing of national black institutions to respond to AIDS, for generally that is what happened, especially in the early years of the epidemic. However, this chapter intends to outline a more complicated picture, one that includes the limited success experienced by some organizations despite a larger overarching framework of denial. Whatever one's view of the response to AIDS on the part of such institutions as the NAACP, the National Urban League, or "the black church," we must use this issue and the examples provided in this chapter to grapple with the larger question: What role should and can such institutions play in the more cross-cutting politics of black communities in the twenty-first century?

National Political Organizations

The roles of national black political organizations such as the National Association for the Advancement of Colored People (NAACP), the National Urban League, and the Southern Christian Leadership Conference (SCLC) in responding to AIDS have been uneven at their best moments and neglectful in their worst. With this judgment already delivered, some would argue that it is unfair to expect organizations pursuing civil rights or economic development agendas to focus their limited resources on an issue such as AIDS that is at best tangentially related to the civil rights of black communities. While this argument might hold some weight in a political system in which the agendas of marginalized groups could be so neatly defined and allocated to different spheres, our political system and the political history of African Americans defy the separation of struggles for civil rights from struggles for access to health care or struggles for people with AIDS. In fact, this recognition has motivated civil rights leaders such as Dr. King, or black power organizations such as the Black Panther Party, and black feminist collectives such as the Combahee River Collective not only to articulate claims or demands around political rights, but also around such quality-of-life issues as jobs, housing, and health care.

National black political organizations, especially the three I have chosen to highlight briefly—the NAACP, the National Urban League, and the SCLC—have taken on the expansive role, be it fair or unfair, of serving as national political advocates for much of what ails black communities. Within the political processes of black communities, if one or all of these organizations deem an issue important to black people and deserving of national attention, then the probability that such an issue will gain recognition on a "black political agenda" is sharply increased. Over the years, as previously discussed, these organizations have gained greater access to and influence in the dominant political system. This is not to say that these national black organizations do not confront barriers when trying to shape policy decisions; however, it would be disingenuous to suggest that they have not experienced any benefits from the formal incorporation of African Americans into the political system. They have acquired "enough" access to guarantee a role, if not influence, in policy and agenda-setting debates of the federal government. For example, Dianne Pinderhughes (1995), comments on the access granted NAACP Washington lobbyist Clarence Mitchell:

> As the first full-time Washington lobbyist for the organization from 1950 through the late 1970s, Mitchell lobbied persistently on behalf of the NAACP and civil rights issues. He made the personal contacts that helped establish the NAACP's organizational and professional credibility, familiarize members of Congress and their staffs with the details and the framework of racial issues, and reshape the legislative environment in a manner more favorable to blacks' interests. Mitchell's effort in this regard strongly influenced the passage of the Civil Rights Act of 1964, the Voting Rights Act of 1965, and other civil rights legislation. He was known popularly among the civil rights lobby and legislators as the "101st Senator"—symbolizing the extent to which he had become a familiar figure on Capitol Hill. (210)

Thus, with influence in policy-making circles already established, we can only imagine how the active participation of black elected officials and national black leaders in legislation and policy debates over such issues as funding for AIDS organizations, representation in clinical trials, or the effectiveness of needle exchange might have changed significantly the response to AIDS in dominant and community institutions.

For national black political organizations, the early pattern of response was first denial and later a focus on service activity and distributional claims. Denial took the form of claims that AIDS was not a priority for black communities or was not directly relevant to the work of these organizations. Rarely did leaders engage in battles to redefine or transform AIDS as a political issue for black communities. Instead AIDS programs and policies were discussed and debated in black communities as they had been developed either by dominant institutions such as the CDC or by (primarily white) gay activists. Missing early in the epidemic, and still not altogether visible, were actions by national black leaders and organizations seeking to reshape the AIDS agenda to one explicitly addressing the unique development of this epidemic in black and Latino communities.[2] Thus the apparent dominance of "the AIDS agenda" (if there were one) by gay and lesbian activists, which many black leaders have complained about, seems to have resulted in part from the political work of mobilized lesbian, gay, and queer activists, but also from the dearth of leadership provided by national civil rights organizations rooted in black communities. When the AIDS policy window opened for input, framing, and decision-making, few if any national black political organizations were anywhere to be found.

NATIONAL ASSOCIATION FOR THE ADVANCEMENT OF COLORED PEOPLE

With a mass-based membership now numbering nearly five hundred thousand, the NAACP has grown into the organization many of its founders envisioned in 1909 (Fullwood 1991). Formed to promote what have been called racial status issues or racial-political goals such as integration, the NAACP has become one of the most widely recognized civil rights organizations in the country (Wilson 1960; Franklin 1980; Pinderhughes 1983). The organization functions through a highly bureaucratic structure that includes regional, state, and local divisions as well as a massive sixty-four-person board of directors. Despite being marred, in recent years, by personnel and financial scandals, the organization is still recognized as a major institution in black communities, engaged in struggles beyond the confines of the civil rights domain. Ironically, during the emergence of AIDS the NAACP was headed for the first time by a minister, Rev. Benjamin Hooks.

Analysis of the work pursued by the NAACP in response to AIDS will be brief, largely because the organization has done so little. Most indicators suggest that AIDS, as it manifested itself in black communities, was simply not a priority for this civil rights organization. Most of the responses to this disease by the NAACP centered around awareness and distributive claims. The first article on AIDS to appear in the *Crisis*, the monthly magazine of the NAACP, was not published until 1989, after nearly 17,000 black Americans had already died from opportunistic infections related to AIDS. This first discussion of AIDS in the pages of the *Crisis* came not in a stand-alone article, but in the publisher's notes (Hooks 1989, 3). This absence of direct attention to AIDS was corrected the next year when an independent article appeared entitled, "Impact of AIDS on the Black Community," written by David Hatchett (1990, 28–30).

The NAACP's slow recognition that AIDS was an issue devastating black communities was reflected not only in the pages of the *Crisis*, but also in the comments of staff members. For example, while Ms.

Mildred Roxborough, Director of Development and member of the National Health Committee of the NAACP, was quick to highlight the activity of the National Health Committee, she also admitted that it "has only been in the last two years (since 1991) that the organization took action beyond the declaration of resolutions" concerning the issue of AIDS.[3] Ms. Roxborough explained that part of the delay had to do with definitions of AIDS that placed it outside the civil rights agenda. She stated, "We are a civil rights organization, and our priorities focus on the denial of opportunity initially. But as the problems of health care increased and affected minorities, we expanded our concern to those areas."

The ability of Roxborough to so clearly distinguish between struggles for civil rights and struggles around HIV and AIDS reflects the bounded political ideology embraced by many civil rights organizations to justify their inactivity in this crisis. These leaders argue that AIDS as a policy issue is outside the domain of civil rights, where their expertise and commitment are rooted. However, the claim seems somewhat disingenuous, since only a few civil rights leaders and organizations have sustained any rigorous participation in legislative battles over the civil rights of gay Americans.[4] The contradiction is especially problematic since these civil rights battles affect segments of African-American communities. Such a declaration of a narrow agenda when it is convenient angers many black AIDS activists. Phil Wilson argues that such boundaries make no sense when people's lives are at stake: "I mean the NAACP and the Urban League talk about they're committed to economic development and that's a real thing. But if you are going to do economic development, there has to be folks that are alive to do the work. And if your community is being decimated by drugs and AIDS and alcohol, you have to confront those issues straight on, and they are not."[5]

In contrast to the ideological distance imposed between the political mission of the NAACP and the political needs of those with AIDS in black communities has been the willingness of national organizations like the NAACP to develop AIDS programs in response to funding initiatives and opportunities. There is little evidence to suggest that organizations such as the NAACP have worked to raise or make available the significant resources needed by community activists to compensate for their exclusion from dominant organizations. Instead, the AIDS work pursued by national organizations like the NAACP only occurred after it was funded by third parties such as the CDC. Michael

Pawlson, former staff member of the AIDS Institute, the funding unit for AIDS programs in the state of New York, explains the leverage that traditional black organizations have in dealing with state and federal agencies:

> Whatever it is [federal agencies like the CDC] are trying to do, they can't do it without us because they have no access. The CDC [Centers for Disease Control and Prevention] needs black people to help out, so they go to recognized black leadership. The same with the state and local level. They go to people they know and feel safe with. The irony is that you can't deal with AIDS safely. If you do it safely, you end up with the status quo. But they want a known quantity.[6]

Gil Gerald presents a more cynical interpretation of funding politics, focusing on the motives of black national organizations towards AIDS:

> During 1987 the Office of Minority Health pulled together a meeting of our leaders, and Carl [Beam] was there, and I was there. And we were down in the Office of Minority Health in this conference room. There was Mrs. Lowrey and Mrs. Benjamin Hooks. It was like who's who. And they were all banging on the table saying, "Why don't we have any money?" And I remember I broke down in tears. I cried out and said, "Which one of you has ever held a person with AIDS in your hands, in your arms?" There was silence in the room. So, you know, I said, "I really believe there needs to be some government resources brought to this issue, but have you ever, ever held a person with HIV in your hands?" I was convinced they were all a homophobic bunch of people who had come to the table for money.[7]

Adolph Reed (1986) argues that this pattern of outside funding of black civil rights organizations is not a new phenomenon:

> The major racial advocacy organizations operate ever more frequently as appendages of state and foundation apparatus, deriving large shares of their budgets from administering public programs as delegate agencies and occasionally as line items in public budgets. Moreover, this administrative function is legitimated ultimately by the civil rights elites' claim to an organic *political* relation to the black population. (7)

The acquisition of funds for AIDS work in black communities seems an important and appropriate task for national black organizations. For as Robert Penn, former minority education director at Gay Men's Health Crisis (GMHC) and interim director of Gay Men of African

Descent (GMAD) notes, it takes a lot of money to do AIDS work.[8] However, the concern of black activists is not that national black organizations are demanding that the CDC and other agencies increase AIDS funding directed toward communities of color. Instead, their anger stems from the fact that black gay men—those who were most active in the first stage of response to AIDS in black communities—were largely closed out of early funding opportunities, as the CDC turned to known quantities like the NAACP. From the viewpoint of many grassroots organizations and activists, these national black organizations, with seemingly little interest and track record in this area, took the money and ran.

When organizations like the NAACP have become involved in addressing the issue of AIDS, it has often been within a well-established yet misguided construction of the disease that views certain segments of black communities as more deserving of help and recognition than others. For example, in the summer of 1992 the NAACP sponsored a Health Summit featuring over one hundred invited guests and specialists. At the conclusion of the summit, a comprehensive policy statement was produced that included recommendations to improve the health of black Americans. The document comprised five specific areas. Surprisingly, one component dealt exclusively with the issue of AIDS. Unfortunately, the content of that policy area was not only incomplete in its attention to the threat posed by AIDS to black communities, it also indicated the pseudo-inclusive construction of the disease many organizations have enacted. Specifically, in this discussion of AIDS, all members of the community are encouraged to respond and help. However, only certain members of African-American communities—often women and children—are mentioned as struggling with the disease. Listed below are the five recommendations developed concerning HIV and AIDS in black communities:

> 1. HIV/AIDS is a public health crisis in the African-American community. African-American leaders should take a stand, address the problem as an epidemic, and declare its urgency. The President, Congress and states must commit resources to the African-American community to battle this epidemic.
> 2. Public agencies must fund promising African-American prevention, research, and service projects in order to launch a comprehensive fight against the HIV epidemic by addressing its physical, mental, and social aspects with special emphasis on the needs of women and children.

3. All African-American organizations, including civil rights groups, must join forces to speak out and develop strategies and programs to address HIV/AIDS. Religious institutions must take a vigorous role in preventing the spread of HIV. In order for the "at-risk" population to clearly understand and benefit from HIV prevention messages, the advertising and community education messages must be explicit and clear to the intended audience and must be presented repeatedly in various forms and during appropriate times to reach the intended audiences.

4. In order to meet the special threat HIV poses to African-American women and to address the absence of women in research, service, and education programs, the federal, state and local governments must "partner" with the NAACP and other national, membership-based, conventional, African-American organizations at the national, state, and local levels.

5. In partnership with African-American organizations, federal, state and local governments should establish a longitudinal, comprehensive, HIV prevention, detection and treatment program for each person under the jurisdiction of the criminal justice system . . . from initial arrest to final release, whether institutionalized or not, and including probationers and parolees.[9]

Not one of the points in the document speaks explicitly (despite the insistence in point 3 that discussions and messages about AIDS be explicit) to the condition of black gay men or injection drug users as they struggle through the AIDS epidemic. Instead, only women and children are highlighted in this document, except for a vague reference to "at-risk" populations. Although we can give NAACP officials the benefit of the doubt, assuming that by "at-risk" populations they meant black gay men, black men who have sex with other men, and black injection drug users, we must question why the organization did not mention these groups specifically. Once again, it seems that black leaders are choosing to ally themselves with those thought to be innocent and legitimate victims of AIDS in black communities.

Yet another problem with this document is that none of these points discuss AIDS as a political issue of primary importance to African Americans. There is no request for more funding for drug treatment programs. There is no discussion of needle-exchange programs and the possibility of curbing rates of transmission among injection drug users. There is no discussion of homophobia and the impact of stigma in and out of the community on inhibiting frank and *explicit* discussions of AIDS and HIV. Instead, the policy recommendations are service-oriented and center on the universal need for more programs, more money, and more attention. And while the statement hints at the unequal distribution of money and services for "minority" communities, the next step in transformational leadership, that of redefining AIDS into a political issue and addressing the political, economic, and moral marginalization confronting most people with HIV and AIDS in black communities, is nowhere to be found in this document.

One can discern who the NAACP sees as worthy of struggle not only by examining this Health Policy Statement, but also by surveying the program initiatives generated by the organization. For example, the national AIDS program initiative that members of the organization seemed most proud of, possibly because it was the only one as of 1992, was a program aimed at youth. The initiative, entitled " . . . but afraid to ask" is a pamphlet that attempts to answer the questions young people have about AIDS in a language they can relate to and understand. While undoubtedly an admirable program, it can also be seen as an indication of the overall "safe" focus, this time on children, pursued by the organization. Even this pamphlet provides no detailed discussion of drug use or the sharing of needles, the transmission route accounting for the largest percentage of cases of HIV among black Americans. The organization's strategy apparently seeks to circumvent controversial discussions and debates about issues of homosexuality and drug use, allowing instead familiar patriarchal frameworks of innocent children and victimized women to dictate the terms of the debate.

It would be unfair to represent the actions of the national office as the sum total of the organization's activity regarding AIDS. In fact, local NAACP chapters exhibit varying levels of AIDS program activity. For example, under the leadership of executive director Roger Vann and health committee chair Dr. James Rawlings, the New Haven, Connecticut, chapter of the NAACP has offered numerous programs on HIV and AIDS.[10] In 1996 the health committee structured all of its programs around the topics of HIV and AIDS. Again, while this work does not reflect the effort from the national office, nor the response from most local chapters—especially in the early years of the epidemic—it does suggest that with transformational, grassroots leadership and community support, new and innovative programming can be implemented and sustained.

Unfortunately, it seems that in the case of AIDS such leadership and vision has come almost exclusively from the bottom up. Both Vann and

Rawlings indicated that their local activities had little or nothing to do with the national NAACP's agenda, since they had never received any national directive indicating that HIV or AIDS was a priority for the organization. This example underscores the heterogeneity of political agendas and interests to be found among the local leaders and chapter members of most national black political organizations, including the NAACP. Struggles around the political decisions of the national office and the different desires of local chapters have increasingly found their way into national newspapers. Recent positions by the national office on issues such as the nomination of Clarence Thomas to the United States Supreme Court and the Million Man March sparked great debate and dissension among local chapters and members. While members of the New Haven NAACP have taken the lead in awareness activities, attempting to make AIDS a black political issue, not every chapter pursues such politics. For instance, when I asked officials at the New York NAACP chapter about local programs dealing with AIDS in black communities, I was told that the New York chapter "follows the programs developed by the national office." It seems fair to infer from that answer that they have done very little about AIDS.

NATIONAL URBAN LEAGUE

The National Urban League, founded in 1911 through the merger of three organizations (the Committee for Improving the Industrial Condition of Negroes in New York, the Committee on Urban Conditions, and the National League for the Protection of Colored Women), was established to address the social and economic issues of black Americans increasingly concentrated in urban areas (Franklin 1980). Over the years the organization has evolved into one of the most recognized civil rights organizations in the country, focusing primarily on the economic advancement of African Americans. The Urban League has correspondingly developed a reputation for being one of the more conservative civil rights organizations, particularly in comparison to the NAACP. It is especially interesting, therefore, that during the first ten years of the epidemic the Urban League published articles on AIDS more often and earlier than the NAACP. Again, we must view this fact from the proper perspective. Such a distinction does not mean that the Urban League gave sufficient ink to the issue of AIDS; rather, it means they wrote something about AIDS in a somewhat consistent pattern.

As with the NAACP, much of the initial (and late) response from the

Urban League can be classified as awareness activity. For example, the first article on AIDS to appear in *The State of Black America*, the Urban League's yearly report on the status of African Americans, came in 1987. The seven-page article, written by Dr. Benny J. Primm and entitled "AIDS: A Special Report," traced the history of the disease, highlighting its disproportionate impact on black communities. Although the issue was included in the main text of the report, no mention of AIDS was found that year in the list of recommendations the Urban League publishes as strategies for immediate implementation. AIDS would make the annual list of recommendations in 1988. The resolution that year called for increased funding from the government "to combat AIDS and other sexually transmitted diseases." This demand was preceded by interesting language calling for the unified response of the black community to address the issue of AIDS:

> The devastation of AIDS requires that every sector in the community join in a commitment to stop this epidemic. While we must continue to search for a cure, treatment of the victims of this disease must be humane and responsible. The AIDS issue must not be used as an excuse for further victimization of blacks, homosexuals, and other groups.

There are a number of points worth noting in this statement. First the language, similar to that found in the policy statement of the NAACP, calls on everyone in the community to "join in a commitment to stop this epidemic." Thus it seems that each of these organizations increasingly incorporates an apparently inclusive rhetoric when talking about who should respond to this disease, yet they continue to promote an analysis of AIDS that makes those segments of the community most at risk—black gay men and black injection drug users—invisible as group members. Second, note the sentence urging the humane and responsible treatment of AIDS "victims." Again, the discussion of how to deal with those with HIV or AIDS is reduced to individual acts of good and polite behavior. There is no mention of collective action, group mobilization, or even the articulation of demands for the rights of those living with AIDS. Third, the last sentence in this statement finally seems to acknowledge the use of AIDS discourse that results in secondary marginalization, scapegoating the most vulnerable members of oppressed communities. But after calls for unity, the end of the sentence imposes the now familiar dichotomy between blacks and homosexuals, presenting them as two separate groups dealing with this epidemic. This statement, still more forceful and direct than those of most other indigenous organizations, held on to a way of thinking that located the issues and the black bodies of lesbians and gay men as somewhere outside of blackness, as not intrinsic to African-American communities.

The recognition of AIDS in *The State of Black America* would continue. In 1989 the topic of AIDS was again directly mentioned in the list of recommendations found in the publication. In 1990, while not meriting a separate article, the issue of AIDS appeared in the main text of *The State of Black America*. In this instance it was addressed in a section of Dr. LaSalle D. Leffall, Jr.'s article, "The Health Status of Black Americans." And while the issue of AIDS found consistent attention in *The State of Black America*, the first article on AIDS in *The Urban League Review*, the monthly publication of the National Urban League, did not appear until 1991.[11] The only other written discussion of AIDS by the Urban League in the first decade of the epidemic was a thirteen-page pamphlet, "AIDS in the Black Community," part of the New York Urban League's Black Papers series. Thus, while it seems that the Urban League was more willing than other civil rights organizations to engage in awareness activity by writing about the devastating and disproportionate impact on black communities, rarely did that information seek to fundamentally transform and expand the terms of the debate about AIDS in black communities.

Similar to the efforts of the NAACP, and reflecting the general structure of both organizations, most of the Urban League's service efforts targeting HIV and AIDS originated in its 113 local affiliates. Often these programs were developed in response to requests for proposals (RFP) put forth by state or federal agencies distributing money from such sources as the Ryan White Comprehensive AIDS Resources Emergency (CARE) Act of 1990. As discussed earlier, state and federal authorities are much more disposed to give funding, especially among marginal groups, to those organizations with national name recognition, such as the Urban League or the NAACP. Unfortunately, these funds are often granted without any serious assessment of the organization's capacity to reach targeted segments of black communities most in need. Further, programs from larger national organizations frequently concentrate on providing technical assistance and coordinating the efforts of smaller, community-based organizations involved in the direct provision of services, rather than on providing services for or mobilizing the members of black communities living with AIDS.

For example, the New York Urban League currently runs a program called the Central Harlem HIV Network. As described in a pamphlet, "The Central Harlem HIV Care Network [a coalition of organizations involved in the provision of AIDS care] is one of seven HIV Care Networks in New York City." The program "is funded to develop and coordinate comprehensive services for people affected by HIV and AIDS. . . . The Network provides *services coordination* and is not involved in direct client services (emphasis added)." The resources for this initiative came from funds allocated to New York City through the Ryan White CARE Act.

Probably the most well-known AIDS program/organization to originate through the Urban League, at least in New York, has been the Black Leadership Commission on AIDS (BLCA). BLCA, established in 1987 through a two-day leadership session sponsored by the New York Urban League, has become one of the most powerful "minority" AIDS organizations in New York. Debra Frazier-Howe heads this organization, which is directed by a board comprised of a virtual "Who's Who" of traditional and elected black elite in New York, including former Mayor David Dinkins. The most successful programs of the organization have focused on providing technical assistance to community-based organizations, as well as developing education and prevention programs targeting primarily black clergy. Other programs of BLCA included "The Lifestyle Genesis Learning Series," described as "an Afrocentric self-empowerment program for African-American gay men," and the Community Education Unit, which is committed to increasing awareness of AIDS through such vehicles as public service announcements using black celebrities. It seems that, in particular, "The Lifestyle Genesis Program" was met with much less enthusiasm than some of their other programs.

Despite the recognition BLCA has garnered from black elites, government officials, and other AIDS organizations, many of the black AIDS activists I talked to seemed quite disgruntled with the work of this organization. They described BLCA as an organization composed of high-level black elites who knew nothing about AIDS or the segments of black communities most at risk. The organization, in their view, has had minimal impact on this crisis and little to show from the government contracts they have been awarded. One activist, who asked not to be identified because he feared possible funding repercussions, called BLCA a "showpiece for a bunch of upper-class blacks who were being pressured to do something about AIDS." He suggested that the organization has been "successful" in part because it fulfills "the needs of state officials who have to give some money to black organizations and don't want to fund black gay activists working with black faggots fucking in the parks." Tracy Gardner-Wright, in a less accusatory tone, suggests that part of the success of BLCA, especially with black clergy is Debra Frazier Howe's identity as "one of the flock," a "normal" middle-class, heterosexual black woman with grandchildren. "That's why it will be a Debra Frazier-Howe who will continue to be able to talk to ministers and to congregations as the good little girl who is doing good things. She is one of our flock, one of our exemplary members of our flock doing good things, taking care [of those in need] and truly carrying out the tenets of good Christianity. But implicit in that is she's not flawed. She's not flawed because she's not a junkie and she's not a dyke. She's one of ours. She could be married. . . . A straight black woman's voice in AIDS is a hot commodity."[12]

Unexpectedly, over the years the National Urban League (or at least its local affiliates) has shown a willingness beyond that of the NAACP to discuss the issue of AIDS in black communities. At the same time, the national office, as with other programs, has devoted relatively few resources to dealing with this disease, relying instead on the ability of local affiliates to raise money for their AIDS programs.[13] Further, any constructive involvement of the organization in struggles around AIDS policy has generally been devoid of an analysis that identifies AIDS as involving a primary *political* battle for black communities. Absent from the Urban League's AIDS agenda have been efforts focused on recognition and redefinition, providing an oppositional framework that reconstructs the AIDS crisis at its core. Neither the NAACP nor the Urban League seems interested in expanding the current conception of AIDS in black communities to one which makes central demands for the right to health care, housing, drug treatment, and gay rights. Neither of these organizations seems interested in challenging the secondary processes of marginalization which so strongly condition their response and the action, or lack thereof, of other black organizations. Neither of these organizations seems interested in engaging in a political battle around AIDS tied to and directly affecting the progress and advancement of all black people, the type of struggle in which we might expect civil rights organizations to play a leading role. In fact, a recent *New York Times* article noted that "the nation's two largest black civil rights groups, the Urban League and the National Association for the Advancement of Colored People, will hold their annual conventions this summer; AIDS is on neither agenda" (Sheryl Gay Stolberg, 29 June 1998, A12).

Instead, the efforts of the Urban League have centered on awareness and service activity, with some attention to distributive claims. The organization has focused on such activity as promoting prevention, building provider networks, or helping black community-based organizations secure government contracts and private funding for service prevention. And while not as forceful and politically minded in their actions as many national (primarily white) gay and lesbian organizations, the Urban League has pursued minimal responses to the AIDS crisis. So as we evaluate the interventions of the Urban League and other national black organizations regarding AIDS, we must be concerned not just with whether the intervention occurred at all, but also with the nature and content of the activity. Specifically, to what extent do these efforts promote a more expansive, transformative notion of AIDS and those with AIDS in black communities? The Urban League was apparently content to work within an established political framework, accepting the exclusion of some, and participating only at the margins.

SOUTHERN CHRISTIAN LEADERSHIP CONFERENCE

Established in 1957 in the aftermath of the Montgomery Bus Boycott, through the work of activists such as Bayard Rustin, Ella Baker and Stanley Levison, and the leadership of ministers such as Dr. Martin Luther King, Jr., Rev. Ralph D. Abernathy, and Rev. Joseph E. Lowery, the Southern Christian Leadership Conference (SCLC) has always been a civil rights organization led by and focused on black clergy (Fairclough 1987). Unlike Ms. Roxborough of the NAACP, Rev. Lowery believes that the work of the SCLC and other civil rights organizations stretches beyond a narrowly defined civil rights agenda. "Our movement since the days of Martin Luther King and before has always been not just civil rights but also the total well-being of all Americans" (Page 1991, 18). Thus the SCLC is an exception to the patterns described above. It initiated one of the first AIDS programs to target black communities. Beginning in 1984, under the direction and motivation of Mrs. Evelyn Lowery, the SCLC began holding workshops in black communities, drawing attention to and educating members about the threat of HIV and AIDS. Moreover, according to Quimby and Friedman (1989), the SCLC was one of the first traditional black organizations to hold a national conference (in 1987) on AIDS in the black community.[14] It was not until 1988, however, that the SCLC received major funding from the CDC to develop and implement educational and prevention programs specifically for black communities (Holman et al. 1991). The resulting program, with outposts in five cities—Atlanta, Charlotte, Detroit, Kansas City, and Tuscaloosa—was one of thirty-three programs funded by the CDC to "prevent and control the spread of HIV infection among racial and ethnic minority populations in the United States" (Holman et al. 1991, 688).

In 1990 the SCLC decided to continue its awareness activities, this time relying directly on its history of leadership in the black religious community. Believing that its history of church-based civil rights struggle gave it an advantage in reaching black clergy, the SCLC decided to refocus its efforts and to engage in AIDS education with members of the black church. The goal of the program was to set up AIDS ministries in black churches around the country. Magie A. Shannon, Atlanta director of the SCLC program, explained back in 1991 "that it has been difficult getting into many churches."[15] Many churches, regardless of the reputation of the SCLC, were still not receptive to discussions of AIDS. As we might expect, one area that made church officials reluctant to tackle the issue of AIDS was its association with the topic of homosexuality. Shannon indicated that when dealing with black clergy on the issue of homosexuality, she pursued a strategy which emphasized the concept of Christian equality, reminding ministers that "we are all children of God and need to be loved." She went on to say, "I'm not condoning homosexuality, but everybody knows there are homosexuals in the church."

The work of the SCLC provides yet another example where the issue of AIDS, even among those committed to a more inclusive agenda, is constructed to fit a narrow and conservative ideology, in this case that of the black church. The SCLC has always seen its natural constituency as black clergy and black churchgoers, and its history of both adherence to and promotion of a black, Christian, middle-class moral framework has provided them entry to the community of black clergy. However, this same deference to the moral codes of the black church has limited significantly the educational message that SCLC workers put forth concerning HIV and AIDS. Thus, while the SCLC was willing to make the education of black clergy and church members central to its efforts, it was unwilling to directly challenge churches to radically reevaluate their thinking on the issue of homosexuality and consequently AIDS. Ms. Shannon and the SCLC chose a strategy of constructive engagement, believing it more important to have the church involved in the response to AIDS in black communities than to risk alienating black clergy and church members by explicitly talking about and fighting for the recognition of all those with AIDS.

The very limited framework through which the SCLC pursued its AIDS work angered some black AIDS activists. In particular, they were greatly concerned about the SCLC's inability or unwillingness to openly discuss and recognize black gay men as empowered and worthy members of black communities struggling against AIDS. Phil Wilson comments,

> This is probably going to be an unpopular thing to say, but so be it. I think that some of the things that the SCLC did were particularly problematic because they pretend to do something. They created an AIDS program and put themselves out there as a leader on this issue and then did not lead. . . . The joke goes like this: A guy loses his keys, and he is looking for his keys, and he's on the street and running up the street looking for his keys, and a friend comes up and he says, "What are you doing?" He says, "I'm looking for my keys." His friend says, "Well, where did you lose them?" The guy says, "Over there." [And the friend asks] "Well why are you looking over here?" [And the guy says], "Because the light is better over here." That is what the SCLC did. AIDS is over there, and they are doing work over here.[16]

Gil Gerald confirms Wilson's assessment of the limited framework of the SCLC, providing a more generous account of their successes and failures:

> The SCLC did a lot of conferences. They were [out there] speaking about AIDS. They provided some educational information, and that is remarkable and important. But I think it was coming largely from a very middle-class framework. They had real difficulties dealing with some of the issues like gay sexuality. Mrs. Lowry was a major spokesperson because it was the SCLC women who organized around this. . . . I remember one time we were speaking at the Joint Center for Policy Studies—a black think tank. They had a workshop at their annual conference. She [Mrs. Lowrey] gets up and she says the only context that [we] could talk about black men having sex with men was in prison.[17]

Again, it was the exclusion of black gay men, black men who sleep with men, injection drug users, sex workers, and other marginal subjects in black communities from public discussions of AIDS sponsored by national black political organizations that prompted activists to contest their claims of leadership and action.

Despite the many obstacles and the criticisms aimed at the work of the SCLC, workers like Ms. Shannon continued to try to serve and educate people with AIDS in black communities. One of the most important reasons for Ms. Shannon's commitment to her work is her strong belief that black people should take care of their own. She declares, "They [white people] live in their communities and want to bring meals to our people. We must do it ourselves." This idea that black people are better able to help and care for other black people seems to guide not only the work of Ms. Shannon, but also the programmatic and funding plans of dominant institutions like the CDC. Holman et al. (1991) write as follows:

> Responding to the facts that (a) the AIDS epidemic is occurring among black and Hispanic populations disproportionately to their percentage of the U.S. population and (b) effective human immunodeficiency virus (HIV) prevention programs are racially, ethnically, and culturally relevant and sensitive, CDC in 1988 initiated a five-year grant program for HIV prevention efforts *by national racial and ethnic minority organizations and regional consortia of racial and ethnic minority organizations. . . .*
>   As a result of these grants, substantial resources are being invested in prevention programs *developed by and for racial and ethnic minorities.* (emphasis added, 687)

Interestingly, a number of these early programs targeted not the most vulnerable in African-American communities, but the middle-class professionals such as clergy, dentists, doctors, and social workers presumed to be in contact with and servicing those with AIDS. As noted earlier, the financial assistance and awards provided by government agencies have often facilitated the programmatic efforts of national black organizations. Without directly questioning the motivation of these organizations in pursuing AIDS programming, we must grapple with the question of whether all black organizations should be included in the response to AIDS, regardless of the sexism, drug phobia, classism, or homophobia that may exist in them. Again, dominant public health officials, having little familiarity with African-American communities, develop outreach strategies that involve nationally recognized black organizations. However, the limited public dollars available for black communities might be more effectively used by local organizations that serve and organize a more diverse constituency through a more inclusive moral and political framework. These local organizations may be better able to empower the most marginal in black communities. Clearly, culturally sensitive and indigenously controlled services have been proven to increase the effectiveness of educational and preventive programs, but significant differences exist among African Americans—especially as their behavior puts them at risk for HIV and AIDS—that may make such broad public health strategies ineffective at best and insulting at worst. Specifically, when trying to develop and fund culturally sensitive programs, which and how many characteristics of "the community" do we prioritize? Is it enough that black organizations provide services to black people with AIDS, even if those organizations are enmeshed in moral codes that condemn the behavior and choices of many of those they are supposed to serve?

In attempting to provide needed services to their own, the SCLC has taken the "lead" among civil rights organizations in educating members of black communities about AIDS, at times using indigenous resources to provide for the basic needs of those in the community with AIDS. In doing so, the SCLC seems to have stood largely alone among traditional civil rights organizations. Ms. Shannon has noticed the absence of other major civil rights organizations consistently implementing AIDS programs in black communities:

> I work in a community of AIDS educators, we all know each other. If the NAACP or the Urban League is doing anything then I don't know about it. I'm not trying to say anything bad about the NAACP or the Urban League, but I think the SCLC is the only civil rights organization with a concrete plan and a history of doing something.[18]

But is a concrete plan and the history of service professed by the SCLC enough to qualify as truly effective, even transformative, AIDS work? While organizations such as the SCLC were willing to use their resources (and gain new ones) to preach a message of education and prevention, they often shied away from seeking to influence policy decisions and lead political battles for the rights of individuals living with HIV or AIDS. Thus in many ways the SCLC seems to follow the Christian directive that so many churches have adhered to in dealing with the AIDS crisis: "Love the sinner and hate the sin." Through such a framework the organization can actively work to increase awareness and provide services, while avoiding questions that challenge fundamental thinking about AIDS. Through such a framework black leaders can choose to respond to this crisis, yet cautiously refrain from redefining AIDS as a political issue that demands the attention and action of those in and outside of African-American communities.

"The Black Church"

Activists and scholars have often focused on the activity of what is called "the black church" to understand and explain the political, social, and cultural behavior of African Americans. This attention stems undoubtedly from the recognition and the larger than life "mythology" that the black church has served repeatedly as the glue and motor of black communities (Reed 1986). If any activity was expected to touch every segment of the group, it was assumed that such efforts would be based in the black church. The work of scholars ranging from Gunnar Myrdal (1996) to Aldon Morris (1984) and to Lincoln and Mamiya (1990) provide multiple examples of the role this institution has played, or was thought to play, in struggles for the liberation and rights of African Americans. For instance, Adam Fairclough (1987), commenting on the importance of black clergy and the black church to the Montgomery Bus Boycott, writes, "In a city with neither a black radio station nor a widely read black newspaper, the church provided the information network. It also provided the meeting places, the fundraising machinery, and the means of organizing an alternative transportation system" (17).

Even prior to the civil rights movement the black church was used to build movements for freedom among black people. The black church was a rare center of economic, social, and political independence in black communities, operating with the autonomy to tackle the most sensitive of issues (Mays and Nicholson 1969). It was the black church that acted as meeting space, school, health care facility, and distributor of food from slavery through Reconstruction, through the decades of Jim Crow rule, through the years of northern migration, and now in the post-segregation era. Lincoln and Mamiya (1990) in their national study of black churches from the seven historically black denominations find that nearly 70 percent (67.9 percent) of the black ministers sampled reported that their churches "cooperated with social agencies or other nonchurch programs in dealing with community problems" (220). Hollie I. West (1990), in her article on the new social role of black churches, comments, "African-American churches have traditionally served as a refuge from a hostile white world, beehives of both social and political activity" (51).

Before proceeding I want to note that the "mythology," as Reed (1986) calls it, surrounding the black church has been disputed by numerous scholars (Bunche 1973; Frazier 1964; and Drake and Cayton 1993). These researchers have commented on the passivity and assimilationist tendencies of the black church. In fact Reed reminds us that Dr. Martin Luther King, Jr. also complained about "the apathy of the Negro ministers" (quoted in Reed 1986, 44). It would therefore be a mistake to homogenize and collapse the varying levels of political activism and community involvement to be found in different black churches. For example, Lincoln and Mamiya find that larger black churches are more likely to sponsor community outreach programs. The authors explain: "Larger black churches tend to have more financial resources and facilities, a more highly educated leadership, and more people available to staff their programs" (188). Similarly, both Thomas et al. (1994) and Rubin, Billingsley, and Caldwell (1994), using data from the Black Church Family Project (BCFP), find that churches that have existed longer, that have larger congregations, that have a majority of members from the middle class, that own their building, that have more paid clergy and other staff, or that are led by ministers with more years of formal education were most likely to offer community outreach programs.

In addition to the role of some black churches in civil rights activities and general community outreach programs, the church is also reported to have a long history of responding to the health needs of African-American communities. Thomas et al. (1994) inform us that

> the church has a long history of addressing unmet health and human service needs of the Black community. As long ago as the 1920s, Mays and Nicholson conducted a study of 609 urban churches and 185 rural churches. The authors found that community outreach programs included various activities aimed at addressing health needs, such as (1) programs to feed the unemployed, (2) free health clinics, (3) recreational activities, and (4) child care programs. . . .
>
> Historically, the Black church has been used by public health and medical professionals to gain access to those Blacks who are more difficult to reach through mainstream systems. The National Negro Health Movement, 1915 to 1950, represents the

best historical example of how the Public Health Service utilized the church in a national strategy to bring modern public
health practices to Blacks. (576)

Assumptions about the importance of the black church and religion
to African Americans seem to be supported by the data. Billingsley
and Caldwell (1991) report that 84 percent of black adults responding
to the National Survey of Black Americans said that they were religious, 70 percent identified themselves as members of a church, and
71 percent reported attending church regularly (428). The authors also
suggest that from 65,000 to 75,000 black churches of various denominations currently exist in the United States (432). They note that "we
have also been advised that this number would increase dramatically
if 'storefront churches'—small, independent churches not associated
with major denominations that are located in renovated store sites or
houses—were taken into consideration" (432). Finally, Lincoln and
Mamiya (1990) gauge black church membership at approximately 24
million (xi).

In spite of such significant numbers, other trends, such as the advent
of AIDS, drug epidemics, and increasing poverty and stratification
within black communities, are beginning to make some activists question the central authority given to the church. Grassroots organizers in
black communities wonder what role the church will and can play in
a new political era where increasingly the issues publicly confronting
black communities are cross-cutting and marked by stigma. Specifically, they suggest that while the church is involved in service activity,
these efforts focus primarily on mainstream topics such as family and
marital relationships. For example, using data generated through the
Black Church Family Project, Thomas et al. (1994) find that 67 percent
of the black churches surveyed have at least one community outreach
program, with 54 percent operating two or more programs, and nearly
41 percent sponsoring three or more activities (576). Billingsley and
Caldwell (1991), using preliminary data from the Black Church Family
Project, report that "by far, the largest category of programs offered is
family support and family assistance programs. Forty-two percent of all
programs offered are for family-oriented community outreach programs. These include family support programs such as basic assistance
with food, clothing, and shelter as well as emergency financial aid"
(435).

Despite the high levels of family-oriented service activity reported
above, Rubin et al. (1994, 254), in an analysis of youth programming

reported in the BCFP, discover that of the 176 (28 percent) churches sponsoring youth programs, "the least common programs were youth AIDS support programs (3 percent) and youth health-related services (2 percent)." In contrast to the minuscule number of church youth programs dealing with more stigmatized issues such as AIDS, the two most popular youth initiatives were "teen support programs, which are provided by 39 percent of the churches," and "sports activities" offered by 31 percent of the churches involved in youth programming (254). The authors conclude that "some of the most prominent issues facing African-American youth are not being adequately addressed by black churches. Among these are health-related services and AIDS support programs, with practically no churches reporting their existence. Substance abuse programs are being provided by only 27 churches. Parenting and sexuality programs are also offered in only 27 churches. . . . These findings are of particular concern because social and behavioral science literature indicates that community institutions play important roles in the socialization of youth" (258–60).

Hollie I. West (1990) also suggests that part of the problem is that AIDS is a controversial or cross-cutting issue, pulling the church in two directions. She argues that AIDS triggers two traditions in the black church, one centered around the provision of services and care to those in need, the other based in teaching the Christian scripture. While researchers and activists focus increasingly on the secular activities of the black church, the mission of leading the spiritual development of a wayward congregation still largely guides the decisions and programming of black churches. Thus, within a socially conservative ideology, in which "moral" behavior is the primary standard by which Christianity is judged, the church cannot and will not ignore the presumed "sinful" behavior of many with AIDS in black communities. West writes, "Some clergymen privately acknowledge the dilemma. They recognize the need to confront AIDS and drugs, but conservative factions in their congregations discourage involvement" (51).

AIDS, of course, is not the first issue that has confronted the black church with what appears to be a choice between adherence to moral Christian tenets or the service and counsel of community members in need. Concerns over "out-of-wedlock births" (especially among teenagers) and drug use in black communities are just two examples that have long challenged the moral framework of black churches. As Gail Walker reminds us, "The dual and contradictory legacy of the African-American church is that it has been among the most important instruments of African-American liberation and at the same time one of the most conservative institutions in the African-American community" (1992, 10). Thus a conservative ideology, based on strict norms of "moral" behavior, has often framed at least the church's rhetorical response to many of the controversial social issues facing black communities. However, even within the framework of Christianity based on severe moral judgment, members of black churches have usually found ways to serve their "fallen" brothers and sisters.

It is the contradictory nature of the church, however, that continues to frustrate many AIDS activists who looked to it for a swift, compassionate, and empowering response. Activists and those providing services claim that the church did little or nothing early in the epidemic. Further, they argue that when the church did begin to mobilize, it was with judgment and pity. Articulated concerns with the response of the black church to AIDS have taken at least four forms: (1) questions about whether the black church is really following the Christian teaching it holds so dear; (2) arguments that the black church will never be able to forcefully deal with AIDS until it takes on the issue of sexuality generally, and gays and lesbians in black communities more specifically; (3) claims that the church is only willing to provide services to certain segments of black communities, neglecting AIDS as a political issue for all members of black communities; and (4) concerns that too much attention is being paid to the church, since it has limited influence with the individuals at greatest behavioral risk in black communities.

Dr. Marjorie Hill, former director of New York City's Office of Lesbians and Gay Concerns under Mayor David Dinkins and current board member for the Gay Men's Health Crisis (GMHC), believes that the black church, in avoiding association with this epidemic, may be neglecting the teachings of Christ. She explains that the lessons she learned in the Baptist church dictate a different response to AIDS than that demonstrated by black churches so far:

> Historically, activism in the Black community has come from the church. However, the reluctance of the church to respond to AIDS means they are not following the mission of Christ. I was taught in the Baptist church that Christ took care of the sick. Because the Black church has not taken care of gays, lesbians, and IV drug users, who are definitely in need, they are not fulfilling the mission of Christ. The church has not dealt

with the issue of homosexuality. Many have gays sing in the choir and play the organ, and that is fine until they need the church's help and recognition. . . . Denial only works for so long; the reality of gay men and women will eventually have to be dealt with.[19]

In contrast to Dr. Hill's opinion, some church members suggest that black churches are in fact making progress. For their part, church members point to the numerous AIDS ministries that have been established to deal with AIDS in black communities. They highlight what seem like revolutionary strides in the ability of black ministers to even mention AIDS from the pulpit. Cynthia Kirkwood (1992), discusses the different perceptions of activists pushing the church to move forward:

Many AIDS activists cite denial and disapproval of homosexuality, bisexuality, and intravenous drug use as well as the weight of other social problems as reasons for the turned heads, closed ears, and blinded eyes, even as the fatal disease ravages the black community.

Other activists insist that black churches are not ignoring AIDS; it has become an integral part of their lives. Ministers have buried children and their parents with AIDS, and ministers themselves have gotten sick. These activists feel that the church is being criticized for its methods of responding to the AIDS crisis. Most churches, for example, have not taken a stand supporting distribution of clean needles to injection drug users, a stance that many AIDS activists advocate. (306)

The same debate over the activity or inactivity of the church has been waged in New York City. While some argue that the black church has been neglectful, others suggest that it is progressing slowly, largely at the urging of black AIDS organizations like the Black Leadership Commission on AIDS (BLCA) or The Balm in Gilead. Greg Broyles, formerly of the BLCA, comments,

Sure, the church was slow to respond. But churches are now looking for ways to respond. BLCA has had a lot to do with this. Maybe black gay men were not the people to push the church to respond. They seem to do better when one of their peers challenges them. Rev. James Forbes of Riverside Church told ministers that they needed to respond to everyone. They can't turn anyone away. He is going to be much more effective than others of us.[20]

Another project initiated in New York that has been extremely effective in motivating black clergy to get involved in AIDS ministries is The Balm in Gilead, begun in 1989 by Pernessa C. Steele as the Harlem Week of Prayer for the Healing of AIDS. This event designated one week in the fall of each year to bring together clergy, their congregations, and the community for education, support, and prayer about AIDS. Ms. Steele, who has seen the participation in this event grow exponentially, explains the willingness of clergy to participate by the fact that "black churches didn't know what to do; . . . calling this the Harlem Week of Prayer for the healing of AIDS, they found their language" (Kirkwood 1992, 308). Since her 1989 beginning as the founder and organizer of the Harlem Week of Prayer, Ms. Steele has built a larger organization called The Balm in Gilead. This organization revolves around a number of programs focused on AIDS in black communities, including the Black Church National Day of Prayer for the Healing of AIDS, the Black Church National Education and Leadership Training Conference on HIV/AIDS, and the African-American National Clergy summit on HIV/AIDS, held at the White House in 1995. Additionally, this organization has probably been the beneficiary of more high-powered celebrity fund-raisers than any other black AIDS organization in New York—although BLCA would run a close second. Numerous celebrities like opera diva Jessye Norman have donated their time and talent to raise funds for The Balm in Gilead.

The importance of organizations like BLCA or The Balm in Gilead in constructing an environment where black clergy feel "safe" to take a role in the response to AIDS should not be devalued. As with most stigmatized and controversial issues, few individuals—including clergy—want to be the first to step forward to confront a new challenge. Organizations targeting the education of black clergy have been able to facilitate some association with the issue of AIDS by bringing together clergy and building coalitions capable of sharing both the glory and the wrath of speaking out about and serving those with AIDS in black communities. And while Dr. Marjorie Hill, also a former member of the BCLA board, believes that black churches in the community have progressed slowly, she attributes much of any movement witnessed among black clergy to BLCA's ability to "get influential ministers to say AIDS is our responsibility." Others like Tracy Gardner-Wright point to Pernessa Steele's ability to slowly bring ministers along as a fundamental reason for her success:

I think history will show that Pernessa Steele made some inroads in a way that isn't grand or out there. She's not screaming
at the top of her lungs. It's very slow, methodical. She brings
on folks slowly, but surely. Harlem Week of prayer is becoming, will become an institution. It is a vehicle. I think it is
a very effective vehicle. . . . But you have to build and culti-
vate. When I was working at the [Minority] Task Force [on
AIDS], . . . at 92 St. Nichols, and this whole notion of the Harlem Week of Prayer [was developing] and people were just
kind of oh, what is this, or yeah it's a good idea but what's this.
And this woman would go out to individual ministers talking
to them, sitting down, addressing their fears, very calmly, pro-
fessionally. She knew the church. She knew the book. She
could banter with them back and forth and that is also why I
say it may need to be straight women. Just this whole notion
of one of the flock comes to us wanting to do the good Christian thing makes it harder to turn her away.[21]

Thus, in spite of the other criticisms of BLCA, namely its conservative
and seemingly self-serving agenda, it and other clergy-focused organizations like The Balm in Gilead have facilitated some activity from
black churches around AIDS in New York City. But the question still
remains, Is the church ready to engage in more inclusive and transformative work around this issue? If, as Gardner Wright hypothesizes,
the success of these two women is based in part on their heterosexual
identity, then the answer seems to be no.

So, while many of the service and awareness efforts of black ministers and those working with the black church around AIDS have been
somewhat effective, there is still little activity aimed at full recognition
and redefinition. AIDS organizers in black communities point to the
general reluctance of black churches to fully engage in political battles
rooted in a more expansive understanding of who exactly in black
communities is living with AIDS. The overwhelming condemnation of
the needle-exchange program by most black clergy is offered as but
one example of the expendable positioning of some community members as dictated by the "moral" framework of Christianity. It seems
that only when dealing with the "innocent victims" of the epidemic
are black churches fully prepared to embrace the political struggles of
people with AIDS.

It is not surprising that black ministers have been reluctant to embrace what is seen as the stigmatizing and immoral behavior associated with the transmission of HIV. This distancing from AIDS can be

understood through a self-interest, rational-choice model of behavior, since it has been the public appearance of conforming to Judeo-Christian values and American ideals that has won the church its standing or cultural capital both inside and out black communities. AIDS activists argue that a moral framework, rooted in middle-class values of assimilation and dominant ideas of Christianity, has been used to justify the church's condemnation of both black gay men and black injection drug users. This same moral framework structures the church's understanding and reaction to AIDS in black communities. Further, while there is no denying the stigma of drug addiction in black churches, organizers suggest that distinctions between what clergy deem the "sick" behavior of drug users and the "sinful" behavior of homosexuals have also influenced and differentiated the response each group receives from the church. Neither behavior or lifestyle is condoned by the church, but drug use is seen as a temporary "condition" that black clergy can acknowledge, talk about, and most importantly, develop programs for. Homosexuality, on the other hand, is viewed as sinful behavior, not to be acknowledged or accepted.

The position of the black church on the issue of homosexuality has seemed fairly straightforward, but in fact it has both public and private dimensions. In accordance to the teaching of most organized religions, members of black churches assert that homosexual behavior is immoral and in direct contrast to the word of God. Black ministers have consistently spoken out, preached about and taken action against the perceived immorality and threat posed to the community by gays and lesbians. For example, in 1993 black ministers from numerous denominations in Cleveland, Ohio, organized in opposition to federal legislation to include gay men and lesbians under the protection of the 1964 Civil Rights Bill. These ministers, representing themselves as "true leaders" of the black church, wrote as follows in the local black newspaper, the *Call and Post:*

> We as members and representatives of African-American protestant congregations reaffirm our identity as THE BLACK CHURCH. . . .
> We view HOMOSEXUALITY (including bisexual, as well as gay or lesbian sexual activity) as a lifestyle that is contrary to the teaching of the Bible. Such sexual activity and involvement is contrary to the pattern established during creation. Homosexual behavior in the Bible is forbidden and described as unnatural and perverted. . . .

> Our attitude toward any individuals that are involved in/
> with a HOMOSEXUAL LIFESTYLE is expressed through tolerance
> and compassion. The church's mission is to bring about RESTO-
> RATION. (Matthews 1993, 5C)

Even though condemnation of gay and lesbian sexual behavior is a staple of the black church, it is also well-known that black gay men, in particular, can be found in prominent positions throughout the church. Thus, black gay men involved in the activities of black churches are faced with a familiar dilemma: they have the choice of being quietly accepted as they sing in the church choir, teach Sunday school, and in some cases even preach from the pulpit, or they can be expelled from the church for participating in blasphemous behavior. Nowhere in this choice does the idea of inclusion as fully recognized and empowered members exist. Thus, according to religious doctrine, black lesbian and gay members of the community are to be embraced and taken care of in a time of need. However, their gay identity places them outside the indigenously constructed boundaries of both Christianity and black-ness as defined by the church.

Again it seems that the saying, "Love the sinner, hate the sin," is paramount in understanding the limited response of black clergy to black gay men and lesbians. Gay men are to be loved and taken care of when they are sick, but their loving relationships are not to be recognized nor respected. Most individuals affected by this disease can tell at least one story of going to a funeral of a gay man who died from AIDS and never hearing the acronym mentioned. Family members and ministers are all too willing to grieve the loss of a son or church member, without acknowledging the total identity of that loved one. Lost to AIDS is not only the son missed so dearly, but the totality of his life, which included lovers and gay friends who also grieve for their loss.

We must not lose sight of the fundamental obstacle to the church's wholehearted response to AIDS: its adherence to or reliance on a strict Christian code which views behavior that transmits the virus as im-moral and sinful. Thus, until church leaders are ready to discuss issues of sexuality, drug use, and homosexuality in an inclusive and trans-formed discourse, their ability to serve the entire community as well as to confront, instead of replicate, dominant ideologies will be severely inhibited. Rev. James Forbes of Riverside Church, an interracial and progressive church in New York City's upper west side, has been one of the few black clergy who has publicly called on the church to open its dialogue and redefine the parameters of its thinking about AIDS. In a keynote address at the 1991 Harlem Week of Prayer, Rev. Forbes declared that until the black church deals with fundamental issues such as sexuality, in an inclusive and accepting manner, it will never be able to adequately deal with the AIDS epidemic in black communities.

While ministers like Rev. Forbes preach the need for the church to reevaluate its stance on fundamental judgments of human behavior, others believe that we may have seen the church move about as far as it is going to go. Except for those exceptional congregations committed to a liberation theology, the provision of services for those with AIDS may be the extent of the church's response, because for many clergy there is no way to reconcile behavior that can lead to the transmission of the virus to the doctrine of the Christian church. Rev. Calvin Butts of Abyssinian Baptist Church in Harlem discusses the progress and limits of the church's response:

> The response of the church is getting better. At one time the church didn't respond and when the church did respond it was negative. Ministers thought that a negative response was in keeping with the thinking that AIDS was transmitted by homosexual transmission, drugs, you know. But as more thoughtful clergy became involved, issues of compassion entered the discussion and we used Jesus' refuge in the house of lepers as an example. People became more sympathetic when people close to the church were affected. Also the work of BLCA brought clergy together to work on our response. Unfortunately, there are still quite a few who see it as God's retribution. But we will get through this and the leadership will come from the church working with doctors and organizations like BLCA. There won't be any ACT UP in my church; the work will come out of BLCA.[22]

In an environment, however, where their identity is contested and their full rights and connection with black communities is negated, many black lesbian and gay leaders are actively developing ways to ignore the dictates and challenge the power of the church, especially as it affects AIDS organizing. One such strategy has involved black gay and lesbian leaders as well as AIDS activists in identifying ways to do effective work in black communities without the help of the church. Some suggest that it does not matter whether the church responds to AIDS because the church no longer touches those parts of black communities most at risk for this disease. Colin Robinson, director of the Community Partnership Initiative of GMHC and former executive director of Gay Men of African Descent (GMAD), explains that "the church is still hooked on sin, but compromised by sin. They will take care of you when you get sick, but they won't talk about it, and that is no way to provide effective education."[23] George Bellinger, Jr., a board member of GMAD and former Education Director of the Minority Task Force on AIDS in New York suggests that "we put too much status in the church. They aren't connected to the affected populations, and they bring with them all kinds of middle-class values."[24] Lincoln and Mamiya (1990) reiterate this point with a focus on class divisions in the black church:

> The gradual emergence of two fairly distinct black Americas along class lines—of two nations within a nation—has raised a serious challenge to the Black Church. The membership of the seven historic black denominations is composed largely of middle-income, working-class, and middle-class members, with a scattering of support from poorer members, especially those in southern rural areas who tend to be among the most loyal members. But black pastors and churches have had a difficult time in attempting to reach the hard-core urban poor, the black underclass, which is continuing to grow. In past generations some of the large urban black churches were one of the few institutions that could reach beyond class boundaries and provide a semblance of unity in black communities. The challenge for the future is whether black clergy and their churches will attempt to transcend class boundaries and reach out to the poor, as these class lines continue to solidify with demographic changes in black communities. (384)

Whether the barriers to active participation by black churches in the fight against AIDS be class divisions or moral judgment, activists continue to work independently of the church. Some in black communities have developed AIDS education strategies that do not depend on or include the black church. Others are engaged in strategies that directly challenge the teaching of the church about homosexuality, especially as black gay identities are offered in contrast to the indigenous constructed image of "good black Christian folk." Black gay activists understand that to engage the black community on the issue of AIDS as well as lesbian and gay rights, they must contest and challenge the church's declaration and labeling of gay and lesbian lifestyles as immoral. In response to this challenge, they have taken on the task of redefining themselves as integral, connected, and contributing members of the community, invoking such noted figures as James Baldwin,

Bayard Rustin, Langston Hughes, Bessie Smith, and Audre Lorde to "prove" that one can be black and gay and committed to the advancement of black people.

Part of this contest to be viewed as full members of "the community" includes seeking out leaders inside the religious community, like Rev. James Forbes, who have publicly challenged the representations of more conservative clergy. In the absence of such traditional leaders, black gay activists have begun to build their own religious institutions, like Unity Fellowship, located in such cities as New York, San Francisco, Atlanta, Washington, DC, and Los Angeles. These new black religious institutions frequently replicate the general structure of traditional black churches; however, they offer an interpretation of biblical scripture that embraces the idea of an empowered black lesbian and gay community working with other marginal segments of black communities to build the transformative movement necessary for the cross-cutting politics of the twenty-first century.

Conclusion

National black organizations and leaders have demonstrated a conflicted response to AIDS. A few organizations have used indigenous resources to educate black communities about AIDS. A few black political leaders have consistently worked to redefine the community's understanding of AIDS. However, the majority of groups and elites has chosen either to define AIDS as an issue outside of their domain or to engage in service-oriented programming, where they develop and implement education, prevention, and treatment programs within traditional frameworks. Overall there has been very little reframing of AIDS to awaken the consciousness of black communities and mobilize their political strength in response to this epidemic. Instead, AIDS has most often been represented as an individual medical/moral problem caused, depending on your perspective, by bad people or salvageable individuals engaged in bad behaviors.

Some may argue that the responses I detail in this chapter are biased because they focus on the activities of large civil rights organizations and not those national black organizations concerned with health and health care. However, even when we turn our attention to a national black health organization like the National Medical Association, we find limited and constrained activity. The National Medical Association (NMA), founded in 1895 in response to the racial segregation mandated in the American Medical Association (AMA), continues to call upon its members to do more in the fight against AIDS.[25] In a 1996 address from the President of the NMA, reprinted in the *Journal of the National Medical Association* (1996), Dr. Randall C. Morgan, Jr. suggests that all segments of black communities must do more around AIDS. However, in making this appeal Dr. Randall falls into the familiar rhetoric of highlighting the "innocent victims" of the epidemic: "Males of color are infected with the HIV virus primarily through sex with other men or injection drug use. Women of color, on the other hand, are infected by sex with men or injection drug use. The *most unfortunate* group are those children of color who are infected during the intrauterine period by the mother" (emphasis added, 16).

In addition to assessing the impact of AIDS on black communities through a predictable and divisive framework, Dr. Morgan goes on to list some of the policy positions taken by the NMA concerning AIDS. In this section, which reports on the NMA's efforts to fight AIDS, Dr. Morgan begins with what can only be described as a severe underreporting of the multiple government grants and contracts received by the NMA and its members to develop and implement primarily service and awareness efforts targeting black physicians. Dr. Morgan then moves on to describe the "bold" policy stances of the organization:

> The NMA has been on the frontline of the advocacy efforts for our patients who have HIV/AIDS. We have many clinical experts across the United States who *developed grants for education of providers,* and who have published extensively on HIV and AIDS.
>
> In 1987, the NMA House of Delegates passed a broad resolution that:
>
> - endorsed the efforts of federal, state, and local public health officials to develop health education programs to increase knowledge on the part of the public on how to prevent the transmission of AIDS,
> - strongly supported increased government funding and support for basic clinical research into the causes, prevention, and treatment of AIDS in the black community,
> - supported efforts to disseminate educational information on AIDS to physicians, particularly black physicians, and to the public through publications, information packages, and educational programs, and
> - endorsed an expansion of health education and preventative programs, especially to communities of color, to reduce the spread of AIDS.

In 1990, the NMA opposed testing for AIDS of selective ethnic groups based solely on race. The Association has supported mandatory blood testing for exposure to AIDS in: (1)
blood donors, (2) military personnel, and (3) immigrants. All
other blood testing for exposure to the AIDS virus should be
voluntary.

Finally, the NMA firmly supports the reporting of cases of
HIV infection to the local department of health, with the
knowledge of the patient. The patient also should be encouraged to notify at-risk partners. (emphasis added, 16)

Dr. Morgan's address provides us with yet another example of a national black organization—this time one focused on health and health
care—that has found ways to garner public funds for AIDS education,
yet makes no direct mention in the above text of needle exchange,
the mandatory testing of pregnant women for AIDS—women who are
disproportionately black and Latina—nor the homophobia and heterosexism faced by black gay men in their fight against AIDS. Further, this
organization, which represents black physicians, notes with apparent
pride that they have supported the indiscriminate testing of immigrants. The officials of the NMA seem oblivious to the fact that immigrants are being tested because of their secondary status as immigrants and not because they are necessarily behaviorally at risk. The
NMA's policy supports the testing of all immigrants, including Afro-
Caribbean and other black immigrants. Thus, when we turn our attention to national medical organizations based in black communities, we
find these organizations engaged in traditional interventions meant to
serve, but never to transform or lead.

Finally, earlier in this chapter I raised the question of what role established organizations could and should play in the cross-cutting black
politics of the twenty-first century. It would be presumptuous of me to
argue that traditional leaders and organizations have no role at all.
From the brief examination presented here, it seems that national leaders and organizations have the reputation and familiarity with government and private sources to acquire some of the resources needed to
respond to and mobilize around crises facing black communities. Further, black clergy, while working from a religious framework that inhib-
its their willingness to advocate politically for all in black communities, do control institutions and resources that can be used for the
political mobilization of African Americans. Thus, in an advanced state
of marginalization, where African Americans have been formally incorporated into the political system, it is hard to deny that there exist

some resources available to black communities to mobilize around such crises as AIDS.

However, while formal incorporation has produced greater mobility, resources, and cultural capital for some black elites, these advancements have not trickled down to the masses of black people. And while securing resources for political mobilization will always be a concern in black communities, the more pressing question facing black people may now be how to reflect the differential life experiences and interests among black Americans, while preserving some unified constituency available for mobilization. Further, we need to recognize that not all black institutions can effectively organize the most vulnerable, alienated, and stigmatized groups of African Americans. Established organizations and leaders such as the NAACP and the National Urban League may be so distanced—physically, culturally, and normatively—from certain subpopulations in black communities, that the provision of truly inspired transformative leadership may be beyond their reach. Moreover, traditional leaders, incorporated into dominant institutions to fulfill, in part, managerial roles, may view the transformational demands of those in the second tier of black communities as working against their specific interests and mobility. Manning Marable (1991) suggests that black middle-class leaders may be unable to envision a transformed progressive society:

> The black middle class's failure, in brief, has been one of ideology and historical imagination. The elite constantly maneuvers, responding to minor political crises, but it is unable to project a constructive program for *transforming* society as a whole. It is a failure within qualified and truncated success. As the century moves toward its conclusion, the elite's limited capacity for creative vision or historical consciousness has clearly generated a barrier between its own political objectives and the material needs and aspirations of the exploited black majority. . . .
>
> The impasse within the black freedom movement during the post-reform era will not be transcended unless a new, more creative leadership emerges to raise fundamental questions concerning ideology, politics, and the future of African-Americans' consciousness and identity. (emphasis added, 226–27)

As I have argued throughout this book, marginal groups look inward to find the needed resources and oppositional ideologies necessary to challenge dominant practices of marginalization. However, if this strategy for mounting resistance is available only to certain segments of black communities, under specific conditions, and around particular issues, then it may necessitate the reevaluation of black communities' reliance on linked-fate political mobilization strategies. Specifically, all those concerned with promoting a more expansive notion of blackness as we approach the twenty-first century, be it through contests around nation, gender, or sexuality, must pay attention to the politics national black organizations either produce, challenge, or legitimate.

This examination of the response to AIDS among established black institutions and organizations is not meant to suggest that traditional leadership has no role in the politics of black communities. Instead the lesson to be learned is that expanding and bifurcating African-American communities demand an enlarged, diversified, and democratized political community of transformative leaders, activists, organizers, and organizations. Cross-cutting issues like AIDS necessitate a political strategy which is not driven by simple identity politics, replicating the idea that we can only work for and receive leadership from "one of our own." They necessitate, instead, a political analysis that makes central the differential interests that define the complex politics of black communities. This strategy will need to produce multiple organizations and leaders attending to the specific needs of different segments of black communities. Again, it would be a mistake to devalue the previous significant and sometimes transformational struggles that have been won by mobilized and radicalized black communities and leaders. However, in acknowledging past consensus victories, the forceful emergence of more cross-cutting issues requires a new movement built on the differential, yet intersecting, experiences with marginalization and resistance encountered by African Americans, poor people, and other people of color.

CHAPTER NINE

Women, Children, and Funding

Ronald Johnson, former director of the Minority Task Force on AIDS and "AIDS Czar" for New York City under Mayor David Dinkins, was quoted in a 1990 *New Republic* article as saying, "There's not one black or Hispanic legislator who has done a goddamned thing about AIDS in this city, state, or country. And that's disgusting" (Sullivan 1990, 23). Later, after being confronted with complaints over his outspokenness, Johnson revealed in an interview that

> after my statements [on the inaction of black legislators] were made public, I received a slap on the wrist from officials in the black community. But I told them, I'll retract the statement if you prove me wrong. . . . I don't know what will spur the community. These incremental advances will never get to a political mass that pushes toward a movement; just look at the AIDS statistics in Central Harlem, and we do nothing. We rely on the state's and city's benevolence to fund our programs. I have seen the leaders sitting around the table for two to three years, and there hasn't been one member of the Black Caucus there. In the New York State Legislature Assembly, member Arthur Eve has given one speech in one and a half years. All the legislative allies are white. The legislative heroes for the Ryan White Care Bill were all white.[1]

Mr. Johnson's comments, while clearly very damning, are not unique. Repeatedly, when talking to black AIDS activists, the question of leadership from black elected officials, is one that haunts those struggling against AIDS in African-American communities. Service providers, activists, and African Americans with AIDS question what appears to be a lack of interest or commitment to this issue on the part of black leaders. Keith Cylar, director of Housing Works, a program that secures housing for HIV-positive individuals, and former staff member of the Minority Task Force on AIDS, suggests that black elites have not only been ineffectual in their response to AIDS, but have more generally allowed the decay of health care systems in most black communities:

Health care generally has failed in the black community. Black officials have to take responsibility for the lack of quality health care in our communities. We have accepted this level of service because we have no political will. We hide behind the nationalism of racism. We don't hold our leaders accountable. They pursue an integrationist policy that allows them to control the masses.[2]

The lack of political will Cylar mentions is remarkably difficult to prove. As discussed in chapter 3, politicians have found low-cost ways to provide at least the appearance of being involved in political struggles concerning AIDS, increasing their association with this crisis over the years. Black congressional, state, and city officials have sponsored community meetings, written guest editorials in black newspapers, mentioned AIDS in their speeches, even voted for and cosponsored AIDS-related legislation. As a result, black elected officials challenge claims of inaction like those of Mr. Johnson and Mr. Cylar by pointing (usually around election time) to such efforts as proof that they have attended to the AIDS crisis in African-American communities.

Political practices such as these have long been identified by congressional scholars as low-cost ways for officials to act on an issue without too closely associating themselves with it, especially those issues perceived as controversial or costly (Hall 1996; Fiorina 1974; Miller 1964). While actions such as talking about the affect of AIDS on women and children may be cost-effective for black political leaders, they did little to redefine how the country, and specifically African Americans, understood the manifestation of AIDS in black communities. In light of this, AIDS activists have struggled, usually unsuccessfully, to push black representatives into doing more—authoring bills and becoming legislative leaders in the fight against AIDS. The data indicate however, that while many black officials were holding public meetings to inform the community of the pervasiveness of this epidemic—an important task—these same leaders shied away from major legislative action around AIDS, especially as it affected African-American communities. The issue, it seems, is not whether black elected officials have done anything about AIDS, but whether black elected officials have provided leadership, in particular transformative leadership, in the fight against AIDS in African-American communities. Phil Wilson, a well-known black AIDS activist and former co-chair of the National Black Lesbian and Gay Leadership Forum, argues that merely voting "the right way" does little to help black communities. What is needed, Wilson states, is visibility and leadership:

> They all vote the right way. Almost to a member they have stellar voting records. Do you know who benefits by that? White folks benefit by that. White gay men benefit by them voting the right way. If they want to save black lives, their voices, their visibility, that's what is going to save us. Without the visibility, without the voices, you know, being present and accounted for, the money isn't going to come to our community. I mean this whole notion of follow the money—if Ryan White was doing what it should be doing, you know, the money would be following the proportions of the epidemic, and it is not. . . .
>
> There are a number of people who are great people and they are there when we call them. And they do what we ask them to do when they are in Washington. I'm told that just last week Rangel did a great thing on needle exchange, you know, and I think that is wonderful. But I could give a flying fuck what they do in Washington to be completely honest with you. What I want Rangel to do, I want him to be in his district, talking to black folks about AIDS. I want there to be an AIDS appointment on his schedule every month in his district. I want him to do substantive speeches on AIDS in his district to black folks. If there was not a dime involved, and they did it on a consistent basis, this would be a very, very different epidemic. But as long as it is not on their front burner, the people who follow them, the people who look to them for leadership, it's not going to be on their front burner either.[3]

As discussed in chapter 2, this focus on the work of black elected officials—expecting them to lead the fight against AIDS in black communities—results in part from a history of marginalization, one in which group members come to believe that other marginal group members are more likely to understand their needs and thus advance their battles. Believing that they share a lived experience, marginal group members concentrate their expectations and hopes for progress in the actions of indigenous leaders and organizations. Again, this linked-fate philosophy of struggle and representation has fueled legislative and legal battles to create, maintain, and expand majority black voting districts, as well as to elect black mayors and city council members. In the case of AIDS, it has been the unrealized expectation, held by many black AIDS activists, of an indigenous and "authentically constructed" response to AIDS on the part of black elected officials that continues to frustrate these organizers. This chapter explores what these activists call the "on-again, off-again" political response to AIDS among black elected officials. Specifically, I am interested in the following question: To what extent and in what form did black elected officials *publicly* respond, embrace, and redefine AIDS as an issue for African-American communities? Most of this chapter focuses on black elected officials in Congress. The conclusion, however, turns to the local level, revisiting the response by black New York City elected officials to a proposed needle-exchange program.

Congress

Early in the epidemic, Congress was left to fill the funding and leadership gap left by President Ronald Reagan. Fortunately, Congressmen Weiss (D–NY) and Waxman (D–CA) took the lead in shaping the congressional response to AIDS, sponsoring the first hearings dealing with the AIDS epidemic. In 1982 Congressman Henry Waxman, with the significant help of congressional staffer Tim Westmoreland, held the first congressional hearing on what was then known as "GRID" at the Gay and Lesbian Community Services Center in Hollywood, California. The hearing included testimony by Dr. James Curran (then head of the CDC's Kaposi's Sarcoma and Opportunistic Infection Task Force), who attempted to evade questions concerning the effect of Reagan administration budget cuts on AIDS funding.

Recognizing the need for increased AIDS funding, especially in response to Reagan Administration policies, Congress—the few in Congress who were interested—focused their committees on overseeing and increasing spending for AIDS research. Interestingly, this drive to appropriate more funds was not accompanied by the usual clamor by members trying to specify who would and would not be receiving funding. Instead, it seems the unspoken assumption was that gay men would be the beneficiaries of this effort. This apparently untargeted funding drive was indeed contradictory to the normal operation of Congress, where members often fight to ensure that their constituencies, groups, or geographical locations are included in assessments of damage and resulting compensation. The stigma surrounding AIDS, however, resulted in most members of Congress demonstrating very little interest in associating their constituencies with this disease. Instead, a few members, usually those from districts with large and visible lesbian and gay communities, consistently pushed to ensure at least minimal amounts of funding and attention. Not until the mid to late 1980s did legislators begin to reconceptualize AIDS as yet another possible funding source in the race to win prizes for their constituents and districts. Not coincidentally, it was during this period that congressional members representing poor urban districts, many harboring disproportionate numbers of people of color with AIDS, began to engage in greater numbers in legislative battles around AIDS.

Funding levels were not all that received the time and energy of congressional members involved in the fight against AIDS; they also tried to oversee the federal government's response to AIDS, especially that emanating from the executive branch. For example, *The Review of the Public Health Service's Response to AIDS*, so often cited by academics and policy analysts, was requested by a coalition of congressional committees—including the Subcommittee on Health and the Environment, the House Committee on Energy and Commerce, the Subcommittee on Intergovernmental Relations and Human Resources, and the House Committee on Government Operations. As was the case in trying to appropriate AIDS funding, congressional staff members received little cooperation from Reagan administration officials as they tried to monitor the implementation of funding decisions and policy initiatives. AIDS experts and activists have suggested that without congressional oversight of the Reagan administration and the Public Health Service, even less would have been done to curb this epidemic (Shilts 1987; Panem 1988).

Often overlooked when reviewing the early activity of congressional members in response to AIDS are the attempts by some legislators to restrict the rights and freedoms of people with AIDS (Tokaji 1994). Numerous amendments and bills were introduced requiring mandatory AIDS testing; the quarantining of those who test positive; and the prohibition of those who are HIV positive from working with children, attending schools, or being employed by hospitals and clinics. Legislation attempting to criminalize those who unknowingly passed on the AIDS virus was also a part of the congressional response to AIDS. Former Surgeon General Koop (1991) recounted a phone call from former California Congressman William Dannemeyer, a leading sponsor of such legislation. Dannemeyer was intent on trying to convince Koop to "decree" that mandatory testing and quarantining would be part of the Administration's response to AIDS. Koop writes,

Dannemeyer advocated mandatory testing for the entire nation, the quarantine of all those who tested positively, and a law that would make it a felony for people to "exchange body fluids" if they were contaminated with the virus.

One evening he [Dannemeyer] called me at home: "Chick, why won't you get on with mandatory testing of the entire country?"

"I've told you, that's not within the power of the Surgeon General, but for reasons I've also explained over and over, I wouldn't do it if I could. But suppose just for the sake of argument, I could and did. Suppose I called you next week and said I now knew who every seropositive person was in the whole United States. What would you do?"

After a long pause, Dannemeyer, as I recall, replied, "Wipe them off the face of the earth!" (208)

Dennis Altman (1987) underscores this point, highlighting the restrictive and often homophobic intentions of some congressional members. Altman notes, in particular, the concerns of Dr. David Sundwall, advisor for the Senate Labor and Human Resources Committee chaired by Senator Orrin Hatch of Utah: "Sundwall says that he and Hatch took pains to make sure that their important Senate health panel did not get its hands on an AIDS funding bill, because of the intensely homophobic make-up of the committee" (115–16).

A review of congressional activity early in the epidemic makes it clear that there was no monolithic, inclusive, and tolerant response to AIDS on the part of Congress. A few congressional leaders attempted to supplement the government's response to the epidemic; however, there were also congressional leaders who, like members of the Reagan administration, viewed AIDS as the fault of "bad people," and deserving of restrictive and repressive policies. In these cases, an ideology that defined gay men, lesbians, and drug users as something less than equal was used to justify an outright attack on members of these groups. More recently, both forms of legislative activity—those which seek to distribute benefits and those which seek to prohibit behavior— have continued to shape the agenda of congressional members. Interestingly, the heterogeneity of communities affected by AIDS also has brought into focus a new issue, namely, the disparities that exist among groups living with AIDS. In trying to ensure that all those who are infected get counted as well as receive their fair share of funds and programs, Congress has had to grapple with an expanding definition of those at-risk and suffering from AIDS. And yet, little of this work has evolved into active challenges to the normative judgments they attach to groups marked by AIDS. While inclusive in the benefits they bestow, much of the discussion on the floor and in hearings reiterates the familiar dichotomy between innocent victims and those who brought this disease upon themselves. The response from congressional members representing marginalized groups disproportionately affected by AIDS seems largely to mirror the activity seen in the rest of the Congress, with the actions of these members being more conciliatory than challenging over the years.

Within black communities, the role played by black elected officials in responding to AIDS is generally perceived by activists as being at best minimal and at worst nonexistent.[4] In this characterization, activists do acknowledge that AIDS now appears on the long list of ills confronting black communities recited by black leaders. Further, AIDS has also been incorporated into the speeches and guest editorials by black elected officials. And more often than not, black elected officials vote for and occasionally sponsor bills thought to improve the lives of people with AIDS. But in spite of such gains, it is still generally agreed that few black elected officials have used their public status to lead the fight against AIDS in black communities. Recently, Representative Louis Stokes (D–OH), chair of the Congressional Black Caucus's health committee, commented that AIDS is an issue that "black leadership has shied away from" (Stolberg, *New York Times*, 29 June 1998, A12).

In African-American communities the silence and stifled actions of congressional leaders is especially troubling when one recognizes the community's marginal status and general mistrust of the government in conjunction with the elevated status of indigenous leaders. As noted in chapter 3, the formal political incorporation of black voters through the passage of the Voting Rights Act in 1965 initiated the second influx of black Americans into public office, including the Congress. The first formal election of substantial numbers of black officials occurred during Reconstruction and officially ended in 1901, when George H. White, "the last black congressman of the post-Reconstruction era," left Congress (Bennett 1984). Despite the legacy of Jim Crow, increasing numbers of black Americans have secured the vote late in the twentieth century and we can, consequently, trace a parallel increase in the number of blacks elected to office (L. Williams 1987; E. Williams 1982). For instance, in 1981, when AIDS first emerged into the public view, there were nineteen black members of Congress. By the final session of Congress under review in this analysis (1993–94), the number of black con-

Table 9.1   Number and percentage of black Americans serving in Congress during
the AIDS epidemic

Congressional session	Years	Number of black congressional members	Percentage of black House members	Percentage of black Senate members
97	1981–83	19	4.4	0
98	1983–85	21	4.8	0
99	1985–87	21	4.8	0
100	1987–89	23	5.3	0
101	1989–91	25[a]	5.7	0
102	1991–93	28[b]	6.4	0
103	1993–95	41[c]	9.2	1

Source: Data from Congressional Research Service.

[a]Representative Mickey Leland (D–TX) was killed in a plane crash on 7 August 1989.
He was replaced in the 101st Congress by Craig Washington. Therefore, while twenty-
five blacks served in the 101st Congress, only twenty-four served at any one time.

[b]Representative William Gray, III (D–PA) resigned during the 102nd Congress and
was replaced by Representative Lucien Blackwell. Also Eva Clayton (D–NC) was
elected on 5 November 1992 to the 102nd Congress to fill the vacancy caused by the
death of Representative Walter Jones. Therefore, while twenty-eight Blacks served in
the 102nd Congress, only twenty-seven served at any one time.

[c]Representative Michael Espy (D–MS) resigned on 25 January 1993 to become
secretary of agriculture. He was replaced by Bennie Thompson. Therefore, while forty-
one blacks served in the 103rd Congress (including Senator Carol Moseley-Braun),
only forty served at any one time.

gressional members had increased to forty-one, as table 9.1 shows. It
is also obvious from table 9.1 that while blacks may have made inroads
into Congress, their relative power—in terms of pure demographic par-
ity—still remains suppressed.

Numerous questions or doubts arise about the substantive and symbolic importance of having increasing numbers of African Americans
in Congress. For example, Carol Swain (1993) suggests that black
Americans may be equally well served, at least in terms of voting records, by liberal whites as by blacks in Congress. Thus, according to
Swain, we need not concern ourselves with the election of more black
officials from predominately black districts. On a different note, Lani
Guinier (1994) argues that concern over the statistical representation
of blacks in Congress has diverted attention from the more substantive
goals of transforming institutions to produce "fairness in the competition for favorable policy outcomes" and leaders committed to the empowerment of "the dispossessed (69–70)." Despite this recent scholar-
ship, I would dare say that most African Americans still believe that
black representatives are needed in Congress because they are more

attentive to the needs and concerns of black communities (Hall 1996; Stevens, Mulhollan, and Rundquist 1981; Barnett 1977). This sentiment is illustrated in a joint statement by members of the Congressional Black Caucus, prior to a meeting with President Nixon: "Our concerns and obligations as members of Congress do not stop at the boundaries of our districts; our concerns are national and international in scope. We are petitioned daily by citizens living hundreds of miles from our districts who look on us as congressmen-at-large for black people and poor people in the United States" (Barnett 1977, 4). This line of thinking would lead one to expect that black congressional members—those representatives more in tune with the needs of African-American communities—would recognize the devastation of AIDS upon black communities and lead the legislative and public relations fight against this scourge. Why then did we not see this type of leadership on the question of AIDS?

Using a number of legislative research tools, I examined the political actions of black congressional members in response to AIDS.[5] Legi-Slate, an electronic research tool reporting on legislative activity, allowed me to compare the general participation patterns of black congressional members around the topics of health and AIDS. Specifically, I wanted to know whether the legislative activity of black members looks generally the same across these areas and if it has intensified or lessened over the course of the AIDS epidemic. In this part of the analysis I focus on those bills or amendments in which black members were primary sponsors.[6] We must note that a number of the bills identified through a general search of the subject area "acquired immune deficiency" may be only tangentially related to the subject of AIDS—such as much larger appropriation bills that include only a small section dealing with the funding of AIDS programs. Therefore, we must be very cautious when using the sponsorship of this type of legislation to infer a representative's direct connection and commitment to the issue of AIDS.

To gain a deeper understanding of a black member's willingness to commit political resources to the issue of AIDS, I turned to a more limited set of AIDS votes. By AIDS votes I mean those *recorded* (roll call) votes that were specifically in reference to a piece of legislation or amendment dealing *only* or *predominantly* with the issue of AIDS. For example, votes on amendments focusing on AIDS are included in this set; however, a final bill which may include the amendment as the only section of the bill dealing with AIDS would not be included. As a result, votes on omnibus bills, especially budget bills, were eliminated. Additionally, any bill or amendment dealing specifically with AIDS but decided by voice vote was also deemed ineligible for this set of votes, since voice votes did not allow me to track the specific behavior of each congressional member. Using the *Congressional Quarterly Weekly Report*, the *Congressional Quarterly Roll Call*, the *Congressional Information Service/Annual Legislative Histories*, the *Congressional Record* and Legi-Slate, I identified a set of forty recorded AIDS votes.

Congressional scholars will undoubtedly recognize the limitations of even this more topic-specific analysis. Examination of votes and floor participation, while conveying part of the picture on the interest and effort of legislators, misses numerous other opportunities for House and Senate members to influence AIDS legislation (Hall 1996; Rieselbach 1990; Oppenheimer 1985; Price 1972). For example, this type of analysis will never tell us what happened during the subcommittee and full committee markup of AIDS bills (Hall 1996). Also unaccounted for are the efforts of representatives to influence the rules committee or the witness list for public hearings (Sinclair 1994). Lost to my analysis are the "Dear Colleague" letters and other informal methods congressional members use to influence the outcome of legislative initiatives. Floor debates also can be dominated by minority party members who have less power in the committee structure, so paying attention to floor activity alone may bias our understanding of which individuals are most active around an issue. Finally, and possibly most important, we know that most roll call votes are largely influenced by the member's party affiliation (Kingdon 1981; Clausen 1973; Mayhew 1966). Thus, roll call votes in some cases can be understood as largely symbolic and partisan acts that do not begin to represent the behind-the-scenes dealings where legislators truly exert political power and resources.

Even with all of its limitations, however, analysis of roll call votes and accompanying floor activity can begin to sketch a more accurate picture of the observable and publicly documented political actions of elected officials around controversial issues as well as the ways an issue or policy agenda evolves over time (Sinclair 1982; Brady 1978). This analysis can tell us who were the primary sponsors and cosponsors of AIDS specific bills and amendments; it allows us to see who made a statement during floor debates or who inserted comments later into the *Congressional Record* through the extension of remarks. It also presents us with the opportunity to see which black members voted against their party and under what circumstances. One must not forget that the stigma associated with AIDS made many congressional members reluctant to engage in even symbolic acts that could be perceived as benefiting the most vilified groups with AIDS—gay men and drug users. It would, therefore, be a mistake to think of acts such as voting for or sponsoring a piece of legislation dealing with AIDS as merely symbolic acts without real consequences for legislators. Thus, with all of its limitations, this data begins to outline how, when, and in what form black congressional members chose to intervene in legislative debates around AIDS.

Finally, after reviewing the voting patterns and legislative efforts of black congressional members, I tried to gain a bit more specificity by examining the political activity of black members in response to one specific bill—the Ryan White Comprehensive AIDS Resources Emergency (CARE) Act of 1990, considered by many as one of the most important pieces of AIDS legislation to be approved during the epidemic. I was interested in the role black elected officials played in its initiation, redesign, passage, and implementation. By focusing on the legislative history of this bill and a few other selective public hearings, I examined more closely the full array of interventions marshaled by black congressional members to shape this legislation. Such an examination also allowed me to explore the rhetorical framing of AIDS by black members. Which groups living with AIDS in African-American communities were most often referred to as a reason to act? Were women and children, in tandem, mobilized, as they have been by other institutions and leaders in black communities, to justify the minimal attention devoted to injection drug users, while leaders continued to ignore the plight of black gay men?

A cursory look at the data presented in tables 9.1 through 9.4 begins to sketch out black legislative activity around AIDS and other health issues. Tables 9.1 and 9.2 indicate that the legislative activity of black congressional members, at least in the form of sponsoring bills, has increased almost as steadily as the number of blacks elected to Congress has increased.[7] A similar pattern is evident in table 9.3 regarding the introduction of bills dealing with health and AIDS. As we might expect, the period that corresponds with the AIDS epidemic, has seen continuous growth in the attention paid to the issue of health by the entire Congress—at least as attention is signified in the number of bills being introduced—culminating with the national debate over, and the eventual defeat of, the Clinton health plan. In congruence with their

Table 9.2   Health bills sponsored by black members of Congress during the
AIDS epidemic

Congressional session	Total number of bills sponsored by black members	Health bills sponsored by black members	Total health bills sponsored during session	Percent of health bills sponsored by black members
97	261	39	1,847	2
98	352	64	2,157	3
99	432	71	2,366	3
100	443	135	3,008	4.5
101	406	131	3,584	3.7
102	431	163	3,923	4.2
103	532	221	3,385	6.5

Source: Legi-Slate.
Note: The term *sponsor* refers to those black members who served as primary
sponsors of legislation.

Table 9.3   AIDS bills sponsored by black members of Congress during the
AIDS epidemic

Congressional session	Total numbers of bills sponsored by black members	AIDS bills sponsored by black members	Total AIDS bills sponsored during session	Percent of AIDS bills sponsored by black members
97	261	0	0	—
98	352	0	11	0%
99	432	2	29	6.9
100	443	9	130	6.9
101	406	10	123	8.1
102	431	6	152	3.9
103	532	13	152	8.5

Source: Legi-Slate.
Note: The term *sponsor* refers to those black members who served as primary
sponsors of legislation.

colleagues, black congressional members have also demonstrated a
nearly steady increase—with the exception of the 101st and 102nd
Congresses—in the number of health bills for which they were the
primary sponsors.

Table 9.3 focuses specifically on AIDS-related legislation and outlines a number of familiar patterns, including an increase in the number of AIDS-related bills introduced and an increase in the percent of
such bills sponsored by black representatives. As with health, the number of bills dealing with AIDS introduced in each successive session
of Congress has generally increased over the course of the epidemic,

Table 9.4   Categories of sponsorship for AIDS-related bills by black
congressional members

	Sponsor new program or grant that is AIDS-related	Sponsor AIDS-specific amendment to established program	Sponsor large appropriation bill that includes money for AIDS	Sponsor resolution dealing with AIDS	Procedural
Number	13	14	7	5	1
Percent	32.5	35	17.5	12.5	2.5

Source: Legi-Slate.
Note: The term *sponsor* refers to those black members who served as primary
sponsors of legislation.

except for the 101st Congress. The most dramatic increase is between
the 99th and 100th Congresses, when the number of bills introduced
jumped from 29 to 130. Through the 100th to the 103rd Congresses,
the number of AIDS bills introduced remained relatively constant, averaging in the mid-hundreds. Interestingly, the percentage of AIDS
bills sponsored by black congressional members showed no corresponding increase, moving only slightly between 7 and 8 percent. Thus
in the 99th Congress, when 29 bills dealing with or including AIDS
were introduced, 6.9 percent of them had a black member as the primary sponsor, and in the 100th Congress, when 130 bills dealing with
or including AIDS were introduced, 6.9 percent of those bills also had
a black primary sponsor. In fact, the constant level of black sponsorship is one of the interesting patterns to be found in table 9.3.

The types of AIDS-related bills sponsored by black members are outlined in table 9.4. Sponsorship of bills dealing with AIDS has come
predominately in three forms. The first is the introduction of bills seeking to establish new programs or grants that would include attention
to AIDS. This path, which accounts for nearly a third (32.5 percent) of
all sponsorship among black members, includes bills like the Abandoned Infants Assistance Act of 1988 sponsored by Major Owens (D–
NY) or the Intravenous Substance Abuse and AIDS Prevention Act of
1987 sponsored by Charles Rangel (D–NY). The second means of sponsorship works through the introduction of AIDS-specific amendments
to established programs, such as the Public Health Service Act. Often
these amendments seek to expand current programs or restructure
funding plans to include populations living with AIDS. This form of

legislative activity accounts for over a third (35 percent) of all the AIDS-related bills sponsored by black members. The third vehicle through which sponsorship occurs is the introduction of large appropriation bills which include money for AIDS programs and services. This process is what we might call coincidental sponsorship, since often members have no interest in or ownership over the provisions in the bill focusing on AIDS. As noted above, when black members are listed as primary sponsors of large appropriation bills that include funds for AIDS services, programs, or research, the representative may have little or no intent to provide action or leadership on the issue of AIDS. As is noted in table 9.4, this method generated nearly a fifth (17.5 percent) of all AIDS-related bills sponsored by black congressional members.

More data are needed to answer the question of whether black congressional members led the legislative battle around AIDS in black communities. The general outline of sponsorship patterns just detailed above provides at best a mixed picture of black leadership on the issue of AIDS. It would be extremely difficult to base a credible story of sustained leadership by black congressional members on the issue of AIDS from the data in these three tables. However, this initial data seems to suggest that, far from being completely inattentive, black representatives did, possibly at times unintentionally, engage in political activity in response to AIDS—sponsoring legislation that included AIDS, however minimally. More specifically, tables 9.1 and 9.3 directly contradict the idea that black officials have done nothing regarding AIDS. If we compare the percentage of House members who are black and the percentage of AIDS bills sponsored by black members, we find that between 1985 and 1990 black members sponsored a larger percentage of AIDS bills than we might expect merely from their statistical representation in the Congress. On the other hand black representatives seem to have ignored the issue of AIDS during the early years of the epidemic as well as later in the 102nd Congress. No doubt there are very real limits to the conclusions we can draw from this purely statistical comparison of representation, but it does offer low-level support to the contention by black elected officials that they have been active, if even minimally, in response to this crisis.

A more detailed analysis of black congressional members in relation to AIDS-related votes is needed if we want to assess their behavior on the specific issue of AIDS. To begin this task, I analyzed black congressional activity around "AIDS votes" in the House. The initial list of possible AIDS votes was generated by cross-referencing and examining all the AIDS bills and riders identified by a number of legislative research tools and indexes. After eliminating bills not predominantly dealing with AIDS or decided by voice vote, I was able to identify forty recorded AIDS votes covering 1981–94. The data I assembled for this analysis included a description of the bill, amendment, or motion under consideration; the vote of all black members in that specific Congress; if the member voted with the party and in the majority; and whether each representative engaged in a number of other legislative activities such as making a statement about AIDS on the floor, sponsoring an amendment, or entering comments in the extension of remarks.[8]

A review of this data indicates that on most AIDS votes, black members primarily voted with their party. This most often meant that they voted with the other members of the Democratic party and in the majority. This pattern of party loyalty is particularly evident in their voting against a number of restrictive and discriminatory amendments. For example, in 1987 all black House members voted with the majority of other Democrats and in the majority to defeat an amendment introduced by representative Dannemeyer to HR 558, "Urgent Relief for the Homeless." This amendment mandated that all homeless persons receiving medical assistance under the bill be tested for AIDS. Similarly, in the same year all but one black Congressional member, Cardiss Collins (D–IL), voted with the majority of other Democrats, but in the minority, to oppose a Dannemeyer amendment to HR 162, "High-Risk Occupational Disease." This amendment required that all medical professionals and emergency-care workers be warned they were at risk of contracting AIDS.

Interestingly, while this pattern of general black Democratic unity in opposition to restrictive AIDS amendments can be identified throughout the course of the epidemic, the voting solidarity of black members was sometimes broken. The subject of homosexuality, more than any other AIDS-related topic, seemed to generate dissension. While many who focus on what is believed to be the more intense homophobia in black communities might expect black members to break ranks with other black representatives and the majority of Democratic party members to vote for "anti-gay" legislation, in fact we see the opposite. Specifically, we find a few bold, black representatives willing to forego the presumed unity of black members and the voting instructions of the Democratic leadership to oppose largely homophobic legislation. For example, an amendment introduced in 1985 by former Representative Dornan (R–CA) to HR 3424, "Labor, Health, and Human Services, Education Appropriations" authorized the surgeon general to use certain research funds to close or quarantine bathhouses or massage parlors if they are found to facilitate the spread of AIDS. This measure received significant support from Democratic congressional members, receiving 240 out of 246 Democratic votes. However, five of the nineteen black members able to vote that day voted against the amendment. The "no" votes of Representatives William Clay (D–MO), John Conyers (D–MI), George Crockett (D–MI), Ronald Dellums (D–CA), and Mervyn Dymally (D–CA) constituted five of the six "no" votes registered by Democrats that day. Furthermore, the "no" votes of these black representatives represented five of the total eight "no" votes recorded in the Congress as a whole on the proposed amendment.

A similar stance against the majority and other Democrats was staged in 1987, this time by the majority of voting black congressional members. In a motion to HR 3058, "Labor, Health and Human Services, Education Appropriation," Rep. Dannemeyer instructed the conferees on the 1988 Appropriations bill to accept Senate language prohibiting the CDC from funding AIDS education or information activities that "promote or encourage, directly or indirectly, homosexual sexual activities." Again in defiance of the majority, eleven of the eighteen black members voting on this measure voted "no." This time the eleven "no" votes of black congressional members constituted nearly a fourth of the forty-six Democratic "no" votes as well as the final forty-seven "no" votes recorded by the entire Congress. In contrast, black congressional leaders such as current and former Representatives Mike Espy (D–MS), Floyd Flake (D–NY), William Gray (D–PA), Kweisi Mfume (D–MD), Charles Rangel (D–NY), Gus Savage (D–IL), and Alan Wheat (D–MO) all supported this motion.

It would be a mistake to think that the controversy over issues pertaining to homosexuality dissipated as the epidemic raged on. As late as 1994 an amendment to HR 6, "Elementary and Secondary Education Reauthorization" by Representative Hancock (R–MO), as amended by Representative Unsoeld (D–WA), prohibiting education agencies from using federal money appropriated through this bill to distribute material to students that encourages or supports homosexuality as a positive lifestyle, still motivated substantial disagreement among black congressional members. On this specific measure twenty-eight black House members and the sole black Senate member, Carol Moseley-Braun, voted against the amendment, while nine black House members voted with the Democratic and congressional majority in favor of the proposal. Throughout the legislative history of the AIDS epidemic, concerns over gay and lesbian lifestyles have led to tensions and differences among black congressional members rarely found in response to other AIDS policy and legislative initiatives.

While issues relating to gay and lesbian sexuality were more apt to produce marked dissension among black congressional members, other interests, such as a representative's personal opinion about some policy initiative or the concerns of business elites in their districts also seemed to motivate slightly different voting patterns. For example, in 1992 Representatives Charles Rangel (D–NY) and Gary Franks (R–CT) were the only two black members of Congress to vote in favor of a complicated motion to S 1306, "Alcohol, Drug Abuse, and Mental Health Administration Reorganization," sponsored by Representative Newt Gingrich (R–GA). The motion sought to prohibit the use of federal funds to support needle-exchange programs. The votes registered by both Representatives Rangel and Franks were not a surprise since Rangel had long voiced his opposition to needle-exchange programs, and Franks was socially conservative on many issues. In another instance, Representative Mike Espy was the lone black congressional member to vote "yes" with the Republican and congressional majority in support of an amendment to HR 2273, "Americans with Disabilities Act." This amendment allowed employers to move an employee with a communicable disease, such as AIDS, out of a food-handling position. We might guess that the substantial interests of the poultry industry located in Mr. Espy's district possibly figured into his decision to vote for this amendment. Thus, like other congressional members, black representatives take into consideration district and personal concerns when making voting decisions.

Most recently the AIDS vote that prompted the greatest debate and opposition from black congressional members was a rider to the 1993 National Institutes of Health Reauthorization bill HR 4 (S 1), attempting to prevent the permanent immigration of persons infected with HIV. On the specific motion, instructing the House conferees to agree to the Senate amendment to prevent the immigration of HIV-positive persons, twenty-eight of thirty-four black congressional members (including Senator Carol Moseley-Braun) recorded a "no" vote, voting against the Democratic majority and the larger congressional majority supporting this amendment. Black House members made up nearly one half of the 57 "no" votes registered by House Democrats. The story, however, does not end with this vote on the amendment, because in many ways this measure serves as an example of the level of compromise involved in legislative activity. Specifically, it is often an AIDS rider—an amendment that differs substantially from the main body of the legislation under consideration—that best signals a representative's attitudes toward the issue of AIDS. So while most black congressional members voted against the motion detailed above, all black House members voted for the final Reauthorization bill containing the approved amendment.

Again, the AIDS votes detailed above in no way fully describe the activity of black congressional members. Furthermore, from this data we know nothing about other constraints, such as the composition of a district, that might lead a member to vote one way or another. Left uncontrolled for are characteristics such as the percent gay in a district, which might sway a vote here or there. However, even with its limits, this data does suggest that far from being either invisible or leaders in legislative battles pertaining to AIDS, black congressional members might be considered, instead, good foot soldiers in the war against AIDS. They consistently voted—except in a few cases—for legislation which sought to provide resources to protect the rights of and generally empower people with AIDS. Furthermore, in a political environment in which conservative Republicans, through the introduction of extremists measures, made the sponsoring and support of nonpunitive AIDS legislation costly, black members were willing to vote for such measures as well as, on occasion, vote against their party and the majority. This interpretation should not be read as vindication from accusations that black elected leaders have done little or nothing in response to AIDS. Instead, this information begins to clarify the indictment and the actual role of black House and Senate members in congressional struggles over AIDS. From the evidence presented so far, it seems that black leaders have supported AIDS-friendly initiatives, most often introduced by other representatives. However, with this data we can say little about their efforts to redefine and transform thinking about this epidemic, especially as it raged in African-American communities.

For example, in 1987 HR 2881 sought to establish the National AIDS Commission. As we would predict, all black congressional members voted in favor of this bill. However, it was former Representative William Richardson (D–NM), a Latino Democratic member of the House, who requested on the floor "that in the naming of the commission that there be minority representation on the commission, and, second, that there be a detailed study of the AIDS problems of minorities and the preventative steps that might be taken to address minorities as AIDS victims and cures" (*Congressional Record* 1987, 22241). I am not suggesting that black members did nothing to support this effort, but put simply these officials found low-cost ways to participate. Representatives Lewis (D–GA) and Leland (D–TX) were two of the eighty-four cosponsors of the bill. Congressman Rangel (D–NY) entered a statement into the legislative history printed in the *Congressional Record.* However, Congressman Rangel's comments, as chairman of the Select Committee on Narcotics Abuse and Control, focused on the spread of AIDS, in particular to women, by injection drug use—avoiding any direct comment on the impact of AIDS on African-American communities.

Again, my examination of the forty AIDS votes in this sample reveals little evidence to suggest that most black representatives engaged in any public activity beyond voting "the right way." And while far from conclusive, analysis of the floor statements and the extension of remarks surrounding these AIDS votes indicates that most often these efforts were insignificant in shaping either the design of legislation or the congressional and national debate surrounding the AIDS epidemic. Rarely did black legislators attempt to draw attention to the disproportionate impact of AIDS on African-American and other communities of color. In only three of the votes examined did black representatives include as a part of their floor statements or extension of remarks a direct reference to and discussion of the changing demographics of this epidemic—highlighting the increasing manifestation of AIDS among women, black, Latino, and other communities of color. Black legislators instead focused their comments on the merits or liabilities of specific bills. And on those few occasions when black members did engage the question of race, it was most often to highlight the inclusive and equally threatening presence of AIDS across communities. For example, Representative Louis Stokes (D–OH) in a statement made during a floor debate on AIDS federal policy characterizes AIDS as a disease "affecting people of all ages, sexes, and races" (*Congressional Record* 1988, H-8000). Similarly, Representative Donald Payne (D–NJ) articulating the need for the "AIDS Prevention Act (1990)" talks of an inclusive threat from HIV and AIDS: "This killer disease does not respect sex, age, or ethnicity. AIDS and HIV, . . . are found in men and women, adults and children, whites, Latinos, African Americans, and other ethnic groups" (*Congressional Record* 1990, H-3540).

Interestingly, when black representatives did discuss the unique manifestation of AIDS in African-American communities, it was often to highlight the high incidence of transmission through injection drug use as opposed to male-to-male sex. Repeatedly black congressional members chose to ignore the extreme devastation and rates of infection black gay men experienced as they provided the first wave of the response to this disease in black communities. For instance, when Representative Payne (D–NJ) attempted to sketch out the unique development of AIDS in many New Jersey communities as compared to the rest of the country, the one major group missing from his description was gay men:

> Newark and New Jersey are also different from other cities and States in that a majority of our AIDS cases are not related to homosexual activity. Nationally, 67 percent of the reported AIDS cases are among homosexual and bisexual men. The pattern is different in New Jersey, where over 53 percent of AIDS cases are among intravenous drug abusers. . . .
>
> New Jersey also has a relatively high incidence of HIV infection in women, children, and adolescents. One quarter of those who have contracted AIDS through IV drug use are women. . . .
>
> Infants and children with AIDS make up 3 percent of New Jersey's total AIDS cases. This proportion is also larger than any other State. . . .
>
> AIDS is particularly devastating New Jersey's urban minority communities. A black in New Jersey has 12.4 times the chance of contracting AIDS compared to the average white American. (*Congressional Record* 1990, H-3540)

Representative Payne is to be commended for his attention to AIDS in communities of color and especially to its devastating impact on women. However, in naming the multiple groups suffering from AIDS the only group in New Jersey that Rep. Payne does not discuss in detail is gay men, in particular gay men of color. In his description, gay men with AIDS are only offered as a reference point to demonstrate the significant differences in the manifestation of AIDS in New Jersey. Interestingly, while New Jersey did look substantially different from other parts of the United States dealing with AIDS, in 1990 the second largest route of transmission among those classified as having AIDS in New Jersey was male-to-male sex.

It seems that black congressional members like Representative Payne were intent, when possible, on portraying AIDS either as a disease equally threatening to all in the general public or affecting those respectable and innocent segments of communities of color—women and children—that deserved sympathy and support. Disproportionately, black members sought to highlight the plight of "respectable" victims—women and children—living with AIDS, minimizing the attention directed at black gay men and black men who sleep with men. Ironically, the prevalence of HIV and AIDS among black injection drug users was deployed to separate black communities from (white) lesbian and gay communities. Part of the motivation for such actions by black congressional members seems to be tied to the belief, developed through a history of marginalization, that the respectability and progress of African Americans is put at risk every time behaviors labeled "non-normative" or culturally deviant are associated with black Americans. Furthermore, it seems that black elected officials also bought into the idea, articulated in chapter 4 by Dr. James Curran, that as AIDS became known increasingly as a disease of communities of color, support for AIDS programs and funding among the public and elected officials would correspondingly decrease. In response to this threat black officials repeatedly framed AIDS as a plague threatening all Americans and not as a disease devastating black communities. Clearly, both of these images are true, but it was the active choice to promote one image over the other that suggests a fear of greater stigmatization and loss of support if AIDS was marked by a race other than white. Finally, I specifically say threatening to all *Americans,* since very few black congressional members demonstrated any interest in linking the political battles around AIDS in black communities to the development of AIDS in, for instance, central Africa.

Again, one must be cautious in drawing conclusions, since black congressional members participated in numerous ways beyond those presented to this point. For example, table 9.5 provides us with information about the participation of black members in the public hearings associated with the Ryan White CARE Act of 1990. Every major bill, like Ryan White, has as part of its legislative history a number of public hearings sponsored by one or more committees and subcommittees in the House and Senate. These hearings are used to examine public concern surrounding the legislative topic, providing testimony from experts, agency officials, activists, and the affected public. Congressional hearings are thus one more way that members can demonstrate leadership in an issue area that is of substantive importance to them or their constituencies. To explore the role of black congressional members in

Table 9.5 Public hearings listed in the congressional history of the Ryan White Comprehensive Act of 1990

Hearings (Total = 23 dates)	Committee	Date	Black members in attendance	All other members in attendance	Black members on committee
Pediatric AIDS Hearing	Select Committee on Narcotics	7/27/87	Rangel, Towns	Gilman (ranking Rep. on committee), Green (not a committee member), Weiss, D'Amato (Senator)	Chair Rangel, C. Collins, W. Fauntroy, E. Towns
AIDS Crisis in Two American Cities—New York City (held on site)	Subcommittee on Human Resources (Gov Ops)	9/18/87	Conyers (senior ranking Dem.)	Weiss (chair)	Conyers (subcommittee member), C. Collins, Owens, Towns
AIDS Crisis in Two American Cities—San Francisco (held on site)	Subcommittee on Human Resources (Gov Ops)	11/23/87	Conyers	Weiss (chair) Pelosi Boxer	Conyers, C. Collins, Owens, Towns
Children and HIV Infection (Part 1)	Subcommittee on Human Resources (Gov Ops)	2/22/89	Payne	Weiss (chair), Waxman (D–CA), Pelosi (D–CA), L. Smith, P. Smith	Conyers (Chair), C. Collins, Owens, Towns, Payne (subcommittee member)
Children and HIV Infection (Part 2)	Subcommittee on Human Resources (Gov Ops)	2/23/89	Payne	Weiss (chair) Waxman Pelosi P. Smith	Conyers (Chair), C. Collins, Owens, Towns, Payne
AIDS Epidemic in Newark (held on site)	Subcommittee on Human Resources (Gov Ops)	3/27/89	Payne (D–NJ), Conyers (chair, Gov Ops, MI)	Weiss (chair)	Conyers (Chair), C. Collins, Owens, Towns, Payne

AIDS Epidemic in Detroit (held on site)	Subcommittee on Human Resources (Gov Ops)	4/24/89	Payne, Conyers (Chair, Gov Ops)	Weiss (chair)	Conyers (Chair), C. Collins, Owens, Towns, Payne
AIDS Issues (Part 1): AIDS Update	Subcommittee on Health (EC)	4/4/89	None	Waxman (chair), Rowland (D–GA), Dannemeyer (R–CA), Bliley (R–VA)	M. Lelard, C. Collins (both subcommittee members)
AIDS Issues (Part 1): AIDS and Other Epidemics	Subcommittee on Health (EC)	4/5/89	None	Waxman (chair), Rowland (D–GA), Dannemeyer (R–CA)	M. Leland, C. Collins
AIDS Issues (Part 1): Needle-Exchange Programs	Subcommittee on Health (EC)	4/24/89	None	Waxman (chair) Rowland Neilson	M. Leland, C. Collins
AIDS Issues (Part 1): Needle-Exchange Programs	Subcommittee on Health (EC)	7/19/89	Leland	Waxman (chair) Dannemeyer, Rowland, Neilson, Scheuer, Bruce	M. Leland, C. Collins
AIDS Issues (Part 2): Clinical Drug Development	Subcommittee on Health (EC)	7/20/89	None	Waxman (chair), Rowland, Whittaker, Neilson	M. Leland, C. Collins
AIDS Issues (Part 2): Confidentiality of AIDS Information	Subcommittee on Health (EC)	9/18/89	None	Waxman, Dannemeyer	C. Collins (subcommittee member)

(continued)

Table 9.5 *(continued)*

Hearings (Total = 23 dates)	Committee	Date	Black members in attendance	All other members in attendance	Black members on committee
Treatment and Care for Persons with HIV Infection and AIDS	Subcommittee on Human Resources (Gov Ops)	7/28/89	Payne	Weiss (chair) Pelosi, L. Smith, P. Smith	Conyers (Chair), C. Collins, Owens, Towns, Payne
Treatment and Care for Persons with HIV Infection and AIDS	Subcommittee on Human Resources (Gov Ops)	8/1/89	Payne	Weiss (chair) Pelosi, L. Smith	Conyers (chair), C. Collins, Owens, Towns, Payne (subcommitee member)
AIDS and Young Children in South Florida (held on site)	Select Committee on Children	8/7/89	None	Miller, Lehman (D–FL), Durbin (FL)	Wheat
AIDS Funding Issues (held in San Francisco)	Task Force on Human Resources (Budget)	1/16/90	None	Boxer (chair) Buechner	Espy (subcommittee member)
AIDS Funding Issues (held in San Francisco)	Task Force on Human Resources (Budget)	1/17/90	None	Boxer (chair) Buechner, Beilenson	Espy
AIDS Issues (Part 3): AIDS Epidemic and Medicare, HR4080	Subcommittee on Health (EC)	2/27/90	Towns	Rowland, Dannemeyer, Waxman (chair), Scheuer, Neilson	C. Collins, Towns

AIDS Issues (Part 3): Financing Treatment Services, HR4470	Subcommittee on Health (EC)	4/19/90	None	Waxman, Rowland, Dannemeyer, Neilson	C. Collins, Towns
AIDS Funding Issues: Impact Aid, Early Intervention, Research, and Prevention	Task Force on Human Resources (Budget)	3/7/90	Dinkins testifies. No black members attend, but several House members testify, namely, Schumer (NY), Pelosi (CA), Waxman (CA) and Weiss (NY).	Boxer and Panetta co-chairs. Rogers, Guarini, Durbin, Bryant	Espy (subcommittee member)
Pediatric AIDS	Task Force on Human Resources (Budget)	3/13/90	None	Boxer (chair)	Espy
Hospitals in Crisis: Financial Impact of AIDS on NYC's Hospitals	Task Force on Urgent Fiscal Issues (Budget)	4/6/90	None attend.	Schumer (chair)	Espy

the hearing process, I turn to the Ryan White Comprehensive AIDS Resources Emergency Act of 1990 (Public Law 101-381). Again, this bill is considered by many AIDS advocates and activists to be possibly the most important AIDS bill passed by Congress.[9] The bill amends the Public Health Service Act "to provide grants to improve the quality and availability of care for individuals and families with HIV disease and for other purposes" (CIS/INDEX Legislative Histories, January–December 1990, 101st Congress, 2nd session, 143). More specifically, the law established a grant program to cities with the most AIDS cases,[10] to states,[11] to public and private nonprofit entities that delivered primary health care,[12] and for demonstration projects aimed specifically at infants and children with HIV disease.[13] We might expect that a piece of legislation that sought to provide funding for those cities hardest hit by AIDS, usually the same cities disproportionately populated by African Americans and Latinos, would attract the participation of black members, many of whom come from districts located in or around these areas.

Furthermore, data on members' participation in public hearings can help us round out what we know about how members think and talk about particular issue areas. For example, tables 9.6–9.9 tell us that black members voted overwhelmingly in favor of the Ryan White CARE Act (HR 4785). The tables further indicate, however, that black members were only mildly involved in the floor legislative activity concerning this measure. In contrast table 9.5 provides a different (or at least a more detailed) picture of members' activity around this bill—one that highlights the legislative activity of black members before the bill reached the floor. The data in table 9.5 indicate that of the twenty-three House hearings associated with the Ryan White Act, ten of them were attended by at least one black member. A closer look, however, reveals that two representatives in particular, Conyers (D–MI) and Payne (D–NJ), were quite active around this bill, distinguishing themselves from other black legislators. Representatives Conyers and Payne were the only black members in attendance at eight of the ten hearings in which black legislators participated. Representative Conyers was present at four, and Representative Payne was in attendance, remarkably, at six hearings. In part their high rates of participation can be explained by their membership on relevant full committees and subcommittees. As indicated in table 9.5, Mr. Conyers was the chair of the House Government Operations Committee (Gov Ops) beginning in 1989, while Mr. Payne was a member of the Government Operations

Table 9.6 164. HR 4785. AIDS Prevention Act–Ryan White/Rule (1990)

	Actual Vote	Vote with party	Vote with majority	Extension of remarks	Statement during floor debate
164. HR 4785. AIDS Prevention Act/Rule. Adoption of the rule (H Res 408) to provide for House floor consideration of the bill to authorize emergency relief to cities with the largest numbers of AIDS cases, provide grants for health-care facilities to provide AIDS testing and counseling to help prevent the spread of AIDS, create a system to notify emergency workers of possible exposure to infectious diseases, authorize various other grant and demonstration projects, and require certain studies.					
Clay, William (D–MO)	Y	✓	✓		
Collins, Cardiss (D–IL)	Y	✓	✓		
Conyers, John (D–MI)	Y	✓	✓		
Crockett, George (D–MI)	NV				
Dellums, Ronald (D–CA)	NV				
Dixon, Julian (D–CA)	Y	✓	✓		
Dymally, Mervyn (D–CA)	Y	✓	✓		
Espy, Mike (D–MS)	Y		✓		
Flake, Floyd (D–NY)	NV				
Ford, Harold (D–TN)	Y	✓	✓		
Gray, William (D–PA)	Y	✓	✓		
Hawkins, Augustus (D–CA)	NV				
Hayes, Charles (D–IL)	Y	✓	✓		
Lewis, John (D–GA)	Y	✓	✓		
Mfume, Kweisi (D–MD)	Y	✓	✓		
Owens, Major (D–NY)	Y	✓	✓		
Payne, Donald (D–NJ)	Y	✓	✓		
Rangel, Charles (D–NY)	Y	✓	✓		
Savage, Gus (D–IL)	Y	✓	✓		
Stokes, Louis (D–OH)	Y	✓	✓		
Towns, Edolphus (D–NY)	Y	✓	✓		
Washington, Craig (D–TX)	NV				
Wheat, Alan (D–MO)	Y	✓	✓		✓

House Vote: 308–109
Democratic Party Vote: 247–0
Republican Party Vote: 61–109

Source: *Congressional Quarterly Roll Call*, 1990
Note: All members eligible to vote are listed. This list does not represent the total number of black members serving this Congress.

Table 9.7 166. HR 4785. AIDS Prevention Act–Ryan White/Name reporting, Rowland (1990)

	Actual Vote	Vote with party	Vote with majority	Extension of remarks	Statement during floor debate
166. HR 4785. AIDS Prevention Act/Name Reporting. Rowland, D–GA., substitute to the Dannemeyer, R–Calif., amendment to state that nothing shall be construed to require or prohibit a state from reporting to public health authorities identifying information about people testing positive for HIV, the virus that causes AIDS.					
Clay, William (D–MO)	Y	✓	✓		
Collins, Cardiss (D–IL)	Y	✓	✓		
Conyers, John (D–MI)	Y	✓	✓		
Crockett, George (D–MI)	Y	✓	✓		
Dellums, Ronald (D–CA)	Y	✓	✓		
Dixon, Julian (D–CA)	Y	✓	✓		
Dymally, Mervyn (D–CA)	Y	✓	✓		
Espy, Mike (D–MS)	Y	✓	✓		
Flake, Floyd (D–NY)	Y	✓	✓		
Ford, Harold (D–TN)	Y	✓	✓		
Gray, William (D–PA)	Y	✓	✓		
Hawkins, Augustus (D–CA)	NV				
Hayes, Charles (D–IL)	Y	✓	✓		
Lewis, John (D–GA)	Y	✓	✓		
Mfume, Kweisi (D–MD)	Y	✓	✓		
Owens, Major (D–NY)	Y	✓	✓		
Payne, Donald (D–NJ)	Y	✓	✓		
Rangel, Charles (D–NY)	Y	✓	✓		
Savage, Gus (D–IL)	Y	✓	✓		
Stokes, Louis (D–OH)	Y	✓	✓		
Towns, Edolphus (D–NY)	Y	✓	✓		
Washington, Craig (D–TX)	Y	✓	✓		
Wheat, Alan (D–MO)	Y	✓	✓		

House Vote: 312–113
Democratic Party Vote: 242–10
Republican Party Vote: 70–103

Source: *Congressional Quarterly Roll Call*, 1990
Note: All members eligible to vote are listed. This list does not represent the total number of black members serving this Congress.

Table 9.8   167. HR 4785. AIDS Prevention Act–Ryan White/Name reporting, Dannemeyer (1990)

	Actual Vote	Vote with party	Vote with majority	Extension of remarks	Statement during floor debate
167. HR 4785. AIDS Prevention Act/Name Reporting. Dannemeyer, R-Calif., amendment to allow states to decide whether to establish a reporting system for entities performing HIV testing to confidentiality report to public health officials identifying information about people testing positive for HIV. Before being amended by Rowland, D-Ga., the Dannemeyer amendment would have required states to set up a reporting system before they could receive federal grants.					
Clay, William (D–MO)	Y	✓	✓		
Collins, Cardiss (D–IL)	Y	✓	✓		
Conyers, John (D–MI)	Y	✓	✓		
Crockett, George (D–MI)	NV				
Dellums, Ronald (D–CA)	Y	✓	✓		
Dixon, Julian (D–CA)	Y	✓	✓		
Dymally, Mervyn (D–CA)	Y	✓	✓		
Espy, Mike (D–MS)	Y	✓	✓		
Flake, Floyd (D–NY)	Y	✓	✓		
Ford, Harold (D–TN)	Y	✓	✓		
Gray, William (D–PA)	Y	✓	✓		
Hawkins, Augustus (D–CA)	NV				
Hayes, Charles (D–IL)	Y	✓	✓		
Lewis, John (D–GA)	Y	✓	✓		
Mfume, Kweisi (D–MD)	Y	✓	✓		
Owens, Major (D–NY)	Y	✓	✓		
Payne, Donald (D–NJ)	Y	✓	✓		
Rangel, Charles (D–NY)	NV				
Savage, Gus (D–IL)	Y	✓	✓		
Stokes, Louis (D–OH)	Y	✓	✓		
Towns, Edolphus (D–NY)	Y	✓	✓		
Washington, Craig (D–TX)	Y	✓	✓		
Wheat, Alan (D–MO)	Y	✓	✓		
House Vote: 422–1					
Democratic Party Vote: 251–0					
Republican Party Vote: 171–1					

Source: *Congressional Quarterly Roll Call, 1990*
Note: All members eligible to vote are listed. This list does not represent the total number of black members serving this Congress.

Table 9.9   168. HR 4785. AIDS Prevention Act-Ryan White/Passage (1990)

	Actual Vote	Vote with party	Vote with majority	Extension of remarks	Statement during floor debate	Offered an amendment
168. HR 4785. AIDS Prevention Act/Passage. Passage of the bill to authorize $2.76 billion over five years for emergency relief to cities with the largest numbers of AIDS cases and grants for health-care facilities to provide AIDS testing and counseling to help prevent the spread of AIDS and to help implement a system to notify emergency workers of possible exposure to infectious diseases, authorize various other grant and demonstration projects, and require certain studies.						
Clay, William (D–MO)	Y	✓	✓			
Collins, Cardiss (D–IL)	Y	✓	✓			
Conyers, John (D–MI)	Y	✓	✓			
Crockett, George (D–MI)	Y	✓	✓			
Dellums, Ronald (D–CA)	Y	✓	✓			
Dixon, Julian (D–CA)	Y	✓	✓			
Dymally, Mervyn (D–CA)	Y	✓	✓			
Espy, Mike (D–MS)	Y	✓	✓			
Flake, Floyd (D–NY)	Y	✓	✓			
Ford, Harold (D–TN)	Y	✓	✓			
Gray, William (D–PA)	Y	✓	✓			
Hawkins, Augustus (D–CA)	NV					
Hayes, Charles (D–IL)	Y	✓	✓			
Lewis, John (D–GA)	Y	✓	✓			
Mfume, Kweisi (D–MD)	Y	✓	✓			
Owens, Major (D–NY)	Y	✓	✓			
Payne, Donald (D–NJ)*	Y	✓	✓		✓	
Rangel, Charles (D–NY)	NV					
Savage, Gus (D–IL)	Y	✓	✓			
Stokes, Louis (D–OH)	Y	✓	✓			
Towns, Edolphus (D–NY)	Y	✓	✓			
Washington, Craig (D–TX)	Y	✓	✓		✓	
Wheat, Alan (D–MO)	Y	✓	✓			

House Vote: 408–14
Democratic Party Vote: 249–0
Republican Party Vote: 159–14

Source: *Congressional Quarterly Roll Call, 1990*
Note: All members eligible to vote are listed. This list does not represent the total number of black members serving this Congress.
*Member(s) who co-sponsored this AIDS bill.

Committee and its Subcommittee on Human Resources. The Subcommittee on Human Resources sponsored eight of the twenty-three House hearings included in the legislative history of Ryan White.

In contrast to the work of Representatives Payne and Conyers is the absence of other black members at these hearings, especially those who served as members on relevant full committees. Only three other black congressional members—Representatives Rangel (D–NY), Towns (D–NY), and former Representative Leland (D–TX)—who served on a full committee with jurisdiction over a subcommittee sponsoring a hearing on Ryan White, attended any of the House hearings listed in the legislative history of the Act.[14] Moreover, each of these members participated in only one hearing. Representatives Collins (D–IL), Owens (D–NY), Wheat (D–MO), Fauntroy (D–DC), and Espy (D–MS) attended no hearings, even though they were all members of full committees with jurisdiction over subcommittees sponsoring hearings on Ryan White. Even more egregious, however, was the absence of black congressional members from an 18 September 1987 hearing on the AIDS crisis in New York City. This absence is especially troubling in the case of Representatives Owens and Towns, both black congressional members from New York who were members of the Government Operations Committee—the full committee with jurisdiction over the Subcommittee on Human Resources sponsoring the hearing. As a point of comparison, I should note that *none* of the congressional members from New York participated in this hearing. Instead, the hearing, which was held on site in New York City, was chaired by Representative John Conyers, chair of the Government Operations committee. The practice of not attending the hearings of subcommittees of which one is not a member has long been in place. However, if a representative wanted to demonstrate leadership around a specific issue area, participation in subcommittee hearings is one established and recognized method.

Again, in no way does this data prove a member's commitment to or dismissal of AIDS as a political issue. Instead the data in table 9.5 provide additional information so that we might make informed judgments and distinctions between those few black members for whom AIDS was a priority and the rest, who seemed willing to support the efforts and leadership of others. Only on those issues dealing explicitly with gay men and homosexual "lifestyles" was there any significant voting defection among black members from what might be considered a liberal and redistributive understanding of the government's responsibility to deal with AIDS equally and fairly. Even on those votes concerned with controversial and racially charged programs such as needle exchange, most black members voted in support of at least the investigation of these programs. Thus we once again face a picture which supports the claims of action by black officials, while also signaling the general failure of leadership noted by activists.

Beyond merely counting the number of black members who participated in hearings on Ryan White, an examination of the actual statements made by representatives during these hearings can provide more information. Again, the speeches and comments of black members in attendance at some of these hearings clearly show that black members were extremely reluctant to include in their discussions of AIDS any informed understanding of black, gay male communities and the devastation of AIDS among this group. Instead, black representatives were more apt to mention AIDS among gay men as an illustration of the difference between the development of AIDS in black and white communities. Repeatedly members strove to present a picture of AIDS in black communities largely dominated by women, children, and heterosexual injection drug users. This pattern, while positive in terms of the attention it directed to the increasing numbers of women with AIDS, particularly in black and Latino communities, was at the same time troubling because of the context in which women, children, and heterosexual injection drug users were recognized. Namely, many black legislators instituted a two-tier system of recognition whereby black women and children were used to distract attention from black injection drug users, and black injection drug users were used to distract attention from black gay men and black men who have sex with other men. Through such a process of recognition and attention, rarely was there equal articulation of concern for all segments living with AIDS in black communities. Instead, subgroups were promoted selectively, based on their perceived respectability and empathetic value. Representative Ed Towns, during his opening statement at the Select Committee on Narcotics Abuse and Control Pediatric AIDS Hearings, emphatically stated that "for far too long, too many of us have thought of AIDS as a disease that only affects male homosexuals. But it's not. It affects women. It affects children. How long are we going to wait before we take this disease seriously?" (U.S. House 1987a, 4).

Of course, not all women received equal attention and comment. Most often only those women thought to suffer "innocently" from AIDS—those women infected unsuspectingly from an injection-drug-using male partner—received extended discussion. Furthermore, the impact of AIDS upon women is generally only discussed when women are needed to reflect the distinctiveness of AIDS in black communities, or when the discussion turns to children. Interestingly, in spite of all the articulated concern over the increasing incidence of HIV among women, there is no hearing in the legislative history of the Ryan White Act—at least as indicated by its title—that deals with the impact of AIDS on women, while five of the twenty-three House hearings focused on infants and children with AIDS. The reasons for this are many, but they have primarily to do with the uncomplicated status—in terms of moral codes—of children with HIV and AIDS. For example, Representative Payne in his opening remarks in a 1992 hearing on "Babies without Homes," describes his motivation for being active on this issue as the defense of "these infants—surely the most vulnerable and helpless among us" (U.S. House 1992, 8):

> I have been concerned about abandoned infants and boarder babies throughout my congressional career for two principal reasons. First and foremost, I strongly believe that the United States Congress and this great country have a solemn moral obligation to care for these newborn children. They know nothing about crack cocaine, poverty, drug dealers, and street violence. All they really want is a home and parents to love them. For reasons beyond their control, boarder babies have been cruelly denied even these basics. I am determined, as their representative, to provide for both their care and per-haps—through foster families and adoptive parents—the love and attention they so desperately need. It is an outrage that in the richest country in the world, small children are permitted to reside in hospital nurseries for days, weeks, and even months on end. Indeed, we have lost our moral compass as a Nation if these infants—*surely the most vulnerable and helpless among us*—do not occupy a high priority in our society. (emphasis added, 8)[15]

Without minimizing the concern most individuals share for the well-being of children, we might ask whether the United States also has a moral obligation to women without children or to black gay men or to injection drug users. Through the frame of children, representatives were able to work on the issue of AIDS without the baggage that traditionally comes with this issue. David Dinkins, then Manhattan Borough President, in his testimony during a 1987 hearing on Pediatric AIDS, comments on the more politically attractive and noncostly status of children. He astutely urges public officials willing to look the other way as AIDS kills drug users and gay men, to take action on behalf of our children: "If some of our nation's leaders have found it impossible to find the compassion in their hearts to deal constructively with the health crisis which appears to them to deal death to drug users and gay men, let them consider carefully the problems of these children and think twice about dismissing this snowballing human catastrophe" (U.S. House 1987a, 51).

Unlike children, women as a group were constructed not only as "innocent victims," but also as spreading the virus to the "real" victims of the epidemic, their children. Thus, in a political calculation whereby members were looking for issues with which they could win—those issues and groups whose negatives were low—certain women, those who inject drugs, found only qualified support from black officials. Black AIDS activist Robert Penn describes the binary construction of women in response to AIDS: "It's socially acceptable to take care of women. It is not socially acceptable to take care of people who have a sexually transmitted disease. A female prostitute who is HIV-infected, her female part can be taken care of, her prostitute part can't be taken care of. A female who has a history of intravenous drug use, her female part can be taken care of, but her intravenous drug use part can't be taken care of. Give me a break!"[16] The selective positioning of black women, at once naive victims and the deliverers of a deadly virus to their unborn children, was but one of the AIDS tightropes walked by black members of Congress. They would also have to maneuver around such delegitimizing issues and images as publicly identified black gay men and lesbians, unrepentant injection drug users, and whether AIDS should be represented as a black issue.

When male-to-male sexual transmission of HIV in black communities was discussed, it was often discounted or attributed to circumstances beyond the control (and without the consent) of individual black men, such as forced sodomy in prisons. For example, Representative Rangel, at a hearing he chaired of the Select Committee on Narcotics Abuse and Control on Pediatric AIDS at Harlem Hospital in 1987, repeatedly voiced concern over the spread of AIDS in prisons. Anxiety over the high rates of HIV transmission in the prison system is a concern that Mr. Rangel shared with many AIDS activists. It was Congressman Rangel's framing of male-to-male sex in prison, however, that demonstrated his constrained and judgmental understanding of the conditions and feelings leading to gay sexuality. Specifically, Mr.

Rangel suggested that leaders needed to be concerned with the *sexual assaults* on drug users who would then transmit HIV to the "general community:"

> I wonder whether, in looking at the spread of AIDS as it involves the IV drug users and those that they are having sex activities with, whether or not political and church leaders have looked into sexual activities in the prisons? This is something that of course people don't like to talk about, and we got chaplains in the prison, so if you get into any trouble over this one, you can charge it up to me. We have got Jewish Chaplains, Christian Chaplains, right there where this behavior goes on. We have guards that understand it. We have inmates that are subjected to this type of activity against their will. We have brutality. We have assaults, but now I would think we are having attempted murder if indeed one of these people have AIDS. These people are discharged, they are rotated. They come back to the general community, and they are involved in sexual activity. (U.S. House 1987a, 27)

Mayor Ed Koch, during his testimony before the committee, reminded Congressman Rangel that it was most often consensual sex that took place in the prison system: "We know that consensual sodomy takes place in prison. And anybody who doesn't believe that has their head in the sand. We are not talking about assaults. That takes place regrettably too, but not as often as people think. Consensual [sex] does take place regularly, we are sure" (U.S. House 1987a, 27).

The discounting of AIDS cases among black gay men and at times the seeming exaggeration of the percentage of transmission cases among African Americans through injection drug use was also evident in the testimony of individuals serving black communities. For example, at a 1987 hearing examining the manifestation of AIDS in New York City, Dr. Adaora Adimora of Harlem Hospital states that very few of her patients are gay: "About 75 percent of the people whom we see are IV drug users. The other 25 percent are others such as homosexuals, sexual partners of IV drug abusers, and other people who have gotten AIDS through indeterminate means" (U.S. House 1987b, 135–36). The relatively small percentage of Dr. Adimora's patients who are gay (some small part of the remaining 25 percent) is especially surprising when one considers that in 1991—four years after Dr. Adimora's testimony and after a major explosion in the classification of AIDS cases among injection drug users in black communities—when the first quarterly *AIDS Surveillance Update* was published by the Office of

AIDS and HIV Surveillance in the New York City Department of Health, male-to-male sexual transmission accounted for almost 40 percent of black men classified with AIDS in New York City (New York City Department of Health, 30 April 1991).

Dr. Adimora's testimony about the small numbers of blacks who contract HIV through male-to-male sex stood in contrast to the testimony of Dr. Mindy Fullilove. Dr. Fullilove testified at the corresponding hearing in 1987 examining the impact of AIDS in San Francisco, "The AIDS Crisis in Two American Cities." During her public remarks, Dr. Fullilove reminded the committee that AIDS among black gay men was a serious threat that should not be ignored: "There has been very little attention paid to the specific problems of minority gay men. There are, in fact, not even in San Francisco any specific programs which are reaching out to this group. . . . Most literature has gone through traditional white media. It has not necessarily reached the minority gay communities, which exist somewhat separate from the white gay community here and elsewhere across the country" (U.S. House 1987d, 320). In her prepared statement, Dr. Fullilove elaborates on this point, highlighting the statistics on AIDS among black gay men:

> Bakeman and co-authors have compared the vectors for viral transmission in white, Black, and Latin people with AIDS. They point out that homosexual/bisexual transmission accounts for the largest portion of the AIDS cases in each group. It is important to recognize that 58 percent of Black people with AIDS and 61 percent of Latin people with AIDS acquired the illness through homosexual/bisexual contact. Even in the early publicity of AIDS as "gay" disease, it was presented as a disease of white men. There was little outreach directed at minority gay men, yet the number of cases per million is 1.7 times higher for Black and Latin men than it is for white men. (U.S. House 1987d, 323–24)

Dr. Fullilove was one of the few witnesses who testified at any AIDS hearing to discuss and emphasize the plight of black gay men as a central component of the development of AIDS in black communities. Undoubtedly, her perspective was shaped by the fact that she was in San Francisco, where the numbers of black injection drug users with AIDS in no way paralleled or approached that found in east coast cities like New York or Newark. Despite such locational differences, it seems clear that black congressional members and others in black communities were intent on ignoring the significant numbers of black gay men dealing with AIDS on either coast. Even when congressional members turned to the familiar task of praising small community-based organizations like the Minority Task Force on AIDS in New York City for their effectiveness in responding to AIDS in black communities, the hard work of black gay men and lesbians in organizing this effort was never mentioned. Instead, legislators made black gay men, their work, and their struggles, invisible, choosing to deal with issues and segments of black communities that largely presented few costs to black congressional members—issues such as fairness in funding across communities, and anything that had to do with children.

Despite the tendency for black congressional and elected leaders to distance themselves from more controversial issues and populations surrounding AIDS, there was at least one area in which some black leaders sought to redefine thinking about this disease—namely, the conditions that facilitated the transmission of HIV. While many AIDS activists argued against the use of risk groups, since this categorization was thought to obscure understanding of the direct behaviors that led to the transmission of HIV, a number of black officials engaged in their own effort to emphasize the social, political, and economic context thought to facilitate transmission of HIV, in particular among people of color. In these discussions AIDS was linked to the other crises of health care, poverty, housing, and jobs facing black Americans. AIDS was constructed as a dangerous consequence of desperate conditions found in African-American and Latino communities. Again, David Dinkins, in his testimony during the 1987 hearing on pediatric AIDS, is explicit about the link between AIDS and other urban crises: "As with most crises, AIDS does not exist apart from other chronic problems we face in our cities. The connections among AIDS and poverty, drug abuse, limited access to health care, the housing shortage, discrimination, illiteracy, and other barriers to AIDS prevention and treatment must be acknowledged and explored. Without this perspective, effective measures cannot be undertaken" (U.S. House 1987a, 47).

Later in the same hearing Congressman Rangel reiterates this point, stating that "unless we deal with education, employment opportunities, job training, decent housing, then the problems we are testifying to will always increase. . . . yes, do more to deal with this crisis, but at least go back to Washington with the understanding that it would only be a Band-Aid approach to a much more serious hemorrhage of social and economic problems" (U.S. House 1987a, 51). The tendency to contextualize specific issues within the larger set of crises facing marginal groups is one consequence of marginalization discussed in chapter 2. In this case, the larger environment angle provided black elected officials with another, undoubtedly important, frame for discussing AIDS in black communities that did not specify the behaviors connected to the transmission of HIV—those perceived as controversial and stigmatizing. This frame would continue to be referenced throughout the epidemic by black officials. For example, two years after the preceding comments were made, Representative Conyers during a 1989 hearing on the AIDS epidemic in Newark states that "young people in the minority community, faced with the aspect of poverty, faced with racism, faced with all the negative aspects found in their own community, are reaching out and asking 'What can we do?'. . . We cannot look at AIDS simply as AIDS. We have to look at the social fabric of our society and also the social fabric of our communities and be about the task of changing that" (U.S. House 1989, 82).

This attempt to link AIDS to the other devastating conditions facing black communities was one of the few ways black elected officials sought to redefine the nation's understanding of AIDS. Most often black officials chose to forego positions of leadership around this issue, opting instead to vote with their party and in support of the policy initiatives of other members, although some, like Representatives Conyers, Payne, Rangel, and Owens, offered their own reserved form of leadership around AIDS in black communities. Representative Owens sponsored the Abandoned Infants Act of 1988 (HR 4843), and Representative Payne sponsored the Reauthorization of the Act in 1991 (HR 2722).[17] As the *Congressional Quarterly Almanac* notes, this legislation was largely considered "noncontroversial" and was passed by both the House and Senate, at the same time that "members were reluctant to tackle the politically explosive issues surrounding AIDS in any organized and coherent fashion" (vol. 43, 516).

Similarly, Congressman Rangel also took the early lead among black representatives, sponsoring legislation centered on the issue of AIDS. The group targeted in most of his proposed legislation—injection drug users—was perceived as a much more controversial beneficiary. In response to the stigma surrounding drug users and the damage such attitudes might cause his legislation as well as the representative himself, it is not surprising that the text of his bills often included justifications for the provision of services to injection drug users as being part of a trickle-down intervention that would "protect" women, children, and the larger population of unsuspecting heterosexuals. For example, in the text of the 1989 "Intravenous Substance Abuse and AIDS Prevention Act," sponsored by Congressman Rangel, the threat of AIDS to women and children is highlighted, including a reference in the text of the bill to the fact that "most women with AIDS are in their *childbearing years*, and women infected with HIV may transmit HIV to any of their children born subsequent to the mother's infection" (emphasis added). Once again, as in the pages of the *Amsterdam News*, we are confronted with a focus on women as child-bearers and not as individuals dealing with a life-threatening disease. These women, thus, are not just women but "nation breeders," some type of tainted "race women," responsible for the procreation of "the race." Through such a scenario, the threat of AIDS to this child-bearing population necessitated action on the part of black congressional members, since their fall could signal the fall of "the race."

A comprehensive exploration of the multiple ways in which black elected officials participated in the legislative fight against AIDS is impossible in one chapter. I am particularly burdened by the data available for this chapter, since most of it focused on public demonstrations of leadership. Again, information from the private meetings, negotiations, and dealings in which much of the work of Congress is pursued is simply not available to my research. Those black officials who participated in and led such private proceedings will never show up in my analysis. For example, Representative Stokes (D–OH), a powerful legislator in the area of AIDS, is largely invisible in this chapter. While some of his comments on the floor are available for review, his more substantive work, such as helping to structure the funding formula for the Ryan White CARE Act, happened without official record. Thus I offer conclusions about the overall effort of black elected officials in response to AIDS only with great caution.

Having said that, however, I do believe that the public record suggests a fairly clear delineation between the majority of black congressional members who supported inclusive and nonpunitive efforts in response to AIDS, and the few other black congressional members, such as Payne, Stokes, Rangel, and Conyers, who stepped forward to provide wary leadership in this policy area. These representatives extended benefits to women and children that might never have been won without their efforts. However, the actions of these leaders tended to be tentative, sponsoring needed, yet relatively safe legislation. The majority of black congressional members can point to a mixed record: overwhelmingly voting for those measures that sought to provide

more resources for people living with AIDS, but at the same time operating within a traditional and fairly restrictive conceptualization of
AIDS. It was in transformational leadership that most black congressional members, like their white counterparts, failed. Possibly Congressman Rangel in a 1987 hearing on AIDS and injection drug use
put the challenge and failure of black elected officials best: "Legislation
is, however, only one line of defense against AIDS. To immunize and
protect our communities from the AIDS epidemic, to stop the spread
of this disease in its tracks, we will need the help and support of all
segments of the community—government, business, religious leaders,
educators, the medical profession, and citizens. We in the black community have a special role to play, a vital role to play, because the very
survival of our community depends on how quickly and effectively
we can make AIDS a disease of our past" (U.S. House 1987c, 63). Unfortunately, AIDS is still a disease of our present and we are still search-
ing for truly transformational leadership in black communities.

Conclusion: Needle Exchange (Again)

The first (and maybe only) AIDS-related issue to generate massive response from African-American public officials in New York City was
the needle-exchange program. As discussed in chapter 6, the initial
proposal, which over time would be modified, narrowed, and eventually abandoned, first came to the public's attention in 1986. New York
City Health officials called for the establishment of community-based
centers where drug users could exchange their used needles and syringes ("works") for clean ones (Joseph 1992).[18] The program was defined
as an experiment to see if the provision of clean needles to injection
drug users could lower their rate of HIV infection by reducing the use
of contaminated needles. Needle exchange drew public controversy in
part because the state of New York was one of eleven states in 1986
(plus the District of Columbia) that legally prohibited the possession
of needles and syringes needed for injection drug use.[19] Through the
guise of participation in a study, injection drug users were to be given
an exemption, allowing them to possess and exchange at designated
centers their dirty works for clean needles and syringes. AIDS activists
supporting this program acknowledged that the needle-exchange program did nothing to address the dependency of drug users, yet saw
the program as a first step, keeping injection drug users alive so they
might enter drug rehabilitation programs.

Once the proposed pilot program was made public, it was met with a swift and forceful uproar from black officials. Everyone from then Manhattan Borough President David Dinkins to black Police Chief Benjamin Ward, most of the black ministers, and the board of the Black Leadership Commission on AIDS (BLCA) came out against the program. Their main concerns centered on the idea that somehow the exchange of clean needles for used ones would increase drug use in black communities, signaling, in particular, to black children that it was all right to take drugs. Not lost on anyone involved in or watching the escalating battles around this proposal was the racial dynamic of having white policy-makers import clean needles into largely black and Latino communities. Harlem City Council member Hilton B. Clark called the needle-exchange program a "genocidal campaign" (Page 1991, 17). Others, such as black Police Chief Benjamin Ward, cast the program in the rhetoric of historical plots against black communities, mobilizing memories of the Tuskegee Experiments. He commented that he carried a "particular sensitivity to doctors conducting experiments, and they too frequently seem to be conducted against blacks" (Page 1991, 17). Representative Charles Rangel was also quite vocal, opposing the needle-exchange program on the basis that the "experiment" would encourage and make drug use easy. Even David Dinkins, considered by some to be one of the more responsive African-American officials to the plight of those with AIDS, came out against the proposal. The soon-to-be mayor of New York City suggested that the needle-exchange program would send the wrong message, making injection safer, when we should be trying to stop drug use completely.

The proposed needle-exchange program drew leadership from black communities to the issue of AIDS like nothing else before it. Eventually, as the criticisms voiced by black leaders were joined by the criticisms of Latino leaders, law enforcement officials, ministers, and neighborhood groups, and as the state Health Department imposed scientific restrictions, the initial plan was drastically rescaled. The original design to pass out needles at designated health clinics in communities was scrapped and replaced in 1988 with a plan to distribute clean needles to two hundred injection drug users at the Health Department's downtown government office. Needless to say, in the first few weeks of the program, few injection drug users found their way downtown to pick up needles at a government office near City Hall. However, despite its rather dismal beginning—two participants on the first day—over time the program did attract more participants, and plans for expansion were made. The program, however, hit its greatest barrier, at least temporarily, when in September of 1989 David Dinkins defeated Mayor Ed Koch in the Democratic mayoral primary. Dinkins, along with all the other mayoral candidates except Koch, had pledged to dismantle the program if elected mayor. Consequently, the program was eventually stopped and deemed a failure. Charles Eaton, the person designated at the Health Department to head the program, explained that the central problem Health Department officials had in implementing this program was that they did not know the black community:

> The words and deeds of the black leadership responding to this program put the program in an embattled position. The Department of Health knew nothing about working in the black community, and no one had an inclination to figure it out. Joseph [Stephen Joseph, then Commissioner of Department of Health] said, "Do it quickly and incisively." However, in the battle people got reminded about Tuskegee, and the Department of Health didn't provide an alternative understanding of the program.[20]

This rather quick rendition of the battle over needle exchange in New York City presents us with yet another example of the reactionary participation of black elected officials in the political response to AIDS. Specifically, it seems that black officials have eventually been willing to speak out against policies they deemed destructive to their communities—needle exchange and the unfair distribution of AIDS money to communities of color—however, as is so often the case, these leaders offered no corresponding, proactive plan for dealing effectively with the immediate problem of HIV infection through drug use. Very few officials in their condemnation of the needle-exchange program sponsored legislation to increase funding for drug treatment slots.[21] Furthermore, in the outcry over needle exchange in New York City, black officials seemed to engage in a calculus of human worth, where the lives of "innocent" children and "regular, law-abiding community folk" were designated as more important and worth saving than the lives of black injection drug users. This dynamic of responding to the actions and moral codes of others, often dominant groups, absent any alternative vision of what should be done, seems to be the predominant response to AIDS from many black elected officials. It is not that these leaders vote the wrong way or are totally missing on this issue, as was the case in the first six years of the Reagan administration.

Instead, it is the lack of bold or transformational leadership that seems most troubling when examining the politics of black elected officials as we approach the twenty-first century. Cliff Goodman, a black AIDS activist, questioned the political vision of black leaders, especially those who most readily made claims of conspiracies in talking about AIDS:

> I don't believe AIDS is a conspiracy, but it is possible. But theories like those make Black people seem inferior to the "smart, white, scientific people." But if it is true that we are being attacked, why don't we detail a response. We never hear, "Let's work on a class action suit or go down and protest." We preach and do nothing but hate and fear white people. We give government officials/scientists far too much credit. Our leaders use race to get Blacks in the nationalism mode. That way we trust the person, then we buy whatever they are selling, be it a pill or a political agenda.[22]

Again, it would be inaccurate to suggest that black elected officials have not evolved in their understanding of and relationship to this political issue. In 1992 Mayor David Dinkins, after reviewing the successful operation of a needle-exchange program in New Haven, Connecticut—implemented by John Daniels, the first black mayor of New Haven—reevaluated his stance on needle exchange, vowing that the city would not stand in the way of the implementation of a program funded through private grants. Other black leaders would also follow his lead and alter their positions. The Rev. Calvin Butts of the Abyssinian Baptist Church in Harlem, an early opponent of needle exchange in New York, eventually modified his opposition to the program, noting that we "must keep these people alive, if we are to deal with their other problems."[23]

Over the years of this epidemic, black officials, like most of us affected by this disease, have gotten better in their understanding and response. However, "better" for many of our officials is qualified praise, as their response continues to be both tentative and conflictual. David Dinkins, first as Manhattan Borough President and then as mayor of New York, is one example of the dynamic orientation of black elected officials toward AIDS. Before becoming mayor, Dinkins was very helpful in establishing the Minority Task Force on AIDS. It was his office that sponsored the conference from which the organization began. However, it was also Dinkins who, upon becoming mayor, appointed Woodrow A. Myers, Jr. as Commissioner of the New York City

Department of Health. Many AIDS activists condemned the appointment of Myers who, while Indiana Health Commissioner, supported not only the recording of names of those infected with HIV so their sex partners could be traced, but also the quarantining of those with AIDS who "knowingly" spread the disease. Black officials, however, defended Myers's appointment because they considered him to be one of the outstanding *black* doctors in the country. It was thought that his policies would enhance the condition of the black community; thus his seemingly conservative or reactionary positions about AIDS were to be tolerated. Mayor Dinkins's conflictual response to AIDS is further highlighted when we compare his appointment of Woody Myers to his support for the distribution of condoms in the high schools, a stance many people opposed. It was Mayor Dinkins's appointee to the Board of Education, Dr. Westina L. Matthews, who cast the deciding vote allowing condoms to be available in public high schools in New York City.

The contradictory history of David Dinkins is one that is mirrored by other black leaders. Jesse Jackson has been offered as yet another example of a black official or leader struggling to provide consistent, inclusive, and progressive leadership around the issue of AIDS. His highly publicized work to free the Haitian refugees confined to Guantanamo Bay is just one example of his commitment to the political fight against AIDS. However, Clarence Page (1991) suggests that while Jesse Jackson has been a key celebrity figure in some battles around AIDS, he also suffers from inconsistency in his response to this disease. For example, Page writes that at the funeral of Max Robinson, Jackson's only mention of AIDS was to assure those gathered "that Robinson had told him he caught it from 'heterosexual' promiscuity." Page continues, arguing that "Jackson seemed more concerned with dismissing the notion that his friend was gay than with educating the public" (15–18). Page, in the same article, notes Jackson's apparent mood swings with regard to the attention he pays to AIDS. The author writes that before Magic Johnson's disclosure, when Jackson's media spokesman was asked about the Reverend's activity around the issue of AIDS, he commented, "Well, we haven't led any marches on it." However, Page suggests that a different image was projected the day after the Johnson announcement:

> When I called back the day after Johnson's announcement, Watkins [Jackson's media spokesperson] sounded consider-

ably more enthusiastic about the same issue. "I hope you know
that Reverend Jackson has been in the forefront on this issue
for years, long before many others were," he said. I was then
paged through to Jackson, who explained that he had spent
nights in AIDS hospices in Texas and California during his
1984 presidential campaign, a move he compared in symbolic
value to the way Jesus just before his crucifixion, stayed with
Simon the leper. (Page 1991, 15–18)

While Jackson's inconsistency should not be ignored when assessing
his attention to the issue of AIDS, it may be that such fluctuations stem
more from Jackson's natural sense for following the big story than his
avoidance of the issue itself. For many black officials, this conflict
arises in part because they struggle to hold onto the moral framework
of the black church and its voting constituency, while increasingly facing cross-cutting issues that are not easily understood or responded to
through simple moral categories of "good" and "bad" or "deserving"
and "unworthy." This is not to suggest that every black leader has felt
that AIDS was an issue outside of their domain, responding only when
pushed by activists. However, the legislative or policy initiatives of
these leaders reflect working assumptions that differentiate the needs
of those affected by AIDS from the more general needs of African-
American communities.

By most accounts, one of the most responsible and active leaders
concerned with the issue of AIDS has been Representative Maxine Waters of California. It was Waters who convened a meeting of the Congressional Black Caucus to discuss the role of black legislators in the
fight against AIDS. Waters has also sponsored meetings on the Veteran
Administration's studies identifying disparate effects of AZT on white
and black patients. Furthermore, on more than one occasion Representative Waters has met with black AIDS activists to hear their concerns
and strategize about possible action. Phil Wilson and other black AIDS
activists praise Waters as one example of a new black leader willing
to, as Wilson says "fight for *all* her people."[24]

According to researchers such as Adolph L. Reed, Jr., a hope for a
new type of black leadership—one attentive to all segments of the community, even the most vulnerable of our members—rests in the ever-
widening mechanisms for establishing leadership claims. Reed (1986)
argues that before the 1960s there were few institutional or structural
means, such as voting, to designate and ratify leadership in black communities. Therefore, charismatic behavior and inspiring articulation

often brought notoriety in the community. Since the 1960s, and the passage of the Voting Rights Act, elected black officials have come to increasingly control the mantle of leadership.[25] It is hypothesized that this broadening of avenues to leadership within black communities, beyond traditional paths such as the church, may produce a new generation and gender of leaders, one less constrained by the old tenets and moral codes that historically framed decision making by black elites. Despite such hopes, it has generally been young leaders of the civil rights movement—those who learned about leadership under a less democratic process in black communities—who have won many of the elected positions held by blacks today.

Consequently, the jury is still out on the full impact of the political incorporation of black leaders. Scholars such as Guinier (1994) and Swain (1993) make the argument—from very different political perspectives—that while we have more black elected leaders ratified through a formal institutional process—thereby purportedly increasing accountability—the form of leadership they provide does not look radically different from the leadership of old. This lack of variation is due in part to the institutional structures in which these leaders operate—constraining policy options, legislative action, and radical economic redistribution. However, analysis of black congressional members' response to the AIDS crisis also seems to indicate that part of the consistency between old and new black leadership has to do with the longevity and power of dominant norms and values, acting as tests that marginal groups must pass in their quest for respectability, legitimacy, and equality. Black elected officials thus might see their work as making things better for as many in their communities as possible, without jeopardizing the cultural capital attained by years of black middle-class fortitude. Whatever these officials perceive as their duty, we have now reached a point in black politics where all who proclaim leadership must be held accountable for their actions as well as their silence.

CHAPTER TEN

AIDS and Beyond

AIDS

The manifestations of AIDS in African-American communities have been both devastating and empowering. The loss of group members is a sad and undeniable fact of this disease. Since its formal recognition in 1981, 612,078 individuals in the United States have been classified as having AIDS by the CDC. Of this phenomenal figure, blacks comprised 35 percent of the cases as of June 1997, nearly three times their proportion (12 percent) in the general population. Additionally, they constitute 57 percent of all new infections of HIV. Despite the discovery and incredible benefits of drugs such as protease inhibitors, we know that disproportionately more people of color will continue to be diagnosed with and die from AIDS. The reaction to this incredible loss has ranged from severe grief to extraordinary anger, as every community, group and neighborhood has had to cope with the devastation of this epidemic. And while the political response to AIDS has varied over the course of the epidemic and among groups, consistently it has been the actions and inaction of dominant institutions and indigenous leaders and organizations that have significantly shaped the development and response to this epidemic. Consequently, their actions and inactions as they framed the response to AIDS in African-American communities have dominated the pages of this book.

The responses to this disease from dominant institutions and elites, as noted in chapters 3, 4, and 5, ranged from inadequate to neglectful. The CDC, the President, the U.S. Congress, and the mainstream media all missed or turned down opportunities to portray this epidemic in an urgent and accurate manner that might have saved lives. Throughout this epidemic the response on the part of these institutions has tended either to make invisible or to underrepresent minority groups living with AIDS. Often the poor job of dominant institutions was produced not only by an ideology which defined those with AIDS as less than full citizens, but also by institutional biases and practices that are represented as their standard operating procedures.

For example, the CDC, in the early years of the epidemic, underrepresented and ignored large segments of the drug-using population—primarily people of color—infected with HIV. A significant reason for this neglect stemmed, in part, from the reporting procedures of the CDC, which did not adequately take into account variation in the ability of providers to recognize and report disease among different groups. All medical clinics were expected to report strange infectious occurrences to the CDC, yet doctors in clinics with patients suffering from numerous illnesses and barely able to pay their bills have a difficult time trying to provide proper care, let alone trace the medical histories of their clients and report irregularities to the CDC. Similarly, the mainstream media, with their working assumptions about what kinds of stories their audiences want to read and hear about, what stories will bolster a reporter's career, and what groups are even worthy of being covered, gave only minimal attention to the topic of AIDS in African-American communities, with celebrities largely driving the coverage.

Thus, in the early years of this epidemic, through the actions and ideologies of dominant institutions, AIDS was constructed as a problem of only one group—(white) gay men. If some type of alternative understanding of AIDS in African-American communities was to be offered, it would have to come from the indigenous sources of information within these communities. Furthermore, if some political response were to occur—one that would adequately provide for the needs of African Americans with AIDS, as well redefine the national understanding of this epidemic—most likely it would have to depend on the indigenous resources of these groups.

Initially slow and individualistic, the response to AIDS in African-American communities has evolved over time. In the early years of the epidemic the provision of services was most often accomplished by individual families caring for members who were sick. For example, not until 1986 did New York City have an AIDS organization—Minority Task Force on AIDS—whose focus was explicitly directed toward the needs of people of color with AIDS. When an institutional response did emerge in black communities, most often it came in the form of services and education, with the goal of prevention being primary. This early work was led and staffed mostly by black gay men and lesbians, who demonstrated the same urgency found among many white lesbians and gay male activists. However, in contrast to the more aggressive political tactics of civil disobedience used by predominantly white groups such as ACT UP, the political strategies in African-American communities were much less confrontational, with compromise and education being key.

Not until the mid-1980s did mainstream black organizations and leaders respond in significant numbers, attempting to stem the progression of AIDS through black communities. Often such action came in response to the demands of black AIDS activists and service providers that these leaders do something constructive. Even during this period, however, there was little talk of AIDS as a political issue that threatened to further marginalize significant segments of the community. There was little attempt to pool resources, beyond some minimal provision of services, to be used as a base for organized resistance and mobilization against this disease. Instead, traditional black leaders and organizations often engaged in their own process of secondary marginalization, where dominant discourses which sought to stratify and distinguish between "worthy" and "unworthy" marginal group members were replicated and in some cases adjusted to similarly mark and divide the more vulnerable segments of African-American communities living with AIDS. Ministers, politicians, and others with limited access to dominant resources distinguished between the "innocent victims" of AIDS and those whose "bad" behavior led to their infection. Again, with time this interpretation and discourse would come to include more tolerant portrayals of, for example, injection drug users, but even today remnants of such ideologies still significantly structure the response to AIDS in black communities.

A lack of leadership, in particular transformative leadership, best characterizes the response to AIDS from traditional black organizations and elites. This is not to say that black elected officials and national organizations did nothing. Indigenous institutions and leaders increasingly demonstrated a willingness to fight political battles over nonstigmatized issues such as the fair distribution of AIDS funding, but black officials made few attempts to take on leadership in this area. They made no effort to transform the community's understanding of the fight against AIDS from a social obligation to provide services to an "infected" population to a political fight for the empowerment of the most marginal sectors of black communities. Black elected officials and traditional leaders chose, instead, to mobilize their resources in response to outside initiatives they viewed as threatening to the mainstream of black communities—initiatives such as needle exchange. Black newspapers and magazines rarely made appeals for public confrontation by urging black communities to mobilize around AIDS, unless, of course, such a discussion was connected to genocide and conspiracy theories. In the meantime, black AIDS activists did what they could—distributing education and preventive material, working with indigenous institutions to spur some response, and holding accountable white AIDS organizations that threatened to dominate policy and funding decisions regarding AIDS. However, in an environment where AIDS interacts with poverty, unemployment, a lack of access to health care, and many other issues, a response to this disease without the full weight of community resources and leaders produced only partial victories as the epidemic raged on.

And Beyond

The importance of groups in our political system cannot be denied. In the most generous and passive account of a pluralistic political system, access is usually based on the grouping of individuals with some shared interest, with these individuals pooling resources and influence to affect policy decisions. The role of collective mobilization becomes especially important for marginal groups with a history of being denied full participation in dominant political, economic, and social structures. To complicate matters, recently there has been a transformation in the demographics of the groups we identify as marginal. While the majority of members still remain resource-poor, with very restricted access to and control over dominant institutions, a stratum of marginal group members has emerged with access to dominant resources, institutions, and state apparatuses.

This phenomenon of increasing stratification, and its resulting variation in interests, has affected the ability of marginal groups to define and pursue a unified political agenda. Moreover, this bifurcation in access has also promoted a process of secondary marginalization in these same communities. As stated earlier, consensus issues that dominated the public agenda of black communities in the past are being replaced with cross-cutting issues that draw attention to differences or cleavages among marginal group members. These issues often include or are driven by ideological claims about the material and social divisions seen in black communities. In many cases, cross-cutting issues reinforce and exaggerate in-group differences, facilitating the targeting and scapegoating of the most vulnerable community members. Thus, marginal groups, where stratification and diversity lessen cohesion around interests, face decreasing prospects of being able to mount unified organized resistance. The consequences of such dissension are especially dangerous for the most disempowered marginal group members, who find themselves not only unable to access dominant resources, but they are increasingly denied access to indigenous resources and institutions.

In African-American communities the impact of increasing stratification and heterogeneity is evident in the community's mixed response to AIDS. These effects are also evident in the response of traditional black leaders to any number of other cross-cutting issues dominating the public agenda. For example, the response of traditional black leaders to the push for welfare reform also lends itself to an examination within the framework of marginalization. In the midst of a political battle about substantial reforms that would restructure the lives of numerous poor, African-American women, traditional black leaders were largely ineffective. Unable to mobilize what they considered to be convincing images of black women as innocent victims, many social service agencies and black officials turned once again to the harm such reforms would do to "innocent children." But while nameless black children may be innocent, they were not important enough to significantly alter the dismantling of welfare as we knew it.

Interestingly, in New York City after the proposed legislation was enacted at the national and state levels, a number of advocates for women on welfare promoted the idea that black union leaders would be the next line of defense against workfare, believing these leaders would reject city and state plans to force poor black women to work at substandard wages and under unsafe working conditions. Much to their surprise, black union leaders like Stanley Hill, executive director of District Council 37— the largest union of municipal workers in New York City—far from mounting resistance to the city's and state's proposed workfare programs, entered into an agreement with New York's Republican mayor Rudolph W. Giuliani. Faced with the cross-cutting issue of welfare/workfare, Mr. Hill choose to guarantee the jobs of working-class and middle-class workers, a significant number of them black workers, instead of blocking the city's use of workfare participants. Thus, it seems when black union leaders were faced with what appeared to be conflicting class interests in black communities—between employed middle-class and working-class black people and black women on welfare—they chose to preserve the jobs of their constituencies, leaving poor black women to fend for themselves. Even more disappointing was the willingness of black union leaders to conform to the choices presented by city administrators. There seemed to be little ability (or maybe effort) on the part of union officials to redefine the terms of the debate. Only later would these same officials announce that they would try to organize this newly developing class of workfare workers (Greenhouse 1997). The response to welfare reform by traditional black leaders is yet another example of the conflicting interests and politics to be found in black communities during an era of advanced marginalization and in response to cross-cutting issues. These conflicts require further investigation as we begin to demystify and reconstruct black politics.

Issues such as welfare reform and AIDS all point to the need for a broader framework through which we can analyze the political mobilization of oppressed communities. Marginalization, as used throughout this book, is one framework that can help with this line of study. Specifically, three basic components of this theory make the puzzle of activism among marginal groups, especially the acts of leaders and elites, somewhat clearer.

First, the framework of marginalization models the interactive role that dominant institutions, resources, and groups play in defining the response of marginal groups to political issues. Institutions such as the CDC and the legislative and executive branches of the federal government significantly determined which groups would gain access to dominant resources allocated to deal with the AIDS epidemic. Further, beyond the mere allocation of resources, these same institutions and others, like the mainstream media, played a critical role in developing a dominant discourse which would frame the issues connected to AIDS and set the terms of the political debate. For example, the response of black communities to AIDS was clearly affected by initial CDC and media reports suggesting that AIDS was a disease only of white gay men. Moreover, the promotion of terms like *promiscuous* and *immoral* to characterize those at risk for HIV and AIDS also reinforced the impulse among conservative black institutions to look the other way when confronted with this disease.

Theories of power that focus on the role of dominant or powerful institutions and elites to explain the action or inaction of marginal groups use this approach for valid reasons. However, these theories fall short in explaining why black leaders with limited access to dominant resources, who were provided with alternative information regarding the effect of this crisis on their constituencies, responded slowly to the call for help. This delayed response on the part of black leaders was not just due to the power invested in dominant institutions. Much of their response was determined by the indigenous structures and norms of black communities. It is this gap in the explanatory power of dominant institutional approaches—where powerful and powerless dichotomies fall short—that makes the role of indigenous resources, norms, and values important in explaining the political behavior of marginal groups.

Second, the framework of marginalization emphasizes the role of indigenous resources and ideologies in structuring political actions and attitudes among oppressed people. Specifically, as the material reality or resources available for mobilization change across groups, seemingly similar political issues will, in response, take on a different shape across groups. For example, service providers who work primarily in communities of color, while quick to condemn the overall inaction of black leaders in response to AIDS, were also vehement in pointing out that AIDS is a very different disease in poor black communities than in white gay male communities. In most communities of color AIDS interacts with other crises, such as the lack of health care and education, homelessness, drug addiction, poverty, racism, sexism, and numerous other ills. This is not to suggest that white gay communities do not also have to deal with similar issues, yet few would argue that the magnitude of such concerns is somehow comparable between groups. The general resources afforded to each community for political struggles are also in no way equal. But it would be a mistake to categorize African-American communities as powerless. For while white gay communities include among their ranks men who individually bring economic and political privilege into their battles against this crisis, a number of black communities, while lacking individual resources, have black elected officials at the helm of city resources. Therefore, the form and amount of resources available to marginal groups will vary among groups, influencing the level and type of mobilization arising from each community.

Beyond the specific material conditions of a community are the norms, values, and informal practices that work to construct a group's perception or understanding of an issue. Thus the slow response of black leaders becomes a bit more understandable when one takes into account the presence of institutions such as the black church, which operates from a socially conservative moral framework. These organizations, in the case of AIDS, worked to define certain community members as innocent and worthy of mobilization, while others were labeled deviant, immoral, and bad. Those groups suffering most from AIDS in African-American communities were constructed as standing outside the indigenous moral and racial codes of the community as defined in part by the black church. Members of these subgroups were perceived as a disgrace to "the community" and thus not worth the expense of the limited political capital controlled by black elites. Through the framework of marginalization, the slow and often ineffective response of black leaders, while disheartening, is a bit easier to comprehend. This framework, especially through its attention to secondary marginalization, also prompts the question of whether one can expect a unified, massive response to any stigmatizing, cross-cutting issue when those individuals, leaders, and institutions that control and direct most of the resources of black communities are motivated to protect the cultural capital of the middle class, as well as their own mobility and status.

This question of how marginal communities will build for mobilization under advanced marginalization is the third contribution of this framework. Understanding the deployment of power within marginal communities forces us to question whether patterns of advanced and secondary marginalization fundamentally limit the utility of race as a basis upon which to build political movements in the twenty-first century. There are some scholars who suggest that race is less meaningful than class in understanding the current life choices and conditions of most black people. These researchers argue that class, as it separates and divides specifically inner-city residents and their behaviors, should be viewed as the more salient variable when trying to explain the "black experience" in the contemporary United States (Loury 1987; Murray 1984; Sowell 1984; W. Williams 1982; Wilson 1980). While I do not believe that race has diminished in importance, I do believe that African Americans face a crisis in linked-fate politics. While multiple social identities have always been a part of black communities, processes of advanced and secondary marginalization have recently given greater weight to other identities, such as those structured around class, gender, or sexuality, in determining the lived experiences of group members. This change is taking place not to the exclusion of race, but in conjunction with race. Characteristics such as class, gender, sexual orientation, geographical location, education, and even one's relationship to welfare all *interact* with one's racial identity to structure life choices. Without increased recognition of the broadening of identities through which people exist in and understand the world, traditional black leaders and scholars may end up so out of touch with the differing experiences of multiple segments of black communities that they fill no real function in their communities and thus are left to talk to themselves. The framework of marginalization refocuses our research lens on the contradictions, conflicts, and possibilities that exist within marginal groups as a new generation of indigenous leaders struggles to build principled political movements and identities that are inclusive, empowering, and effective.

NOTES

Chapter One

1. A more detailed account of advanced marginalization appears in chapter 2.

2. Again, a more detailed elaboration of secondary marginalization appears in chapter 2.

3. For example, two general ways to argue for the saliency of some issue to the black community might focus on whether the black community was thought to suffer disproportionately from the issue and whether large segments of the community were affected by the issue.

4. As I highlight the stratification and difference evident in marginal groups and cross-cutting issues, I must also note the significant stratification and diversity present among white dominant group members. Along any and every dimension there is variation. Thus, in theoretically deploying the concept of dominant groups, institutions, and norms, I do not mean to erase the very substantial variation that shapes the divergent experiences and behaviors of white Americans.

5. *New York Times*, 25 January 1991; U.S. Department of Health and Human Services, Centers for Disease Control, *HIV/AIDS Surveillance Report*, February 1993.

6. Throughout this book, I will use the terms *gay community, traditionally recognized gay community,* and *predominately white lesbian and gay community* to symbolize those segments or members of lesbian and gay communities who have been politically active regarding AIDS. These terms or identities are not meant to negate the presence and activism of lesbian, gay, bisexual, two-spirit, and transgender people of color. Further, these representations are not meant to perpetuate stereotypes that "homosexuality" is somehow endemic only to the white communities. Instead, I use these terms to indicate that people whose primary political work regarding AIDS is rooted in the institutions of lesbian and gay communities have been, at least early on, predominately white. In contrast, many of the lesbian, gay, bisexual, two-spirit, and transgender people of color whose work includes lesbian and gay issues and who may be affiliated with lesbian and gay institutions, generally focus their AIDS work on the way this crisis affects communities of color. Finally, the AIDS work of some people spans an entire spectrum of concerns. My analysis, however, requires highlighting the different interests of each community, especially as they were played out early in the epidemic.

7. "Phone zaps" are planned attacks on a target's communication system. Members of the protesting group are asked to continuously call and fax the business, organization, or agency, demanding that they respond to some issue. The aim is to disable the communication system for some undetermined amount of time.

8. Centers for Disease Control, *HIV/AIDS Surveillance Report* (January 1991).

9. Other communities of color are also experiencing increased numbers of AIDS cases. The specific increase is difficult to ascertain since Asian and Pacific Islanders as well as Native Americans are often underrepresented in the official counts of the Centers for Disease Control, as are all communities of color. See, for example, Lindan et al. 1990.

10. Centers for Disease Control and Prevention, *HIV/AIDS Surveillance Report* 7, no. 2 (1995).

11. Centers for Disease Control and Prevention, *HIV/AIDS Surveillance Report* 10, no. 1 (1998).

12. Some scholars who study power explain the process of marginalization in more formal language, arguing that through any number of strategies of marginalization, A limits or excludes B from gaining access to, participating in, or controlling those social mechanisms—institutions, ideologies, social relationships—that determine B's life chances. Through the systematic implementation of strategies of exclusion, B is relegated to a position of marginality. Targeted or marginal groups are thus left vulnerable to the control and oppression of others more dominant in society. Again, note that while oppression, especially in a more sustained form, has come primarily from dominant groups and individuals, control is also exerted by other more privileged marginal group members. See, for example, Dahl (1957), Bachrach and Baratz (1962), and Lukes (1974).

13. I want to thank Victoria Hattam for reminding me that black elites might also be concerned with other forms of cultural capital. For instance, indigenous cultural capital might exist within marginal groups that is generated not from adhering to dominant norms, but from being viewed (and represented by mainstream media) as determined to challenge dominant norms and vehicles of oppression. Thus, militant leaders who are feared, harassed, and sometimes killed by dominant institutions, can be loved and revered by other members of their marginal group as well as sympathetic dominant group members. I suspect that many African-American leaders try to walk a tight political line—attempting to generate and manage both indigenous and dominant cultural capital. In this study, however, my focus is on the constraints and benefits of dominant cultural capital.

14. Although the majority of the interviews used in the book took place between 1990 and 1993, about a third of them were conducted between 1995 and 1997.

15. New York City Department of Health, *AIDS Surveillance Update, 3rd Quarter 1997* (issued January 1998).

16. New York City Department of Health, *AIDS Surveillance Update, 1st Quarter 1997* (issued April 1997).

17. U.S. Department of Commerce. *1990 Census of Population, General Population Characteristics: New York*, Section 1 of 2, (1990CP-1-34).

18. *New York Times*, "U.S. Reports AIDS Deaths Now Exceed 100,000," 25 January 1991, A: 18; also figures from New York City Department of Health.

19. New York City Department of Health, *AIDS Surveillance Update, 3rd Quarter 1997* (issued January 1998). Again, we must remember that other communities of color are also being devastated by AIDS. For example, Latino/a adults constitute 18 percent of all adult AIDS cases, double their 9 percent share in the general population. Latina women account for 20 percent of female AIDS cases; Latino men constitute 17 percent of all male adult cases, and Latino/a children represent 24 percent of all pediatric AIDS cases (CDC, HIV/AIDS Surveillance Report 9, no. 1 [1997]).

20. Individuals were chosen to be interviewed because (1) of their obvious association with the response to this disease (i.e., staff members at the only Minority AIDS Organization in Harlem); (2) their names came up repeatedly in conversations with other interviewees or other people consulted on who should be interviewed; (3) they are known leaders in African-American communities, black lesbian and gay communities, or the larger lesbian and gay community. As we might expect, availability and willingness also significantly determined who was interviewed.

21. Thus, in the same way that those who study voting behavior quite often compare white and black Americans with regard to their voting choice or rate of turnout, recognizing and acknowledging differences in the composition and location of these two

groups, I too engage in a set of analyses which recognize and incorporate the differences of these groups in my analyses, while using their shared experience of marginalization and oppression, undoubtedly manifested in different ways as a basis of similarity that allows for comparison across groups.

Chapter Two

1. In contrast to the contention that black communities are "more" homophobic is the counterargument that marginal groups, either because of an understanding of the outsider position or a lack of power to enforce their prejudices, have been more inclusive and accepting of lesbian and gay members relative to other groups rooted in dominant society.

2. We need only remember the overwhelming denunciation of a proposed needle-exchange project in New York City by most black and Latino/a leaders for proof of their disdain for black and Latino/a injection drug users.

3. The "hidden transcript" includes those discourses, plans, actions, and cultural practices developed by oppressed or marginal group members outside of the gaze and earshot of the dominant group. Access to the hidden transcript is thought to provide greater clarity about the consciousness and intent of marginal group members.

4. The designation of marginal groups as "outsiders" does not imply any lack of participation on the part of marginal group members in dominant institutions and systems. As enslaved black people experienced categorical exclusion from control over or access to decision making in dominant institutions, they nevertheless were forced to "participate" in economic and social life under slavery. Thus, marginal group members are often forced to "participate," providing the base or foundation for those institutions and systems which formally exclude and oppress them.

5. The malleability of dominant norms is especially relevant to the institution of marriage. The sanctity of heterosexual marriage, which has often been presented as the state's sanctioning of the "natural" union of one man and one woman, has been used historically to promote white supremacist ideas of citizenship and economic labor relations.

6. In arguing that many Irish and Italian Americans live with a self-imposed or self-selected ethnicity, I do not mean to discount those instances when stereotypes such as alcoholism among the Irish or mafia connections among Italians are deployed to limit the opportunities and benefits available to group members. However, I do believe that the marginalization of people of color and lesbians and gays is more pervasive and systemic, in terms of its detrimental effects, within this society.

7. Some scholars contend that Marx developed at least two theories of ideology (Abercrombie, Hill, and Turner 1990).

8. I employ a "bottom-up" view of power, where the consequences experienced by marginal groups are the subject of examination, as opposed to the motivation or conscious intent of those exercising power. This perspective is in direct opposition to Rae (1988) and to other researchers who contend that the exercise of power necessitates some conscious action. In the framework I propose, a correlative oppressor need not be identified for every marginalized group to suggest that power is a determining factor in a situation. Instead only the strategies and consequences of marginalization, insofar as they are linked to the status or position of some marginal group, must be identified.

9. For earlier thoughts on this subject among political scientists, see, for instance, Paul F. Lazarfeld, Bernard Berelson, Hazel Gaudet, Angus Campbell, Philip E. Converse, Warren E. Miller, Donald E. Stokes, Sidney Verba, Norman H. Nie, Robert Dahl, Raymond E. Wolfinger, Richard Brody, Steve Rosenstone, Michael Dawson, Hanes Walton, Jr., Catherine Tate, Diane Pinderhughes, and Linda Williams.

10. I use the term *collaboration* cautiously because quite often we assume free will and

deliberate choices when speaking of a strategy of collaboration. Jim Scott (1990) informs us that collaboration can also mask practices of resistance made evident through the hidden transcript.

11. Although there are other paths to indigenous power and indigenous cultural capital, this analysis centers on dominant cultural capital and access.

12. Interview with Keith Boykin.

Chapter Three

1. Data from the Joint Center for Political Studies' *National Roster of Black Elected Officials* (Washington, DC: Joint Center for Political Studies, 1993).

2. The bifurcation in income between middle-class and poor blacks is also a gendered phenomenon: female-headed households constitute an increasingly larger percentage of black families in poverty (Jaynes and Williams 1989). Whatever one thinks of female-headed households, we cannot talk about class differences among African Americans without making gender a significant category of analysis.

3. The expansion of both of these groups came at the expense of a shrinking black working class (Hacker 1995).

4. The long and rich history of black women who write and organize around their specific concerns includes the work of women such as Maria Stewart, Anna Julia Cooper, Sojourner Truth, and Nannie Burroughs. Recent articulations of demands specific to the needs of women and poor people continued this tradition during the 1970s and 80s in the form of organizations such as the National Welfare Rights Organization, the National Black Feminist Organization, and the Combahee Women's Collective.

5. Interview with Gil Gerald.

6. Interview with Phil Wilson.

7. Interview with Phil Wilson.

8. The conference was organized "with the assistance of the city health department and the University of California" (Quimby and Friedman 1989, 405).

9. Personal communication from Gil Gerald. Mr. Gerald gave me a copy of his welcoming remarks from the conference held on 18 July 1986.

10. Interview with Gil Gerald.

11. Interview with Colin Robinson.

12. Interview with Dr. Billy Jones.

13. Interview with Dr. Billy Jones.

14. I discuss the controversy over needle exchange in more depth in chapters 6 and 9.

15. Interview with Dr. Billy Jones.

16. Chapter 4 discusses the perceived conflict in mission between the Centers for Disease Control (CDC) and the National Institute of Drug Abuse (NIDA). In this instance NIDA saw their focus as drug abuse and thus relegated responsibility for investigating and educating addicts about the connection between drugs and AIDS to the CDC. Unfortunately the CDC, having little or no experience with the drug-using population, was unable and unwilling to fulfill these externally imposed goals.

17. Interview with Phil Wilson.

18. Interview with Joe Presley.

19. Interview with Joe Presley.

20. Interview with Gil Gerald.

21. I use the word *primarily* to underscore the fact that while almost every traditional white gay AIDS organization has some people of color working on staff and serving as volunteers, the majority of their employees are white.

22. Undoubtedly, part of the reason some of these organizations were reluctant to involve themselves in politics has to do with the restrictions that come with certification as a not-for-profit (501-C3) organization.

23. Information for this section on United for AIDS Action came from my attendance at most of these meetings as a representative of the organization Black AIDS Mobilization (BAM!), and from literature I collected and interviews I conducted.

24. I use the terms *minority* and *white* AIDS organization to represent the racial staffing and client patterns evident in these organizations.

25. As the percentages of African Americans and Latinos/as classified with AIDS increased, elected officials from these communities sought to have government agencies examine the level of services available in these communities when making funding decisions.

26. Interview with Dr. Billy Jones.

27. Interview with Gil Gerald.

28. There are conflicting views on the effectiveness of GMAD during the AIDS crisis. Some argue that in a crisis of this proportion GMAD should be a leader, holding programs whenever possible. Other GMAD members suggest that there are more dimensions to the lives of black gay men than just the threat of AIDS; thus GMAD should provide a supportive environment in which black gay men can discuss and work on all the opportunities and obstacles that structure their lives.

While this debate will probably not be settled any time soon, I still believe, every time I see seventy-five black gay men at one of their meetings, that this is an example of the success of struggle—in need of work and adjustment, but still a success.

29. *Two-spirit* is a term used in Native American communities to represent those who embody both "masculine" and "feminine" traits and sexual desires.

30. Information on the Audre Lorde Project comes from my personal knowledge as a board member of the organization, as well as printed material detailing the history and current projects of the organization.

31. The Audre Lorde Project is one of the few truly multiracial gay organizations in New York and the country.

32. The lack of jobs or unemployment is most often named by African Americans as the most important problem facing black communities (Dawson 1994).

Chapter Four

1. Centers for Disease Control and Prevention, *HIV/AIDS Surveillance Report* 9, no. 1 (1997). As early as April 1986, data from a Gallup poll indicated that over 95 percent of blacks and whites had heard about "a disease called AIDS" (Thomas 1989).

2. I use the term *nonwhite* since in some surveys the operating racial classifications are white and nonwhite.

3. Throughout this analysis, I use the word *disease* when referring to AIDS because it has become a part of the public definition and articulation of this crisis, although AIDS signifies a syndrome of numerous opportunistic infections attacking the weakened immune system of someone who is HIV positive.

4. Centers for Disease Control and Prevention, *HIV/AIDS Surveillance Report* 9, no. 1 (1997).

5. I use the term *external institutions* to mark those information sources that, while not necessarily seen as dominant, are clearly external to the indigenous sources of information about AIDS produced in black communities.

6. This definition of the CDC's mission is listed on their web page (http://www.CDC.gov/).

7. Much of our knowledge of the details of the early history of AIDS comes from Shilts (1987).

8. Interview with Dr. Kimberly Smith.

9. Dr. James Curran was chosen to head this effort in part because of his background

in studying sexually transmitted diseases. He also had just completed a project in which he worked closely with a number of gay community health leaders and center staff.

10. We must remember that CDC staff members did not construct the details of AIDS in a vacuum; members of the gay community engaged very early in struggles over how AIDS would be defined and represented.

11. The CDC began in 1946 as the Communicable Disease Center. The name was changed in 1970 to the Center for Disease Control and then changed again in 1980 to the Centers for Disease Control. Only later would "and Prevention" be added to its title.

12. Interview with Dr. David Ostrow.

13. Seroprevalence represents the degree of HIV infection found in a designated population.

14. This phrasing is not meant to suggest that the only cases of HIV and AIDS among people of color were appearing in intravenous-drug-using populations. Clearly, black, Latino, Native American and Asian gay men were also living and struggling with being HIV positive and having AIDS in the early years of the epidemic. However, while gay men of color were dealing with this disease, a much larger number of intravenous drug users of color were dying from AIDS without ever being recognized in the official numbers of this epidemic.

15. In 1993 blacks were *four* times more likely to be arrested for possession of cocaine or heroin than were whites (Day 1995).

16. Latino/a drug users are three times more likely than white drug users to be diagnosed with AIDS (Day 1995).

17. In hectic, overworked medical environments individuals requiring care are often referred to not as patients with a medical history to be concerned with, but instead as one-time "visits" to be counted when making decisions about the allocation of resources.

18. Interview with Keith Cylar.

19. Interview with Dr. David Ostrow.

20. Interview with Dr. David Ostrow.

21. Interview with Dr. Helene Gayle.

22. Interview with Dr. Gerald Friedland.

23. Interview with Dr. Gerald Friedland.

24. Interview with Dr. James Curran.

25. I use the more inclusive (and I believe politically powerful) term *black community* as distinct from more specific African-American or Haitian communities.

26. Because of the CDC's designation of all Haitians as a risk group in the early years of the epidemic, Haitians in the United States have a history of mobilizing around AIDS. In fact, the Haitian community sponsored one of the largest known AIDS protests in 1990. The activities of the Haitian community should not be seen as originating out of the African-American community; the responses from these two distinct communities actually have been very different. Most recently, African Americans demonstrated less than substantial attention and action in response to the plight of Haitian refugees quarantined and imprisoned at the U.S. Naval Base at Guantanamo Bay.

27. While the term *risk group* has clearly been perceived as stigmatizing, we must face the reality that we need ways to communicate or force community ownership of stigmatized issues such as AIDS. In a political world in which an individual's needs and concerns are most often put forth and protected through their group identification, be it gay and lesbian, middle-class or African American, it may be helpful to frame the manifestation of new issues partly in terms of their impact on specific groups in society. Undoubtedly, some will argue that "assigning" disease to subgroups of the population allows most individuals to look the other way. However, I believe that we can develop

frames that highlight the specific manifestation of crises in certain communities, while also imparting a more global responsibility.

28. Interview with Dr. James Curran.

29. Interview with Dr. Helen Gayle.

30. Interview with Dr. James Curran.

31. Interview with Curran.

32. Interview with Curran.

33. Interview with C. Everett Koop.

34. Interview with Koop.

35. Interview with Koop.

36. Interview with Dr. Helene Gayle.

37. Interview with Dr. James Curran.

Chapter Five

1. Centers for Disease Control and Prevention, *HIV/AIDS Surveillance Report* (1992): 1. Hereafter cited parenthetically in text (e.g., CDC, *HIV/AIDS* 1992, 1).

2. The willingness of the media to air or print stories that focused on the "innocent victims" of the epidemic is a phenomenon that can be identified across communities.

3. "New Challenges in Reporting on AIDS," Columbia University School of Journalism, Center for New Media, 11 November 1996.

4. NBC, 17 June 1982, 5:52:20 to 5:54:20.

5. Interview with George Strait.

6. Interview with George Strait.

7. I relied heavily on James Kinsella's *Covering the Plague* (1989) for information on the *New York Times* coverage of AIDS.

8. I do not believe that either Mr. Signorile or the Kaiser report controlled for the differences in the overall number of stories each paper publishes routinely.

9. Interview with Tom Morgan.

10. In detailing the response to biased and racist media coverage from activists of color, I do not want to discount their roles in organizations such as ACT UP and GLAAD. Clearly, black, Latino/a, Native American, Asian, and Pacific Islander activists involved themselves in this issue in numerous ways and through multiple organizations.

11. For this analysis I use the *New York Times Index.* Parts of the *Times,* including letters to the editor, are not indexed. I am assuming that all significant coverage has been indexed and that omissions from the index occur consistently across and within subject matter.

12. As noted in the previous chapter, many AIDS activists concerned with the visibility of women and people of color with this disease fought to have the case definition revised. Activists believed that the pre and post-1987 case definitions were based largely on the research pursued early in the epidemic, focusing primarily on the trajectory of AIDS in white gay men. It was expected that the revised case definition would increase the number of cases among women and people of color. This expectation seems to have been realized, with men of color and women generally experiencing the largest relative jump in the number of newly reported cases of AIDS between 1992 to 1993, and showing the largest holdover or ratio in the number of cases between 1993 and 1994 (table 5.1). This example again illustrates the importance of institutions in constructing the facts and defining the "victims" of a disease.

13. This section never could have been completed without the work of Tamara Jones, Terri Bimes, Jayna Brown, and Sonya Brewer, who helped to examine the Vanderbilt Television Archives Index for 1981–93.

14. No stories from 1981 were included in this sample because no stories on AIDS appeared in 1981.

15. Pediatric AIDS cases are children under thirteen years of age (CDC).

16. Interview with George Strait.

17. Harper (1996) discusses the heterosexual personae of both Johnson and Ashe.

18. Interview with George Bellinger, Jr.

19. Interview with Greg Broyles.

Chapter Six

1. In this project I define the black press as those newspapers and magazines oriented to reporting the news and events of black communities, read primarily by African Americans, and owned or operated generally by black Americans.

2. *Essence* is a magazine that targets black middle-class women.

3. Interview with Linda Villarosa.

4. Interview with Tom Morgan.

5. Interview with Morgan.

6. In 1987 the *Index to the Black Newspaper* changed its name to the *Black Newspaper Index*.

7. As I explained in chapter 1, when appropriate, this analysis will be contextualized by locating the data in New York City.

8. *Ethnic Newswatch* (Stamford, CT: Softline Information, 1997). This is a database on CD-ROM.

9. The actions of the Haitian community were the subject of several articles in many black newspapers. The first story printed on AIDS in the *Amsterdam News* detailed the awarding of a grant to a Haitian group. However, it was the political activity of the Haitian community that gained them notice in 1985. In November 1985 the *Amsterdam News* ran a story by J. Zamgba Browne on the Haitian community's protest of a three-part series on WCBS-TV in New York entitled, "Junkies, Haitians, Homosexuals: Is It Their Problem? Not Anymore. It's Yours, AIDS" (9 November 1985). In the article, organizers of New York City's Haitian community complained about claims made on the program that AIDS originated in Haiti or Africa. They also voiced concern over the absence of any mention that only a few months prior to the airing of the program both the CDC and the New York City Department of Health removed Haitians from the list of high-risk groups.

10. The quotation from Egyir seems to contradict a statement by W. A. Tatum, chairman and editor in chief of the *Amsterdam News,* in an 17 August 1987 *New York Times* article on the black press. In the article, written by Alex S. Jones, Mr. Tatum states that "if blacks are going to make any progress, the media has to reflect who black people are, even with warts." The author goes on to write, "But candor has its limits. Another part of the black newspaper tradition, which is observed at the *Amsterdam News* and most of the city's other black papers, has been observance of an unwritten rule to avoid criticism of black elected officials and leaders."

11. Gary Byrd reportedly read about Kemron in the *New York Native,* an indigenous gay magazine. Byrd has stated that he was alerted to the discovery when walking through the terminals of the Port Authority and saw the headlines "The Cure" and "More on Kenya's Claim to Have Miracle AIDS Drug."

Chapter Seven

1. Circulation figures are taken from the *Media Industry Newsletter* 50, no. 9 (3 March 1997).

2. I used the *Reader's Guide to Periodical Literature* and the *Index to Black Periodicals* to generate the list of AIDS articles published in each of these black magazines.

3. Both Alfred Balk and Roland Wolseley note that *Jet* brought the Emmet Till case and the Montgomery bus boycott to the attention of black Americans (Wolseley 1990, 145).

4. If we figure that *Jet* generally publishes four times as many issues than monthly magazines—holding the size of the magazine and number of articles in each issue constant—we can compare publication records. Of course this says nothing about the content of these articles.

5. Interview with Linda Villarosa.

6. As late as June 1997 heterosexual transmission accounted for 7 percent of AIDS cases among black men and 36 percent among black women. Intravenous drug use and male-to-male sexual transmission accounted for 82 percent of cases among black men, while intravenous drug use accounted for 46 percent of identified AIDS cases among black women (CDC, *HIV* June 1997).

7. In a personal communication, Gil Gerald, one of the men cited in the article, describes what he considers to be the unprofessional tactics used by Randolph in researching and writing this article:

> This was most hurtful to me (The Laura Randolph article) and to others who wrote letters of protest to *Ebony*. In fact as [Randolph] was saying goodbye to me after a very protracted discussion of AIDS, she asked if I had ever slept with women. She had already put away her note pad, and we were engaged in small talk. The article DOES NOT INDICATE THAT I HAD BEEN SEXUAL WITH ONE WOMAN (she [Randolph] could not know because she did not explore) EIGHT TO NINE YEARS PRIOR TO 1981. SHE HAS NO IDEA WHETHER I USED PROTECTION OR NOT—SHE DID NOT ASK (AND I DID)! AND SHE ASSUMES IT WAS A BLACK WOMAN (THAT SHE WAS JAPANESE HAWAIIAN IS ULTIMATELY NOT MATERIAL—SHE IS A HUMAN AFTER ALL—BUT THIS IS ABOUT THE THREAT TO THE BLACK HETEROSEXUAL WOMAN): AND FURTHER IT IMPLIES DUPLICITY—SHE NEVER ASKED OR EXPLORES WHAT MY SEXUAL IDENTITY WAS NINE YEARS PRIOR TO 1981. It still hurts that a slam would be hurled at black gay men—suggesting our total disrespect and disregard for the health and welfare of black women! Neither Craig nor I were closeted, and we both paid dearly for that . . . if she needed such individuals [the dangerous bisexual infector of black women] she was careless in how she constructed and illustrated her case.

8. A significant number of stories printed by black newspapers are generated from or in response to reports, research, or other outside catalysts commenting on black communities. This finding reiterates the importance of dominant institutions such as the CDC in providing information that can then find its way into indigenous information sources.

9. The *Amsterdam News* also printed (some) stories, letters, and editorials attacking homophobia and AIDS phobia as well as highlighting gay and bisexual members of black communities, but those responses were usually written by readers, not staff associated with the paper.

10. Interview with Kimberly Smith.

11. Interview with Tom Morgan.

12. Quote taken off the Internet from the home page of the *Alternative Press Index* (http://www.altpress.org/api.html).

13. Communiqué from Gil Gerald.

14. During the first decade of the AIDS epidemic, the *American Muslim Journal* changed its name several times. In the beginning of the epidemic the paper was known as the *Bilialian News*; in early 1982 the name was changed to the *World Muslim News*; and by the end of 1982 it had taken the name *American Muslim Journal*. This name would

last through the first ten years of AIDS. Using data from the *Index to Black Newspapers* I explore the AIDS coverage in the *American Muslim Journal*. I could not locate an index to the *Final Call*, making a systematic examination of its AIDS coverage more difficult. The analysis of the *Final Call* relies on those stories on AIDS identified by research assistants and myself based on available copies of the paper published between 1981 and 1993.

Chapter Eight

1. Interview with Gil Gerald.

2. The demand for equity with regard to AIDS has recently found its way into the vocabulary of black legislators and national organizations.

3. Interview with Mildred Roxborough.

4. For example, on 15 September 1997 the National Gay and Lesbian Task Force (NGLTF) honored Coretta Scott King for her commitment to fighting for the civil rights of lesbian and gay people. In her acceptance of the award Mrs. King said, "I accept this award as a reaffirmation of my commitment to carry forward the unfinished work of my husband, Martin Luther King, Jr. My husband understood that all forms of discrimination and persecution were unjust and unacceptable for a great democracy. He believed that none of us could be freed until all of us were free, that a person of conscience had no alternative but to defend the human rights of all people." She continued, "I want to reaffirm my determination to secure the fullest protection of the law for all working people regardless of their sexual orientation . . . it is right, just, and good for America (NGLTF Press Release, 15 September 1997).

Black civil rights leaders have endorsed the idea of gay rights at other times, but all too often that support has come after significant negotiations to push black elected officials and traditional leaders to this position. For instance, Gil Gerald (1987) details the difficult and time-consuming efforts he and others engaged in to force organizers of the "Jobs, Peace, and Freedom" March, a march in honor of the twentieth anniversary of the March on Washington in 1963, to agree to have an openly lesbian or gay speaker at the march (Audre Lorde). Again, this example is not offered to discount the hard work of black legislators such as Maxine Waters or John Lewis who have shown leadership around both lesbian and gay rights as well as AIDS issues. However, most activity from black officials on the topic of AIDS or gay rights can be characterized as voting the right way but showing little leadership. I deal with this topic extensively in chapter 9.

5. Interview with Phil Wilson.

6. Interview with Michael Pawlson.

7. Interview with Gil Gerald.

8. Interview with Robert Penn.

9. Ms. Roxborough informed me that the entire policy proposal was submitted to the Clinton transition team as *the* blueprint for the improvement of black health and health care in the United States. Maybe this explains the Clinton Administration's record on AIDS, especially in black communities.

10. Interview with Dr. James Rawlings.

11. This was the first article according to the *Index to Black Periodicals.*

12. Interview with Tracy Gardner-Wright.

13. In their edited volume *A Common Destiny: Blacks and American Society* (1989), Jaynes and Williams note that "unlike the NAACP, the Urban League has never been a mass membership organization, although it is organized into local affiliates (about 100 branches) that conduct the bulk of its programmatic activities" (185). They go on to comment on the financial stability of the organization: "As of 1985, the National Urban League far surpassed all other black organizations in terms of donations and program

expenditures; its outside revenues totaled $23,573,000, compared with $7,686,000 for the NAACP" (186).

14. The date of the first national conference on AIDS sponsored by the SCLC has been disputed. Some claim that a SCLC conference in 1986 was national in focus.

15. Interview with Magie A. Shannon.

16. Interview with Phil Wilson.

17. Interview with Gil Gerald.

18. Interview with Magie A. Shannon.

19. Interview with Dr. Marjorie Hill.

20. Interview with Greg Broyles.

21. Interview with Tracy Gardner-Wright.

22. Interview with Rev. Calvin Butts.

23. Interview with Colin Robinson.

24. Interview with George Bellinger, Jr.

25. The National Medical Association was founded in 1895 under the name the National Association of Colored Physicians, Dentists, and Pharmacists. The organization changed its name to the National Medical Association at its second national meeting at Meharry Medical College in Nashville, Tennessee, in 1903 (http://www.natmed.org/about.html).

Chapter Nine

1. Interview with Ronald Johnson.

2. Interview with Keith Cylar.

3. Interview with Phil Wilson.

4. Interviews with Phil Wilson, Gil Gerald, Colin Robinson, Ronald Johnson, Tracy Gardner-Wright.

5. None of the work of this chapter could have been completed without the incredible assistance of Alethia Jones, as well as Terri Bimes, Sonya Brewer, and Alexis McGill.

6. The primary sponsor is the member who signs the bill for its introduction. Often the primary sponsor is expected to guide the legislation through the House or Senate and can be instrumental in soliciting the support and cosponsorship of other members.

7. The number of bills sponsored by black Congressional Members decreased slightly during the 101st Congress.

8. Cost and length constraints prevented me from including tables which detail the data for all forty AIDS votes. These tables can be accessed by contacting the author directly.

9. In choosing which AIDS-related legislation to examine in-depth, my research assistants and I performed an informal survey of AIDS activists to see what they thought was the most important AIDS legislation to be considered during the first thirteen years of the epidemic. Overwhelmingly, the Ryan White Care Act was named most often, followed by the 1993 Reauthorization of the National Institutes of Health (NIH) and the Americans with Disabilities Act.

10. When originally passed, the Act provided emergency funds for metropolitan areas with more than two thousand confirmed AIDS cases or where the per capita incidence of AIDS was .0025. The fifteen cities that had at the time of passage more than two thousand confirmed AIDS cases were Atlanta; Boston; Chicago; Dallas; Fort Lauderdale; Houston; Los Angeles; Miami; New York; Newark; Philadelphia; San Diego; San Francisco; San Juan, Puerto Rico; and Washington, DC. As noted in the *Congressional Quarterly Almanac*, these cities accounted for more than 50 percent of all reported AIDS cases in the United States at that time: "Jersey City, NJ, also qualified for the emergency aid because of the high incidence of AIDS in that relatively small city" (1990, 582).

One other significant part of the Ryan White Act was that it required cities to establish

HIV health services planning councils. The councils were to include a number of different constituencies working on and living with AIDS: "The council would have to include providers of health care, social services, and mental health services; representatives of community-based and AIDS service organizations; local public health agencies, hospitals or health-care planning agencies; individuals with HIV disease; nonelected community leaders; state government officials . . . (*Congressional Quarterly Almanac* 1990, 584). It was thought that these councils could democratize a process of setting funding priorities for cities and metropolitan areas. As we might expect, these councils, while finding ways to get important work done, have also been the sites of important battles over race and the fair distribution of resources.

11. Some of the provisions in Title II (grants targeted to states) of the Ryan White Act include a set-aside for women and children, requiring states to use 15 percent of the funds received for services for women, infants, children, and families suffering from HIV. This section also requires that charges for services be waived for people below the poverty level and reduced for those with incomes between 100 and 300 percent of the poverty level. Finally, Title II requires matching funds from states.

12. Subtitle 2: Category Grants requires that grants to provide early intervention services for hemophiliacs "be made through the network of comprehensive hemophilia diagnostic and treatment centers" (*Congressional Quarterly Almanac* 1990, 586). This section also provides for reduced charges for low-income patients.

13. Unlike any other segment of the population living with HIV and AIDS, infants and children were singled out as the focus for demonstration projects. As we might expect, through this formulation, funds could go to entities servicing women, but only those that serviced pregnant women. Thus, women gained recognition in Title IV of the Act only as they were understood to serve as possible infectious agents for their children. This section also included a provision that disallowed the use of funds to distribute hypodermic needles or syringes for the use of illegal drugs.

14. I use the terms *attendance* and *participation* loosely, since a representative need only show up for a very short time to be recorded as in attendance at one of these hearings.

15. "Boarder babies" are children who remain in hospitals after it is no longer medically necessary; they have nowhere to go because of parental abandonment, death, inability, or state intervention.

16. Interview with Robert Penn.

17. The original version of this Act authorized $37 million over three years for demonstration projects aimed at finding solutions to the problem of abandoned babies associated most directly with crises of drug use and AIDS (*Congressional Quarterly,* 8 October 1988, 2811). The reauthorization provided $30 million to programs and agencies providing services to this population (*Congressional Quarterly,* 3 August 1991, 2175).

18. Interview with Charles Eaton.

19. Most of the eleven states with such laws were experiencing debilitating problems with intravenous drug use.

20. Interview with Charles Eaton.

21. It is well-known that in New York City there is generally at least a six-month waiting period for anyone interested in residential drug rehabilitation. This wait is, unfortunately, an effective deterrent to rehab; former drug users indicate that when someone using drugs feels ready for rehab, they need to act on that impulse immediately to increase their chance of success.

22. Interview with Cliff Goodman.

23. Interview with Rev. Calvin Butts.

24. Interview with Phil Wilson.

25. I do not want to dichotomize too rigidly the charismatic leadership, noted most often in black ministers, and the structurally based leadership of black elected officials.

Quite often those leaders elected to political positions have gained notoriety and office by their association with the black church. One positive consequence of the development of alternative paths to leadership in black communities has been the increased opportunity for black women to gain publicly recognized positions of leadership. Formerly, with the path to leadership leading straight through the pulpit, a place reserved for men in most black churches, this meant the de facto exclusion of women from public positions of power.

BIBLIOGRAPHY

Abeles, Ronald R. 1976. "Relative Deprivation, Rising Expectations, and Black Militancy." *Journal of Social Issues* 32, no. 2: 119–17.

Abercrombie, Nicholas, Stephen Hill, and Bryan S. Turner, eds. 1990. *Dominant Ideologies.* London: Unwin Hyman.

Adam, Barry D. 1987. *The Rise of a Gay and Lesbian Movement.* Boston: Twayne Publishers.

Adoni, Hanna, and Sherril Mane. 1984. "Media and the Social Construction of Reality: Toward an Integration of Theory and Research," *Communications Research* 11, no. 3 (July): 323–40.

Aguero, Joseph E., Laura Bloch, and Donn Byrne. 1985. "The Relationships Among Sexual Beliefs, Attitudes, Experience, and Homophobia." In *Bashers, Baiters, and Bigots,* edited by J. P. De Cecco. New York: Harrington Park Press, 95–108.

Allen, Richard, Michael Dawson, and Ronald Brown. 1989. "A Schema-Based Approach to Modeling an African-American Racial Belief System," *American Political Science Review* 83, no. 2: 421–41.

Allen, Robert L. 1969. *Black Awakening in Capitalist America.* Garden City, NJ: Doubleday.

Alternative Press Index. 1969–. College Park, MD: Alternative Press Center.

Altman, Dennis. 1986. *AIDS in the Mind of America.* Garden City, NJ: Anchor Books.

Alwood, Edward. 1996. *Straight News: Gays, Lesbians, and the News Media.* New York: Columbia University Press.

Alyson Almanac. 1990. Boston: Alyson Publications.

Amaker, Norman C. 1988. *Civil Rights and the Reagan Administration.* Washington, DC: Urban Institute Press.

Anderson, Benedict. 1991. *Imagined Communities.* London: Verso.

Anekwe, Simon. 1987. City to Spend $42M on Public Education." *Amsterdam News,* 20 June, 36.

Bachrach, Peter. 1969. *The Theory of Democratic Elitism: A Critique.* London: University of London Press.

Bachrach, Peter, and Morton S. Baratz. 1962. "The Two Faces of Power." *American Political Science Review* 56: 947–52.

———. 1963. "Decisions and Nondecisions: An Analytical Framework." *American Political Science Review* 57: 641–51.

———. 1970. *Power and Poverty. Theory and Practice.* New York: Oxford University Press.

Barker, Lucius J. 1988. *Our Time Has Come: A Delegate's Diary of Jesse Jackson's 1984 Presidential Campaign.* Urbana: University of Illinois Press.

Barkley Brown, Elsa. 1994. "Negotiating and Transforming the Public Sphere: African American Political Life in the Transition from Slavery to Freedom." *Public Culture* 7: 107–46.

Barnett, Marguerite Ross. 1977. "The Congressional Black Caucus: Symbol, Myth, and Reality." *Black Scholar* (January/February): 17–26.

———. 1982. "The Congressional Black Caucus: Illusions and Realities of Power." In *The*

New Black Politics: The Search for Political Power, edited by M. B. Preston, L. J. Henderson, Jr., and P. Puryear. New York: Longman, 28–54.

Barrera, Mario. 1979. *Race and Class in the Southwest: A Theory of Racial Inequality.* Notre Dame, IN: University of Notre Dame Press.

Bayer, Ronald. 1983. *Private Acts, Social Consequences: AIDS and the Politics of Public Health.* New Brunswick: Rutgers University Press.

Beach, Stephen W. 1977. "Social Movement Radicalization: The Case of the People's Democracy in Northern Ireland. " *Sociological Quarterly* 18 (summer): 305–18.

Beale, Frances. 1995. "Double Jeopardy: To Be Black and Female." In *Words of Fire: An Anthology of African-American Feminist Thought,* edited by B. Guy-Sheftall. New York: New Press, 146–55.

Beam, Joseph, ed. 1986. *In the Life: A Black Gay Anthology.* Boston: Alyson Publications.

Bell, Inge Powell. 1971. "Status Discrepancy and the Radical Rejection of Non-violence." In *Conflict and Competition: Studies in the Recent Black Protest Movement,* edited by J. H. Bracey, Jr., A. Meier, and E. Rudwick. Belmont, CA: Wadsworth.

Bennett, Lerone, Jr. 1966. *Confrontation: Black and White.* Baltimore, MD: Penguin Books.

———. 1984. *Before the Mayflower: A History of Black Americans.* 5th ed. New York: Penguin Books.

Bentley, Arthur. 1949. *The Process of Government.* Evanston, IL: Principia Press.

Berube, Allan. 1990. "Marching to a Different Drummer: Lesbian and Gay GIs in World War II." In *Hidden From History: Reclaiming the Gay and Lesbian Past,* edited by M. Duberman, M. Vicinus, and G. Chauncey, Jr. New York: Meridian, 383–94.

Biery, Roger E. 1990. *Understanding Homosexuality: The Pride and the Prejudice.* Austin, TX: Edward-William.

Billingsley, Andrew, and Cleopatra Howard Caldwell. 1991. "The Church, the Family, and the School in the African American Community." *Journal of Negro Education* 60, no. 3: 427–40.

Blassingame, John W. 1972. *The Slave Community: Plantation Life in the Antebellum South.* New York: Oxford University Press.

Blauner, Robert. 1972. *Racial Oppression in America.* New York: Harper and Row.

Bobo, Lawrence. 1983. "Whites' Opposition to Busing: Symbolic Racism or Realistic Group Conflict?," *Journal of Personality and Social Psychology* 45: 1196–1210.

Bobo, Lawrence, and James R. Kluegel. 1991. "Modern American Prejudice: Stereotypes, Social Distance, and Perceptions of Discrimination toward Blacks, Hispanics and Asians." Paper presented at the Annual Meeting of the American Sociological Association, Cincinnati, OH, 23–27 August 1991.

Bourdieu, Pierre. 1986. "The Forms of Capital." In *Handbook of Theory and Research for the Sociology of Education,* edited by J. G. Richardson. New York: Greenwood Press, 241–58.

Bowles, Samuel, and Herbert Gintis. 1986. *Democracy and Capitalism: Property, Community, and the Contradictions of Modern Social Thought.* New York: Basic Books.

Bowles, Jacqueline, and William A. Robinson. 1989. "PHS Grants for Minority Group HIV Infection Education and Prevention Efforts." *Public Health Reports* 104, no. 6 (November–December): 552–59.

Bowser, Benjamin P. 1992. "African-American Culture and AIDS Prevention: From Barrier to Ally." *Western Journal of Medicine* 157, no. 3 (September): 286–89.

Brady, D. W. 1978. "Critical Election, Congressional Parties, and Cluster of Policy Change." *British Journal of Political Science* 8: 79–99.

Brandt, Allan M. 1987. *No Magic Bullet: A Social History of Venereal Disease in the United States Since 1880.* New York: Oxford University Press.

Brink, William, and Louis Harris. 1963. *The Negro Revolution in America.* New York: Simon and Schuster.

Broom, Leonard. 1959. "Social Differentiation and Stratification." In *Sociology Today*, edited by R. K. Merton, L. Broom, and L. S. Cottrell. New York: Basic Books, 429–41.

Bunche, Ralph. 1973. *The Political Status of the Negro in the Age of FDR*, edited by D. W. Grantham. Chicago: University of Chicago Press.

Buono, Anthony F., and Judith B. Kamm. 1983. "Marginality and the Organizational Socialization of Female Managers." *Human Relations* 36, no. 12: 1125–40.

Burawoy, Michael, Alice Burton, Ann Arnett Ferguson, Kathryn J. Fox, Johsua Gamson, Nadine Gartrell, Leslie Hurst, Charles Hurzman, Leslie Salzinger, Joseph Schiffman, and Shiori Ui. 1991. *Ethnography Unbound: Power and Resistance in the Modern Metropolis.* Berkeley: University of California Press.

Burns, James MacGregor. 1978. *Leadership.* New York: Harper and Row.

Carby, Hazel. 1987. *Reconstructing Womanhood: The Emergence of the Black Female Novelist.* New York: Oxford University Press.

———. 1992. "Policing the Black Woman's Body in an Urban Context." *Critical Inquiry* 18 (summer): 738–55.

Carmichael, Stokley, and Charles V. Hamilton. 1967. *Black Power: The Politics of Liberation in America.* New York: Vintage Books.

Carter, Erica, and Simon Watney. 1989. *Taking Liberties: AIDS and Cultural Politics.* Great Britain: WBC Print, Ltd.

Chauncey, George, Jr. 1989. "Christian Brotherhood or Sexual Perversion? Homosexual Identities and the Construction of Sexual Boundaries in the World War I Era." In *Hidden From History: Reclaiming the Gay and Lesbian Past*, edited by M. Duberman, M. Vicinus, and G. Chauncey, Jr. New York: Meridian Books, 294–317.

———. 1994. *Gay New York: Gender, Urban Culture, and the Making of the Gay Male World 1890–1940.* New York: Basic Books.

Chirimuuta, Richard, and Rosalind Chirimuuta. 1989. *AIDS, Africa, and Racism.* London: Free Association Books.

Clausen, A. R. 1973. *How Congressmen Decide: A Policy Focus.* New York: St. Martin's Press.

Cohen, Anthony P. 1985. *The Symbolic Construction of Community.* London: Routledge.

Cohen, Cathy J. 1996a. "Contested Membership: Black Gay Identities and the Politics of AIDS." In *Queer Theory/Sociology*, edited by S. Seidman. Oxford: Blackwell, 362–94.

———. 1996b. "The Price of Inclusion in the Marriage Club." *Gay Community News* 24, nos. 3–4: 27, 37–38.

———. 1997. "Straight Gay Politics: The Limits of an Ethnic Model of Inclusion." In *NOMOS 39: Ethnicity and Group Rights*, edited by I. Shapiro and W. Kymlicka. New York: New York Univesity Press, 572–616.

———. 1997a. "Punks, Bull Daggers, and Welfare Queens: The Radical Potential of 'Queer' Politics." *GLQ* 3: 437–65.

Cohen, Cathy J., and Michael Dawson. 1993. "Neighborhood Poverty and African-American Politics." *American Political Science Review* 87, no. 2: 286–302.

Cohen, Cathy J., Kathleen Jones, and Joan Tronto, eds. 1997. *Women Transforming Politics: An Alternative Reader.* New York: New York University Press.

Colby, David C., and Timothy E. Cook. 1991. "Epidemics and Agenda: The Politics of Nightly News Coverage of AIDS." *Journal of Health Policy and Law* 16, no. 2: 215–49.

Collins, Patricia Hill. 1990. *Black Feminist Thought: Knowledge, Consciousness and the Politics of Empowerment.* New York: Unwin Hyman.

Conyers, J. E. and W. L. Wallace. 1976. *Black Elected Officials: A Study of Black Americans Holding Governmental Office.* New York: Russell Sage.

Conover, Pamela Johnston, Ivor Crewe, and Donald D. Searing. 1996. "Institutions and Political Learning: Contextual and Developmental Models." Paper prepared for Annual Meeting of the American Political Science Association, San Francisco.

Cook, Fay Lomax, Tom R. Tyler, Edward G. Goetz, Margaret T. Gordon, David Protess, Donna R. Leff, and Harvey L. Molotch. 1983. "Media and Agenda Setting: Effects on the Public, Interest Group Leaders, Policy Makers, and Policy." *Public Opinion Quarterly* 47: 16–35.

Cook, Timothy E. 1989. *Making Laws and Making News: Media Strategies in the U.S. House of Representative.* Washington, DC: Brookings Institution.

Cook, Timothy E., and David C. Colby. 1992. "The Mass-Mediated Epidemic: The Politics of AIDS on the Nightly Network News." In *AIDS: The Making of a Chronic Disease,* edited by E. Fee and D.M. Fox. Berkeley: University of California Press, 84–122.

Cooper, Peter A. 1988. "Community under Seige: The AIDS Epidemic in Harlem." *Amsterdam News,* 30 July, 4 and 36.

Cornish, Rev. Samuel, and John Brown Russwurm. 1827. *Freedom's Journal.* Malvern, PA: Accessible Archives.

Cose, Ellis. 1993. *The Rage of a Privileged Class.* New York: HarperCollins.

Cott, Nancy F. 1987. *The Grounding of Modern Feminism.* New Haven: Yale University Press.

Cox, Oliver. 1970. *Caste, Class, and Race.* New York: Modern Reader.

Crenshaw, Kimberle. 1989. "Demarginalizing the Intersection of Race and Sex: A Black Feminist Critique of Antidiscrimination Doctrine, Feminist Theory, and Antiracist Politics." *University of Chicago Legal Forum, 1989,* 139–67.

———. 1992. "Whose Story Is It Anyway? Feminist and Antiracist Appropriations of Anita Hill." In *Race-ing Justice, En-gendering Power: Essays on Anita Hill, Clarence Thomas, and the Construction of Social Reality,* edited by T. Morrison. New York: Pantheon Books.

Crenson, Matthew A. 1971. *The Un-Politics of Air Pollution: A Study of Non-Decision-Making in the Cities.* Baltimore and London: John Hopkins Press.

Crimp, Douglas, ed. 1989. *AIDS: Cultural Analysis, Cultural Activism.* Cambridge: MIT Press.

Crimp, Douglas, and Adam Rolston. 1990. *AIDS demo graphics.* Seattle: Bay Press.

Cruikshank, Margaret. 1992. *The Gay and Lesbian Liberation Movement.* New York: Routledge.

Curry, Leonard P. 1981. *The Free Black in Urban America, 1800–1850: The Shadow of the Dream.* Chicago: University of Chicago Press.

D'Emilio, John. 1983a. *Sexual Politics, Sexual Communities: The Making of a Homosexual Minority in the United States, 1940–1970.* Chicago: University of Chicago Press.

———. 1983b. "Capitalism and Gay Identity." In *Powers of Desire: The Politics of Sexuality,* edited by A. Snitow, C. Stansell, and S. Thompson. New York: Monthly Review Press, 100–113.

———. 1992. *Making Trouble: Essays on Gay History, Politics, and the University.* New York: Routledge.

D'Emilio, John, and Estelle B. Freedman. 1988. *Intimate Matters: A History of Sexuality in America.* New York: Harper and Row.

Dahl, Robert A. 1957. "The Concept of Power." *Behavioral Science* 2: 201–5.

———. 1958. "A Critique of the Ruling Elite Model." *American Political Science Review* 52: 463–69.

———. 1961. *Who Governs? Democracy and Power in an American City.* New Haven: Yale University Press.

———. 1967. *Pluralist Democracy in the United States.* Chicago: Rand McNally.

———. 1985. *A Preface to Economic Democracy.* Berkeley: University of California Press.

Dahrendorf, Ralf. 1959. *Class and Class Conflict in Industrial Society.* Stanford: Stanford University Press.

Dalton, Harlon L. 1989. "AIDS in Blackface." *Daedalus* 118, no. 3: 205–27.

Dalton, Harlon L., Scott Burris, and the Yale AIDS Law Project. 1987. *AIDS and the Law.* New Haven: Yale University Press.

Dates, Jannette L. 1990. "Print News." In *Split Images: African Americans in The Mass Media,* edited by J. L. Dates and W. Barlow. Washington, DC: Howard University Press, 343–87.

Davies, James C. 1969. "The J-Curve of Rising and Declining Satisfactions as a Cause of some Great Revolutions and a Contained Rebellion." In *Violence in America: Historical and Comparative Perspectives,* edited by H. D. Graham and T. R. Gurr. Washington, DC: U.S. Government Printing Office, 690–730.

Davis, Angela. 1981. *Women, Race, and Class.* New York: Random House.

Dawson, Michael C. 1994. *Behind the Mule: Race and Class in African-American Politics.* Princeton: Princeton University Press.

Day, Dawn. 1995. *Health Emergency: The Spread of Drug-Related AIDS among African-Americans and Latinos.* A special report prepared for a consortium of organizations.

De Cecco, John P., ed. 1985. *Bashers, Baiters, and Bigots: Homophobia in American Society.* New York: Harrington Park Press.

Dent, Gina, ed. 1992. *Black Popular Culture.* Seattle: Bay Press.

Des Jarlais, Don C., Samuel R. Friedman, and Jo L. Sotheran. 1992. "The First City: HIV Among Intravenous Drug Users in New York City." In *AIDS: The Making of a Chronic Disease,* edited by E. Fee and D. M. Fox. Berkeley: University of California Press, 279–95.

Dickie-Clark, H. F. 1966. *The Marginal Situation.* London: Routledge & Kegan Paul.

Dobie, Kathy. 1989. "Woman of the Year: Yolanda Serrano." In *Ms.* (January/February), 79–83.

Dollimore, Jonathan. 1991. *Sexual Dissidence: Augustine to Wilde, Freud to Foucault.* Oxford: Clarendon Press.

Domhoff, G. William. 1970. *The Higher Circles.* New York: Random House.

Drake, St. Clair, and Horace R. Cayton. 1993. *Black Metropolis: A Study of Negro Life in a Northern City.* Chicago: University of Chicago Press.

Driedger, Diane. 1989. *The Last Civil Rights Movement: Disabled Peoples' International.* New York: St. Martin's Press.

Duberman, Martin. 1991. *About Time: Exploring the Gay Past.* New York: Meridian.

———. 1994. *Stonewall.* New York: Plume.

Du Bois, W. E. B. 1986. *Writings.* Edited by N. Huggins. New York: The Library of America.

Duggan, Lisa. 1996. "The Marriage Juggernaut." In *Gay Community News* 24, no. 3–4 (winter/spring): 5, 26, 34.

Durkheim, Emile. 1964. *The Division of Labor in Society.* New York: Free Press.

Eagleton, Terry. 1991. *Ideology: An Introduction.* London: Verso.

Edelman, Murray. 1971. *Politics as Symbolic Action.* Chicago: Markham.

Eisinger, Peter K. 1973. "The Conditions of Protest Behavior in American Cities." *American Political Science Review* 67: 11–28.

———. 1982. "Black Empowerment in Municipal Jobs: The Impact of Black Political Power." *American Political Science Review* 76: 380–92.

———. 1984. "Black Mayors and the Politics of Racial Economic Advancement." In *Readings in Urban Politics: Past, Present and Future,* 2d ed. edited by H. Hahn and C. N. Levine. New York: Longman.

Elias, Norbert. 1978. *The History of Manners, The Civilizing Process.* Vol. 1. New York: Pantheon Books.

Epstein, Steven. 1996. *Impure Science: AIDS, Activism, and the Politics of Knowledge.* Berkeley: University of California Press.

Fairclough, Adam. 1987. *To Redeem the Soul of America: The SCLC and MLK, Jr.* Athens: University of Georgia Press.

Fanon, Frantz. 1963. *The Wretched of the Earth.* New York: Grove Weidenfeld.

Farley, Reynolds. 1984. *Blacks and Whites: Narrowing the Gap?* Cambridge: Harvard University Press.

———. 1989. "The Quality of Life for Black Americans Twenty Years After the Civil Rights Revolution." In *Health Policies and Black Americans,* edited by D. P. Willis. New Brunswick: Transaction Publishers, 9–34.

Farley, Reynolds, and Walter R. Allen. 1987. *The Color Line and the Quality of Life in America.* New York: Russell Sage Foundation.

Fauci, Anthony S. 1991. "The Human Immunodeficiency Virus: Infectivity and Mechanisms of Pathogenesis." In *The AIDS Reader: Social, Political, Ethical Issues,* edited by N. F. McKenzie. New York: Meridian, 25–41.

Feagin, Joe, and Melvin Sikes. 1994. *Living with Racism: The Black Middle-Class Experience.* New York: Beacon Press.

Fee, Elizabeth, and Daniel M. Fox. 1988. *AIDS: The Burdens of History.* Berkeley: University of California Press.

Fenno, Richard F. 1990. *Watching Politicians: Essays on Participant Observation.* Berkeley: Institute of Government Studies.

Ferguson, Russell, Martha Gever, Trinh T. Minh-ha, and Cornel West. 1992. *Out There: Marginalization and Contemporary Cultures.* Cambridge: MIT Press.

Fields, Barbara J. 1982. "Ideology and Race in American History." In *Region, Race, and Reconstruction: Essays in Honor of C. Vann Woodward,* edited by J. Morgan Kousser and J. McPherson. New York: Oxford University Press, 143–77.

———. 1990. "Slavery, Race, and Ideology in the United States of America." *New Left Review* no. 181 (May/June): 95–118.

Fiorina, Morris P. 1974. *Representatives, Roll Calls, and Constituencies.* Lexington, MA: D. C. Health.

Fiske, Susan T., and Shelley E. Taylor. 1984. *Social Cognition.* New York: Random House.

Fitzgerald, Frances. 1986. *Cities on a Hill: A Journey through Contemporary American Cultures.* New York: Simon and Schuster.

Flacks, Richard W. 1967. "The Liberated Generation: An Exploration of the Roots of Student Protest." *Journal of Social Issues* 23 (July): 52–75.

Fogelson, Robert M. 1971. *Violence as Protest.* Garden City, NY: Doubleday.

Foucault, Michael. 1979. *Discipline and Punish: The Birth of the Prison.* New York: Vintage Books.

———. 1980. *The History of Sexuality.* Vol. 1. *An Introduction.* Translated by R. Hurley. New York: Vintage Books.

Franklin, John Hope. 1980. *From Slavery to Freedom: A History of Negro Americans.* 5th ed. New York: Alfred A. Knopf.

Frazier, E. Franklin. 1957. *Black Bourgeoisie: The Rise of a New Middle Class in the United States.* New York: Collier Books.

———. 1964. *The Negro Church in America.* New York: Schocken Books.

Frazier, E. Franklin, and C. Eric Lincoln. 1974. *The Negro Church in America: The Black Church Since Frazier.* New York: Schocken Books.

Freeman, Jo. 1973. "The Origins of the Women's Liberation Movement." *American Journal of Sociology* 78, no. 4: 792–811.

Freire, Paulo. 1972. *The Pedagogy of the Oppressed.* New York: Continuum.

Frey, Frederic W. 1971. "Comment: On Issues and Nonissues in the Study of Power." *American Political Science Review* 65: 1081–101.

Friedman, Samuel, Jo L. Sotheran, Abu Abdul-quader, Beny J. Primm, Don C. Des Jarlais, Paula Kleinman, Conrad Mauge, Douglas S. Goldsmith, Wafaa El-Sadr, and Robert

Maslansky. 1987. "The AIDS Epidemic among Blacks and Hispanics." *The Miliband Quarterly* 65, suppl. 2: 455–99.

Fulwood, Sam, III. 1991. "The NAACP at the Crossroads." *Emerge* (October): 41–45.

Gaines, Kevin K. 1996. *Uplifting the Race: Black Leadership, Politics, and Culture in the Twentieth Century.* Chapel Hill: The University of North Carolina Press.

Gamson, William A. 1968. "Stable Unrepresentation in American Society." *The American Behavioral Scientist* (November/December): 15–21.

———. 1975. *The Strategy of Social Protest.* Homewood, IL: Dorsey Press.

Garber, Eric. 1990. "A Spectacle in Color: The Lesbian and Gay Subculture of Jazz-Age Harlem." In *Hidden From History: Reclaiming the Gay and Lesbian Past,* edited by M. Duberman, M. Vicinus, and G. Chauncey, Jr. New York: Meridian.

Gates, Henry Louis. 1992. "Two Nations . . . Both Black." *Forbes,* 14 September, 132–35.

Gaventa, John. 1980. *Power and Powerlessness: Quiescence and Rebellion in an Appalachian Valley.* Urbana: University of Illinois Press.

Gay Men's Health Crisis. *The First Ten Years: GMHC 1990–1991 Annual Report.* New York: Gay Men's Health Crisis.

Geertz, Clifford. 1973. *The Interpretations of Cultures.* New York: Basic Books.

Genovese, Eugene D. 1976. *Roll Jordan, Roll: The World the Slave Made.* New York: Vintage Books.

Geschwender, James A. 1971. "Explorations in the Theory of Social Movements and Revolution." In *The Black Revolt,* edited by J. A. Geschwender. Englewood Cliffs, NJ: Prentice-Hall.

Giddens, Anthony. 1968. "Power in the Recent Writings of Talcott Parsons." *Sociology* 2 (September): 257–72.

———. 1973. *The Class Structure of the Advanced Societies.* New York: Harper and Row.

Giddens, Anthony, and David Held, eds. 1982. *Classes, Power, and Conflict: Classical and Contemporary Debates.* Berkeley and Los Angeles: University of California Press.

Giddings, Paula. 1984. *When and Where I Enter: The Impact of Black Women on Race and Sex in America.* New York: Bantam Books.

———. 1992. "The Last Taboo." In *Race-ing Justice, En-gendering Power: Essays on Anita Hill, Clarence Thomas and the Construction of Social Reality,* edited by T. Morrison. New York: Pantheon Books, 441–65.

Gilens, Martin. 1996. "Race and Poverty in America: Public Misperceptions and the American News Media." *Public Opinion Quarterly* 60 (winter): 515–41.

Gilroy, Paul. 1991. *There Ain't No Black in the Union Jack: The Cultural Politics of Race and Nation.* Chicago: University of Chicago Press.

Gitlin, Todd. 1980. *The Whole World Is Watching! Mass Media in the Making and Unmaking of the New Left.* Berkeley: University of California Press.

Goffman, Erving. 1963. *Stigma: Notes on the Management of Spoiled Identity.* New York: Simon and Schuster.

Gordon, Milton Myron. 1964. *Assimilation in American Life: The Role of Race, Religion, and Natural Origins.* New York: Oxford University Press.

Gramsci, Antonio. 1971. *Selections from the Prison Notebooks.* Edited and translated by Q. Hoare and G. Nowell-Smith. London: Lawrence and Wishart.

Greenhouse, Steven. 1997. "Labor Leaders Seek to Unionize Welfare Recipients Who Must Go to Work." *New York Times,* 19 February, A18.

Grmek, Mirko D. 1990. *History of AIDS: Emergence and Origin of a Modern Pandemic.* Translated by R. C. Maulitz and J. Duffin. Princeton, NJ: Princeton University Press.

Grossman, James R. 1989. *Chicago, Black Southerners, and the Great Migration.* Chicago: University of Chicago Press.

Guinan, Mary E. 1993. "Black Communities' Belief in 'AIDS as Genocide': A Barrier to Overcome for HIV Prevention." *Annals of Epidemiology* 3, no. 2 (March): 193–95.

Guinier, Lani. 1994. *The Tyranny of the Majority: Fundamental Fairness in Representative De-mocracy.* New York: Free Press.

Gurin, Patricia, Shirley Hatchett, and James S. Jackson. 1989. *Hope and Independence: Blacks' Response to Electoral and Party Politics.* New York: Vintage Books.

Gutman, Herbert G. 1976. *The Black Family in Slavery and Freedom, 1750–1925.* New York: Vintage Books.

Guy-Sheftall, Beverly, ed. 1995. *Words of Fire: An Anthology of African-American Feminist Thought.* New York: New Press.

Hacker, Andrew. 1992. *Two Nations: Black and White, Separate, Hostile, Unequal.* New York: Ballantine Books.

———. 1995. *Two Nations: Black and White, Separate, Hostile, Unequal.* Expanded and up-dated edition. New York: Ballantine Books.

Hagendoorn, Louk, and Joseph Hraba. 1989. "Foreign, Different, Deviant, Seclusive, and Working Class: Anchors to an Ethnic Hierarchy in the Netherlands." *Ethnic and Racial Studies* 12, no. 4 (October): 441–68.

Hall, Richard L. 1996. *Participation in Congress.* New Haven: Yale University Press.

Hallin, Daniel C. 1989. *The "Uncensored War": The Media and Vietnam.* Berkeley: University of California Press.

Hammonds, Evelynn. 1986. "Missing Persons: African American Women, AIDS, and the History of Disease." *Radical America* 20, no. 6: 7–23.

———. 1992. "Race, Sex, AIDS: The Construction of 'Other'." In *Race, Class, and Gender: An Anthology,* edited by M. L. Andersen and P. Hill Collins. Belmont, CA: Wads-worth, 329–40.

———. 1997. "Toward a Genealogy of Black Female Sexuality: The Problematic of Si-lence." In *Feminist Genealogies, Colonial Legacies, Democratic Futures,* edited by M. J. Al-exander and C. Talapade Mohanty. New York: Routledge, 170–82.

Harper, Philip Brian. 1993. "Eloquence and Epitaph: Black Nationalism and the Homo-phobic Impulse in Response to the Death of Max Robinson." In *The Lesbian and Gay Studies Reader,* edited by H. Abelove, M. A. Barale, and D. M. Halperin. New York: Routledge, 159–75.

———. 1996. *Are We Not Men? Masculine Anxiety and the Problem of African-American Iden-tity.* New York: Oxford University Press.

Harvard AIDS Institute. 1996. "Communities of Color." *Harvard AIDS Review* (spring/summer).

Hatchett, David. 1990. "The Impact of AIDS on the Black Community." in *Crisis* 97, no. 9 (November): 28–30.

Head, Anthony. 1985. "'Village People': Japan's 'Burakumin,'" *Contemporary Review* 246: 74–78.

Hemphill, Essex ed. 1991. *Brother to Brother: New Writings by Black Gay Men.* Boston: Aly-son Publications.

Henry, Charles P. 1990. *Culture and African American Politics.* Bloomington: Indiana Uni-versity Press.

Herek, Gregory M., and John P. Capitanio. 1993. "Public Reactions to AIDS in the United States: A Second Decade." *American Journal of Public Health* 83, no. 4 (April): 574–77.

———. 1994. "Conspiracies, Contagion, and Compassion: Trust and Public Reactions to AIDS." *AIDS Education and Prevention* 6, no. 4: 365–75.

Heyward, William L., and James W. Curran. 1989. "The Epidemiology of AIDS." *The Science of AIDS: Readings from Scientific American.* New York: W. H. Freeman.

Higginbotham, Jr., A. Leon. 1978. *In the Matter of Color: Race and the American Legal Process.* Oxford: Oxford University Press.

Higginbotham, Evelyn Brooks. 1992. "African-American Women's History and the Meta-language of Race." *Signs* 17, no. 2 (winter): 251–74.

———. 1993. *Righteous Discontent: The Women's Movement in the Black Baptist Church, 1880–1920.* Cambridge: Harvard University Press.

Hochschild, Jennifer L. 1995. *Facing Up to the American Dream: Race, Class and the Soul of the Nation.* Princeton, NJ: Princeton University Press.

Holman, Priscilla B., William C. Jenkins, Jacob A. Gayle, Carlton Duncan, and Bryan K. Lindsey. 1991. "Increasing the Involvement of National and Regional Racial and Ethnic Minority Organizations in HIV Information and Education." *Public Health Reports* 106, no. 6 (November/December): 687–94.

hooks, bell. 1984. *Feminist Theory: From Margin to Center.* Boston: South End Press.

———. 1989. *Talking Back: Thinking Feminist, Thinking Black.* Boston: South End Press.

Hooks, Benjamin. 1989. "Editor's Comments." In *the Crisis.* Washington, DC: National Urban League, 3.

Ignatiev, Noel. 1995. *How the Irish Became White.* New York: Routledge.

Index to Black Newspapers. 1981–1993. Woster, OH: Indexing Center, UMI.

Index to Black Periodicals. 1981–1993. Boston: G. K. Hall.

Iyengar, Shanto. 1991. *Is Anyone Responsible? How Television Frames Political Issues.* Chicago: University of Chicago Press.

Iyengar, Shanto, and Donald R. Kinder. 1987. *News That Matters.* Chicago: University of Chicago Press.

Jaimes, M. Annette, ed. 1992. *The State of Native America: Genocide, Colonization, and Resistance.* Boston: South End Press.

James, Joy. 1997. *Transcending the Talented Tenth: Race Leaders and American Intellectualism.* New York: Routledge.

Jay, Karla, and Allen Young, eds. 1992. *Out of the Closets: Voices of Gay Liberation,* twentieth anniversary edition. New York: New York University Press.

Jaynes, Gerald D., and Robin M. Williams, Jr., eds. 1989. *A Common Destiny: Blacks and American Society.* Washington, DC: National Academy Press.

Jenkins, Joseph Craig. 1981. "Sociopolitical Movements." In *Handbook of Political Behavior,* edited by S. Long. New York: Plenum Press.

Jenkins, Joseph Craig, and Charles Perrow. 1977. "Insurgency of the Powerless: Farm Worker Movements (1946–1972)." *American Sociological Review* 42, no. 2: 249–68.

Joint Center for Political Studies. 1993. *National Roster of Black Elected Officials.* Washington, DC: Joint Center for Political Studies.

Jones, Bryan D., ed. 1989. *Leadership and Politics: New Perspectives in Political Science.* Lawrence: University Press of Kansas.

Jones, James H. 1981. *Bad Blood: The Tuskegee Syphilis Experiment: A Tragedy of Race and Medicine.* New York: Free Press.

Jones, Mack. 1978. "Black Political Empowerment in Atlanta: Myth and Reality." In *Annals of the American Academy of Political and Social Science,* edited by J. R. Howard and R. C. Smith, vol. 439 (September): 90–117.

Jordan, Winthrop D. 1968. *White over Black: American Attitudes toward the Negro, 1550–1812.* Chapel Hill: University of North Carolina Press.

Joseph, Stephen C. 1992. *Dragon within the Gates: The Once and Future AIDS Epidemic.* New York: Carroll & Graf.

Kaiser Family Foundation. 1998. *National Summary of African Americans don HIV/AIDS: Summary of Findings/Toplines.* Menlo Park, CA: Henry J. Kaiser Family Foundation.

Karnig, Albert K., and Susan Welch. 1980. *Black Representation and Urban Policy.* Chicago: University of Chicago Press.

Katz, Jonathan Ned. 1992. *An American History: Lesbian and Gay Men in the U.S.A.* Rev. ed. New York: Meridian.

Katzman, David M. 1973. *Before the Ghetto: Black Detroit in the Nineteenth Century.* Urbana: University of Illinois Press.

Katznelson, Ira. 1981. *City Trenches: Urban Politics and the Patterning of Class in the United States*. Chicago: University of Chicago Press.

Kelley, Robin D. G. 1990. *Hammer and Hoe: Alabama Communists during the Great Depression*. Chapel Hill: University of North Carolina Press.

———. 1993. "Kickin' Reality, Kickin Ballistics: The Cultural Politics of Gangsta Rap in Postindustrial Los Angeles." In *Droppin' Science: Critical Essays on Rap and Hip Hop Culture*, edited by W. E. Perkins. Philadelphia: Temple University Press.

Kinder, Donald R. 1987. "Pluralistic Foundations of American Opinion on Race." Paper presented at the annual meeting of the American Political Science Association, Chicago, IL.

Kinder, Donald R., and Lynn M. Saunders. 1996. *Divided by Color: Racial Politics and Democratic Ideals*. Chicago: University of Chicago Press.

King, Deborah. 1988. "Multiple Jeopardy, Multiple Consciousness: The Context of a Black Feminist Ideology, " *Signs: Journal of Women in Culture and Society* 14, no.1 (August): 42–72.

Kingdon, John W. 1981. *Congressmen's Voting Decisions*. 2d ed. New York: Harper and Row.

———. 1984. *Agendas, Alternatives, and Public Policies*. New York: HarperCollins.

Kinsella, James. 1989. *Covering the Plague: AIDS and the American Media*. New Brunswick: Rutgers University Press.

Kirkwood, Cynthia. 1992. "The Black Church and AIDS." *Christianity and Crisis*, 21 September.

Koop, C. Everett. 1991. *Koop: The Memoirs of America's Family Doctor*. New York: Random House.

Kramer, Larry. 1989. *Reports from the Holocaust: the Making of an AIDS Activist*. New York: St. Martin's Press.

Kropi, Walter. 1974. "Conflict, Power and Relative Deprivation." *American Political Science Review* 68: 1571.

Landry, Bart. 1987. *The New Black Middle Class*. Berkeley: University of California Press.

Leffall, LaSalle D., Jr. 1990. "Health Status of Black Americans." In *State of Black America*, ed. Janet Dewart. New York: National Urban League, 121–42.

Leites, Nathan, and Charles Wolf, Jr. 1970. *Rebellion and Authority*. Chicago: Markham.

Leland, John. 1996. "the End of AIDS?" *Newsweek*, 2 December, 64.

Lenin, V. I. 1969. *What Is to Be Done? Burning Questions of our Movement*. New York: International Publishers.

Lester, Calu, and Larry L. Saxxon. 1988. "AIDS in the Black Community: The Plague, the Politics, the People." *Death Studies* 12: 563–71.

Lévi-Strauss, Claude. 1985. *The View from Afar*. Translated by J. Neugroschel and P. Hoss. New York: Basic Books.

Lincoln, C. Eric. 1973. *The Black Muslims in America*. Boston: Beacon Press.

———. 1997. "The Muslim Mission in the Context of American Social History." In *African-American Religion: Interpretive Essays in History and Culture*, ed. T. E. Fulop and A. J. Raboteau. New York: Routledge, 277–94.

Lincoln, C. Eric, and Lawrence H. Mamiya. 1990. *The Black Church in the African American Experience*. Durham, NC: Duke University Press.

Lindan, Christine P., Norman Hearst, James A. Singleton, Alan I. Trachtenberg, Noreen M. Riordan, Diane A. Tokagawa, and George S. Chu. 1990. "Underreporting of Minority AIDS Deaths in San Francisco Bay Area, 1985–86." *Public Health Reports* 105, no. 4 (July–August): 400–404.

Lipsitz, Lewis. 1970. "On Political Belief: The Grievances of the Poor." In *Power and Community: Dissenting Essays in Political Science*, edited by P. Green and S. Levison. New York: Random House, Vintage Books.

Lorde, Audre. 1982. *Zami: A New Spelling of My Name*. New York: Persephone Press.

Loury, Glenn. 1987. "Who Speaks for Black Americans?" *Commentary* 83 (January): 34–38.

Luker, Kristen. 1984. *Abortion and the Politics of Motherhood*. Berkeley: University of California Press.

Lukes, Steven. 1974. *Power: A Radical View*. London: Macmillan.

———. ed. 1986. *Power*. New York: New York University Press.

McAdam, Doug. 1982. *Political Process and the Development of Black Insurgency, 1930–1970*. Chicago: University of Chicago Press.

McBride, David. 1991. *From TB to AIDS: Epidemics among Urban Blacks since 1900*. Albany: State University of New York Press.

McCarthy, John D., and Mayer N. Zald. 1973. *The Trend of Social Movements in America: Professionalization and Resource Mobilization*. Morristown, NJ: General Learning Press.

———. 1977. "Resource Mobilization and Social Movements: A Partial Theory." *American Journal of Sociology* 82, no. 6: 1212–41.

McCombs, M. E., and D. Shaw. 1972. "The Agenda-Setting Function of the Mass Media." *Public Opinion Quarterly* 36: 176–87.

McNeil, William H. 1976. *Plagues and People*. Garden City: Doubleday, Anchor Press.

Manton, Kenneth G., Clifford H. Patrick, and Katrina W. Johnson. 1989. "Health Differentials between Blacks and Whites: Recent Trends in Mortality and Morbidity." In *Health Policies and Black Americans*, edited by D. P. Willis, 129–99.

Marable, Manning. 1983. *How Capitalism Underdeveloped Black America*. Boston: South End Press.

———. 1985. *Black American Politics: From the Washington Marches to Jesse Jackson*. London: Verso Press.

———. 1991. *Race, Reform, and Rebellion: The Second Reconstruction in Black America*. Jackson: University Press of Mississippi.

Marotta, Toby. 1981. *The Politics of Homosexuality*. Boston: Houghton Mifflin.

Martin, J. M., and E. P. Martin. 1985. *The Helping Tradition in the Black Family and Community*. Silver Springs, MD: National Association of Social Workers.

Martin, Louis E. 1984. "What Role for the Black Press?" *Africa Report*, May–June, 51–54.

Marx, Karl, and Frederick Engels. 1972. *Ireland and the Irish Question*. New York: International Publishers.

Massey, Douglas S., and Nancy Denton. 1993. *American Apartheid: Segregation and the Making of the Underclass*. Cambridge: Harvard University Press.

Matthews, Rev. C. Jay. 1993. "The Black Church Position Statement on Homosexuality." *The Call and Post*, 10 June, 5C.

Mayhew. David. R. 1966. *Party Loyalty among Congressmen: The Difference between Democrats and Republicans, 1947–1962*. Cambridge: Harvard University Press.

Mays, Benjamin, and Joseph Nicholson. 1969. *The Negro's Church*. New York: Russell and Russell.

Memmi, Albert. 1965. *The Colonizer and the Colonized*. Boston: Beacon Press.

Merelman, Richard M. 1968. "On the Neo-Elitist Critique of Community Power." *American Political Science Review* 62, 451–60.

Merron, Robert. 1957. *Social Theory and Social Structure*. New York: Free Press.

Miliband, Ralph. 1969. *The State in Capitalist Society: An Analysis of the Western Systems of Power*. London: Weidenfeld and Nicolson.

Miller, W. E. 1964. "Majority Rule and the Representative System of Government." In *Cleavages, Ideologies, and Party Systems*, edited by E. Allardt and Y. Littunen. Helsinki: Westmark Society.

Miller, Arthur H., Patricia Gurin, Gerald Gurin, and Oksana Malanchuk. 1981. "Group

Consciousness and Political Participation." *American Journal of Political Science* 25, no. 3 (August): 494–511.

Mills, C. Wright. 1956. *The Power Elite.* London: Oxford University Press.

Minow, Martha. 1990. *Making All the Difference: Inclusion, Exclusion, and American Law.* Ithaca, NY: Cornell University Press.

Mohr, Richard D. 1988. *Gays/Justice: A Study of Ethics, Society, and Law.* New York: Columbia University Press.

———. 1992. *Gay Ideas: Outing and Other Controversies.* Boston: Beacon Press.

Moore, Barrington, Jr. 1978. *InJustice: The Social Bases of Obedience and Revolt.* Armonk, New York: M. E. Sharpe.

Moore, Charles H., and Patricia Hoban-Moore. 1990. "Some Lessons from Reagan's HUD: Housing Policy and Public Service." *PS Political Science and Politics* 23 (March): 14.

Moraga, Cherrie, and Gloria Anzaldua eds. 1981. *This Bridge Called My Back: Writings by Radical Women of Color.* New York: Kitchen Table, Women of Color Press.

Morgan, Randall C., Jr. 1996. "HIV/AIDS in African Americans: Role of the National Medical Association in Diagnosis, Treatment, and Education." *Journal of the National Medical Association* 89, no. 1: 14–18.

Morris, Aldon D. 1984. *The Origins of the Civil Rights Movement: Black Communities Organizing for Change.* New York: Free Press.

Morris, Aldon D., and Carol McClurg Mueller, eds. 1992. *Frontiers in Social Movement Theory.* New Haven: Yale University Press.

Morris, Glenn T. 1992. "International Law and Politics: Toward a Right to Self-Determination for Indigenous Peoples." In *The State of Native America,* edited by M. Annette Jaimes. Boston: South End Press, 55–86.

Morrison, Toni, ed. 1992. *Race-ing Justice, En-gendering Power: Essays on Anita Hill, Clarence Thomas, and the Construction of Social Reality.* New York: Pantheon Books.

Munson, Danni. 1991. *The Gay and Lesbian Almanac and Events of 1991.* Chicago: Envoy.

Murray, Charles. 1984. *Losing Ground: American Social Policy, 1950–1980.* New York: Basic Books.

Myrdal, Gunner. 1944. *An American Dilemma.* New York: Harper and Row.

———. 1996. *An American Dilemma.* New Brunswick: Transaction Publishers.

Nagel, Jack H. 1975. *The Descriptive Analysis of Power.* New Haven: Yale University Press.

Nelkin, Dorthy, David P. Willis, and Scott V. Parris, eds. 1991. *A Disease of Society: Cultural and Institutional Responses to AIDS.* Cambridge: Cambridge University Press.

Nelson, William E. 1982. "Cleveland: The Rise and Fall of the New Black Politics." In *The New Black Politics: The Search for Political Power,* edited by M. B. Preston, L. J. Henderson, Jr., and P. Puryear. New York: Longman.

———. 1987. "Cleveland: The Evolution of Black Political Power." In *The New Black Politics: The Search for Political Power,* 2d ed., edited by M. B. Preston, L. J. Henderson, Jr., and P. Puryear. New York: Longman.

Nicholas, Lionel J., Colin Tredoux, and Priscilla Daniels. 1994. "AIDS Knowledge and Attitudes toward Homosexuals of Black First-Year University Students, 1990–1992." *Psychological Reports* 75, 819–23.

Nichols, Eve K. 1989. *Mobilizing against AIDS.* Cambridge: Harvard University Press.

Nussbaum, Bruce. 1990. *Good Intentions: How Big Business and the Medical Establishment are Corrupting the Fight against AIDS, Alzheimer's, Cancer and More.* New York: Penguin Books.

Oaks, Robert F. 1985. "Defining Sodomy in Seventeenth-Century Massachusetts." In *The Gay Past: A Collection of Historical Essays,* edited by S. J. Licata and R. P. Petersen. New York: Harrington Park Press, 79–84.

Oberschall, Anthony. 1973. *Social Conflict and Social Movements*. Englewood Cliffs, NJ: Prentice-Hall.

Office of Technology Assessment. 1985. *Review of the Public Health Service's Response to AIDS—A Technical Memorandum*. Washington, DC: Health Program, Office of Technology Assessment, United States Congress. (Distributor: Supt. of Docs., U.S.G.P.O.)

Olson, Mancur, Jr. 1965. *The Logic of Collective Action*. Cambridge: Harvard University Press.

Omolade, Barbara. 1994. *The Rising Song of African American Women*. New York: Routledge.

Omvedt, Gail. 1973. "Towards a Theory of Colonialism." *Insurgent Sociologist* (spring) 1–24.

Opp, Karl-Dieter. 1982. "The Evolution Emergence of Norms." *British Journal of Social Psychology* 21: 139–49.

Oppenheimer, Bruce I. 1985. "Legislative Influence on Policy and Budgets." In *Handbook of Legislative Research*, edited by S. C. Patterson and M. E. Jewell. Cambridge: Harvard University Press, 621–67.

Oppenheimer, Gerald M. 1988. "In the Eye of the Storm: The Epidemiological Construction of AIDS." In *AIDS: The Burdens of History*, edited by E. Fee and D. M. Fox. Berkeley: University of California Press.

———. 1992. "Causes, Cases, and Cohorts: The Role of Epidemiology in the Historical Construction of AIDS." In *AIDS: The Making of a Chronic Disease*, edited by E. Fee and D. M. Fox. Berkeley: University of California Press, 49–83.

Ostrow, David G., Rupert E. D. Whitaker, Kevin Frasier, Cathy Cohen, Jim Wan, Cathy Frank, and Evelyn Fisher. 1991. "Racial Differences in Social Support and Mental Health in Men with HIV Infection: A Pilot Study." *AIDS Care* 3, no. 1: 55–62.

Padug, Robert A., and Gerald M. Oppenheimer. 1992. "Riding the Tiger: AIDS and the Gay Community." In *AIDS: The Making of a Chronic Disease*, edited by E. Fee and D. M. Fox. Berkeley: University of California Press.

Page, Clarence. 1991. "Deathly Silence." *The New Republic*, 2 December, 15–18.

Page, Benjamin I., Robert Y. Shapiro, and Glenn R. Dempsey. 1987. "What Moves Public Opinion?" *American Political Science Review* 81: 23–44.

Panem, Sandra. 1985. "AIDS: Public Policy and Biomedical Research." *Hastings Center Report* 15, special supplement (August).

———. 1988. *The AIDS Bureaucracy*. Cambridge: Harvard University Press.

Parenti, Michael. 1970. "Power and Pluralism: A View from the Bottom." *Journal of Politics* 32: 501–30.

———. 1978. *Power and the Powerless*. New York: St. Martin's Press

Parks, Robert E. 1928. "Human Migration and the Marginal Man." *American Journal of Sociology* 32, no. 6: 892.

Parsons, Talcott. 1957. "The Distribution of Power in American Society." *World Politics* 10, 123–43.

———. 1963. "On the Concept of Influence." *Public Opinion* 27: 37–62.

———. 1967. *Sociology Theory and Modern Society*. New York: Free Press.

Patton, Cindy. 1985. *Sex and Germs: The Politics of AIDS*. Boston: South End Press

———. 1990. *Inventing AIDS*. New York: Routledge.

Perlman, Janice E. 1976. *The Myth of Marginality: Urban Poverty and Politics in Rio de Janeiro*. Berkeley: University of California Press.

Perrow, Charles, and Mauro F. Guillén. 1990. *The AIDS Disaster: The Failure of Organizations in New York and the Nation*. New Haven: Yale University Press.

Perry, Huey L. 1995. "A Theoretical Analysis of National Black Politics in the United States." In *Blacks and the American Political System*, edited by H. L. Perry and W. Parent. Gainesville: University Press of Florida, 11–37.

Perry, Huey L., Tracey L. Ambeau, and Frederick McBride. 1995. "Blacks and the National Executive Branch." In *Blacks and the American Political System,* edited by H. L. Perry and W. Parent. Gainesville: University Press of Florida, 105–29.

Peterson, Paul. 1981. *City Limits.* Chicago: University of Chicago Press.

Phelan, Shane. 1989. *Identity Politics: Lesbian Feminism and the Limits of Community.* Philadelphia: Temple University Press.

Pinderhughes, Dianne M. 1983. "Collective Goods and Black Interest Groups." *Review of Black Political Economy* 12 (winter): 219–36.

———. 1987. *Race and Ethnicity in Chicago Politics.* Champaign: University of Illinois Press.

———. 1995. "Black Interest Groups and the 1982 Extension of the Voting Rights Act." In *Blacks and the American Political System,* edited by W. L. Perry and W. Parent. Gainesville: University Press of Florida, 203–24.

Piven, Frances Fox, and Richard A. Cloward. 1979. *Poor People's Movements.* New York: Vintage Books.

Pocock, J. G. A. 1970. "Ritual, Language and Power." In *Politics, Language, and Time: Essays on Political Thought and History,* edited by J. G. A. Pocock. London: Methuen.

Polsby, Nelson W. 1959. "The Sociology of Community Power: A Reassessment." *Social Forces* 37: 235.

———. 1963. *Community Power and Political Theory.* New Haven: Yale University Press.

———. 1968. "Community: The Study of Community Power." In *International Encyclopedia of the Social Sciences,* vol. 3, 157–63.

Poulantzas, Nicos. 1973. *Political Power and Social Classes.* Translated and edited by T. O'Hagan. London: N. L. B., and Sheed and Ward.

Preston, Michael B. 1982. "Black Politics and Public Policy in Chicago: Self-Interest Versus Constituent Representation." In *The New Black Politics: The Search for Political Power,* by M. B. Preston, L. J. Henderson, Jr., P. Puryear. Pp. 159–86.

Prewitt, Kenneth, and Alan Stone. 1973. *The Ruling Elites.* New York: Harper and Row.

Price, David E. 1972. *Who Makes the Laws?* Cambridge: Schenkman.

Primm, Beny J. 1987. "AIDS: A Special Report." In *State of Black America.* New York: National Urban League, 159–66.

Quimby, Ernest, and Samuel R. Friedman. 1989. "Dynamics of Black Mobilization Against AIDS in New York City." *Social Problems* 36, no. 4 (October): 403–15.

Rae, Douglas W. 1988. "Knowing Power: A Working Paper." In *Power, Inequality, and Democratic Politics,* edited by I. Shapiro and G. Reeher. Boulder: Westview Press.

Reed, Adolph L., Jr. 1986. *The Jesse Jackson Phenomenon.* New Haven: Yale University Press.

———. 1988. "The Black Urban Regime: Structural Origins and Constraints." *Comparative Urban and Community Research* 1: 138–89.

———. 1991. "The 'Underclass' as Myth and Symbol: The Poverty of Discourse about Poverty." *Radical America* 24, no. 1 (January): 21–40.

———. 1994. "Sources of Demobilization in the New Black Political Regime: Incorporation, Ideological Capitulation, and Radical Failure in the Post-Segregation Era." Unpublished paper.

Reich, Michael. 1971. "The Economics of Racism." In *Problems in Political Economy,* edited by D. M. Gordon. Lexington, MA: D. C. Heath.

———. 1991. *Toxic Politics: Responding to Chemical Disasters.* Ithaca, NY: Cornell University Press.

Rieselbach, Leroy N. 1990. "Institutional Factors, Legislative Behavior, and Congressional Policymaking: Developments in the 1980s." In *Annual Review of Political Science,* vol. 3, edited by S. Long. Norwood, NJ: Ablex, 60–197.

Rifkin, Jeremy. 1995. *The End of Work: The Decline of the Global Labor Force and the Dawn of the Post-Market Era*. New York: G. P. Putnam's Sons.

Roediger, David R. 1991. *The Wages of Whiteness: Race and the Making of the American Working Class*. London: Verso.

Rogers, Everett M., and James W. Dearing. 1988. "Agenda-Setting Research: Where Has It Been and Where Is It Going?" In *Communication Yearbook*, vol. 11, edited by J. A. Anderson. Beverly Hills: Sage.

Rose, Tricia. 1992. "Black Noise: Rap Music and Black Cultural Resistance in Contemporary American Popular Culture." Ph.D. diss., Brown University).

———. 1992. "Black Texts/Black Contexts." In *Black Popular Culture*, edited by G. Dent. Seattle: Bay Press.

Rosenstone, Steven J., and John Mark Hanson. 1993. *Mobilization, Participation, and Democracy in America*. New York: Macmillan.

Rubin, Roger H., Andrew Billingsley, and Cleopatra Howard Caldwell. 1994. "The Role of the Black Church in Working with Black Adolescents." *Adolescence* 29, no. 114 (summer): 251–66.

Sabatier, Renee. 1988. *Blaming Others: Prejudice, Race, and Worldwide AIDS*. Washington, DC: The Panos Institute.

Sarte, Jean-Paul. 1948. *Anti-Semite and Jew*. Translated by George J. Becker. New York: Schocken Books.

Savitt, Todd L. 1978. *Medicine and Slavery: The Diseases and Health Care of Blacks in Antebellum Virginia*. Urbana: University of Illinois Press.

Schattschneider, E. E. 1960. *The Semi-Sovereign People: A Realist's View of Democracy in America*. New York: Holt, Rinehart & Winston.

Schuman, Howard, Charlotte Steeh, and Lawrence Bobo. 1985. *Racial Attitudes in America: Trends and Interpretations*. Cambridge: Harvard University Press.

Scott, James C. 1985. *Weapons of the Weak: Everyday Forms of Peasant Resistance*. New Haven: Yale University Press.

———. 1990. *Domination and the Arts of Resistance: Hidden Transcripts*. New Haven: Yale University Press.

Sears, David. 1988. "Symbolic Racism." In *Eliminating Racism*, edited by P. Katz and D. Taylor. New York: Plenum Press, 53–84.

Sears, Stephanie. 1997. "The Woman Question and a Race Problem: Black Women's Support of the Million Man March." Unpublished ms., Yale University.

Sedgwick, Eve Kosofsky. 1990. *Epistemology of the Closet*. Berkeley: University of California Press.

Seidman, Steven. 1993. "Identity and Politics in a 'Postmodern' Gay Culture: Some Historical and Conceptual Notes." In *Fear of a Queer Planet: Queer Politics and Social Theory*, edited by M. Warner. Minneapolis: University of Minnesota Press, 105–42.

Sherrill, Kenneth S. 1991. "Half Empty: Gay Power and Gay Powerlessness in American Politics." Paper presented at the Annual Meeting of the American Political Science Association, Washington, DC, August 1991.

Shilts, Randy. 1987. *And the Band Played On: Politics, People, and the AIDS Epidemic*. New York: Penguin Books.

Shingles, Richard D. 1981. "Black Consciousness and Political Participation: The Missing Link." *American Political Science Review* 75: 76–91.

Shorter, Edward, and Charles Tilly. 1974. *Strikes in France, 1830–1968*. London: Cambridge University Press.

Signorile, Michelangelo. 1992. "Out at the *New York Times*." *The Advocate*, 5 May.

Sinclair, Barbara. 1982. *Congressional Realignment*. Austin: University of Texas Press.

———. 1994. "House Special Rules and the Institutional Design Controversy." *Legislative Studies Quarterly* 19, no. 4 (November): 477–94.

Singer, Eleanor. 1989. "Trends in Public Opinion about AIDS." Paper prepared for delivery to medical center's AIDS Seminar, University of Michigan, 25 July.

Singer, Eleanor, Theresa F. Rogers, and Mary Corcoran. 1987. "The Polls—A Report: AIDS." *Public Opinion Quarterly* 51, 580–95.

Sirgo, Henry B. 1995. "Blacks and Presidential Politics." In *Blacks and the American Political System*, edited by H. L. Perry and W. Parent. Gainesville: University Press of Florida, 75–104.

Skocpol, Theda. 1984. *Vision and Method in Historical Sociology.* Cambridge: Cambridge University Press.

Smith, Barbara, ed. 1983. *A Black Feminist Anthology.* Albany, NY: Kitchen Table, Women of Color Press.

Smith, Robert. 1981. "Black Power and the Transformation from Protest to Politics." *Political Science Quarterly* 96 (fall): 431–43.

Smith, Rogers. 1997. *Civic Ideals: Conflicting Visions of Citizenship in U.S. History.* New Haven: Yale University Press.

Sniderman, Paul M., and Michael G. Hagen. 1985. *Race and Inequality: A Study in American Values.* Chatham, NJ: Chatham House.

Sontag, Susan. 1989. *AIDS and Its Metaphors.* New York: Farrar, Straus, and Giroux.

Sowell, Thomas. 1984. *Civil Rights: Rhetoric or Reality?* New York: Quill.

Stack, Carol B. 1975. *All Our Kin: Strategies for Survival in a Black Community.* New York: Harper and Row.

Staples, Robert. 1976. "Race and Colonialism: The Domestic Case in Theory and Practice." *Black Scholar* (June): 37–48.

Stevens, Jacqueline. 1997. "On the Marriage Question." In *Women Transforming Politics: An Alternative Reader,* edited by C. J. Cohen, K. B. Jones, and J. C. Tronto. New York: New York University Press, 62–83.

Stevens, Arthur G., Jr., Daniel P. Mulhollan, and Paul S. Rundquist. 1981. "U.S. Congressional Structure and Representation: The Role of Informal Groups." *Legislative Studies Quarterly* 6, no. 3 (August): 415–37.

Stevenson, Howard C., and Gwendolyn Davis. 1994. "Impact of Culturally Sensitive AIDS Video Education on the AIDS Risk Knowledge of African-American Adolescents." *AIDS Education and Prevention* 6, no. 1, 40–52.

Stolberg, Sheryl Gay. 1998. "Eyes Shut, but America Is Being Ravaged by AIDS." *New York Times,* 29 June, A1.

Stone, Clarence N. 1987. "The Study of the Politics of Urban Development." In *The Politics of Urban Development,* edited by C. N. Stone and H. T. Sanders. Lawrence: University Press of Kansas.

———. 1990. "Transactional and Transforming Leadership: A Re-examination." A paper prepared for the Annual Meeting of the American Political Science Association, San Francisco, CA.

Stoneburner, Rand L., Mary Ann Chiasson, Isaac B. Weisfuse, and Pauline A. Thomas. 1990. "Editorial Review: The Epidemic of AIDS and HIV-1 Infection among Heterosexuals in New York City." *AIDS* 4: 99–106.

Stonequist, Everett V. 1935. "The Problem of the Marginal Man." *American Journal of Sociology* 41, no. 4 (July): 1–12.

———. 1937. *The Marginal Man: A Study in Personality and Culture Conflict.* New York: Russell and Russell.

Sullivan, Andrew. 1990. "Gay Life, Gay Death: the Siege of a Subculture." *The New Republic,* 17 December.

———. 1996. "When Plagues End." *New York Times,* 10 November, section 6, 52.

Sullivan, Gerard. 1985. "A Bibliographic Guide to Government Hearings and Reports,

Legislative Action, and Speeches Made in the House and Senate of the United States Congress on the Subject of Homosexuality." In *Bashers, Baiters, and Bigots: Homophobia in American Society,* edited by J. De Cecco. New York: Harrington Park Press, 135–90.

Swain, Carol M. 1993. *Black Faces, Black Interests: The Representation of African Americans in Congress.* Cambridge: Harvard University Press.

Tarrow, Sidney. 1989. *Democracy and Disorder: Protest and Politics in Italy, 1965–1975.* Oxford: Oxford University Press.

Tate, Greg. 1992. *Flyboy in the Buttermilk: Essays on Contemporary America.* New York: Simon & Schuster.

Tate, Katherine. 1993. *From Protest to Politics: The New Black Voters in American Elections.* Cambridge: Harvard University Press.

Taylor, Paul. 1929. *Mexican Labor in the United States: Valley of the South Platte, Colorado.* Berkeley: University of California Publications in Economics, vol. 6, no. 2.

Thomas, Rosita M. 1989. "American Public Opinion on AIDS." Report prepared by the Congressional Research Service. Government Division Report no. 89–85.

Thomas, Stephen B., and Sandra Crouse Quinn. 1993. "The Tuskegee Syphilis Study, 1932–1972: Implications for HIV Education and AIDS Risk Education Programs in the Black Community." *American Journal of Public Health* 81, no. 11 (November): 1498–1505.

Thomas, Stephen B., Sandra Crouse Quinn, Andrew Billingsley, and Cleopatra Caldwell. 1994. "The Characteristics of Northern Black Churches with Community Health Outreach Programs." *American Journal of Public Health* 84, no. 4: 575–79.

Thompson, John B. 1990. *Ideology and Modern Culture: Critical Social Theory in the Era of Mass Communication.* Stanford: Stanford University Press.

Tilly, Charles. 1978. *From Mobilization to Revolution.* Reading, MA: Addison-Wesley.

Tilly, Charles, Louise Tilly, and Richard Tilly. 1975. *The Rebellious Century, 1830–1930.* Cambridge: Harvard University Press.

Tokaji, Daniel. 1994. "The Politics of Fear: Attempts to Legislate Against Gays and Lesbians." Unpublished paper.

Treichler, Paula A. 1988. "AIDS, Gender, and Biomedical Discourse: Current Contests for Meaning." In *AIDS, the Burdens of History,* edited by E. Fee and D. M. Fox. Berkeley: University of California Press.

Troop, David. 1992. *Rap Attack 2.* Boston: South End Press.

Truman, David B. 1958. *The Governmental Process.* New York: Alfred A. Knopf.

Tryman, Mfanya Donald. 1995. "Jesse Jackson's Campaigns for the Presidency: A Comparison of the 1984 and the 1988 Democratic Primaries." In *Blacks and the American Political System,* edited by W. L. Perry and W. Parent. Gainesville: University Press of Florida, 50–72.

Turner, John C. 1987. *Rediscovering the Social Group: A Self-Categorization Theory.* New York: Basil Blackwell.

Ulack, Richard, and William F. Skinner, eds. 1991. *AIDS and the Social Sciences: Common Threads.* Lexington, KY: University Press of Kentucky.

United States Department of Commerce. 1990. *1990 Census of Population, General Population Characteristics: United States* (1990CP-1-1). Washington, DC: U.S. Department of Commerce, Bureau of the Census, Data User Services Division.

———. 1990. *1990 Census of Population, General Population Characteristics: New York,* section 1 of 2, (1990CP-1-34). Washington, DC: U.S. Department of Commerce, Bureau of the Census, Data User Services Division.

United States House. 1987a. Select Committee on Narcotics Abuse and Control. *Pediatric AIDS Hearing.* 100th Congress, 1st session. 27 July.

———. Subcommittee of the Committee on Government Operations. 1987b. *The AIDS Crisis in Two American Cities.* 100th Congress, 1st session. 18 September.

————. 1987c. Select Committee on Narcotics Abuse and Control. *Intravenous Drug Use and AIDS: The Impact on the Black Community.* 100th Congress, 1st session. 25 September.

————. 1987d. Subcommittee of the Committee on Government Operations. *The AIDS Crisis in Two American Cities.* 100th Congress, 1st session. 23 November.

————. 1989. Human Resources and Intergovernmental Relations Subcommittee of the Committee on Government Operations. *The AIDS Epidemic in Newark and Detroit.* 101st Congress, 1st session. 27 March.

————. 1992. Subcommittee on Select Education. *Hearing on Babies without Homes: Babies Abandoned at Birth.* 102nd Congress, 2nd session. 28 May.

Urry, John, and John Wakeford, eds. 1973. *Power in Britain: Sociological Readings.* London: Heinemann Educational Books.

Vaid, Urvashi. 1995. *Virtual Equality: The Mainstreaming of Gay and Lesbian Liberation.* New York: Anchor Books.

Waldinger, Roger. 1996. *Still the Promised City? African-Americans and New Immigrants in Postindustrial New York.* Cambridge: Harvard University Press.

Walker, Gail. 1992. "'Oh Freedom': Liberation and the African-American Church." *Guardian,* 26 February.

Walker, Jack L., Jr. 1991. *Mobilizing Interest Groups in America.* Ann Arbor: University of Michigan Press.

Wallace, Deborah, and Rodrick Wallace. 1990. "The Burning Down of New York City: Its Causes and Its Impacts." Paper prepared by the Public Interest Scientific Consulting Service, 256–72.

Walton, Hanes Jr. 1972. *Black Politics: A Theoretical and Structural Analysis.* Philadelphia: J. B. Lippincott.

Washington, Booker T. 1995. *Up From Slavery.* Edited by W. L. Andrews. Oxford: Oxford University Press.

Waters, Mary. 1990. *Ethnic Options: Choosing Identities in America.* Berkeley: University of California Press.

Watney, Simon. 1989. *Policing Desire: Pornography, AIDS, and the Media.* Minneapolis: University of Minnesota Press.

Weber, Max. 1968. *Economy and Society.* Edited by G. Roth. New York: Bedminster.

Weeks, Jeffrey. 1991. *Against Nature: Essays on History, Sexuality, and Identity.* Concord, MA: Paul and Co.

Weinbaum, Eve. 1997. "Successful Failures: Local Democracy in a Global Economy." Ph.D. diss. Yale University.

West, Cornel. 1990. "The New Cultural Politics of Difference." In *Out There: Marginalization and Contemporary Cultures,* edited by R. Ferguson, M. Gever, T. T. Minh-ha, and C. West. Cambridge: MIT Press, 19–36.

————. 1993. *Race Matters.* New York: Beacon Press.

West, Hollie I. 1990. "Down from the Clouds: Black Churches Battle Earthly Problems." *Emerge* (May).

Weston, Guy. 1986. "AIDS in the Black Community." *BLACK/OUT: The Magazine of the National Coalition of Black Lesbians and Gays* 1, no. 2 (fall): 12–15.

White, D. M. 1972. "The Problems of Power." *British Journal of Political Science* 2: 479–90.

White, Evelyn C., ed. 1990. *The Black Women's Health Book: Speaking for Ourselves.* Washington: Seal Press.

Williams, E. 1982. "Black Political Progress in the 1970s: The Electoral Arena." In *The New Black Politics,* edited by M. B. Preston, L. J. Henderson, Jr., and P. L. Puryear. New York: Longman, 73–108.

Williams, Linda. 1987. "Black Political Progress in the 1980s: the Electoral Arena." In *The*

New Black Politics, 2d ed., edited by M. B. Preston, L. J. Henderson, Jr., and P. L. Puryear. New York: Longman, 97–135.

Williams, Sherley Anne. 1992. "Two Words on Music: Black Community." In *Black Popular Culture*, edited by G. Dent. Seattle: Bay Press, 164–72.

Williams, Walter. 1982. *The State against Blacks*. New York: New Press.

Willie, Charles V. 1975. "Marginality and Social Change." *Society* 12, no. 5, 10–13.

Wilson, James Q. 1960. *Negro Politics*. New York: Free Press.

Wilson, William Julius. 1980. *The Declining Significance of Race: Blacks and Changing American Institutions*, 2d ed. Chicago: University of Chicago Press.

———. 1987. *The Truly Disadvantaged: The Inner City, the Underclass, and Public Policy*. Chicago: University of Chicago Press.

Wolf, Michelle A., and Alfred P. Kielwasser, eds. 1991. *Gay People, Sex, and the Media*. New York: Harrington Park Press.

Wolfe, Maxine. 1990. "AIDS and Politics: Transformation of Our Movement." In *Women, AIDS, and Activism*, edited by ACT UP/NY Women and AIDS Book Group. Boston: South End Press, 233–37.

Wolfinger, Raymond E. 1971. "Nondecisions and the Study of Local Politics." *American Political Science Review* 65: 1063–80.

———. 1974. *The Politics of Progress*. Englewood Cliffs, NJ: Prentice-Hall.

Wolseley, Roland E. 1990. *The Black Press, U.S.A.*, 2d ed. Ames: Iowa State University Press.

Woodward, C. Vann. 1974. *The Strange Career of Jim Crow*. Oxford: Oxford University Press.

Wright, Erik Olin. 1976. "Class Boundaries in Advanced Capitalism." *New Left Review* 98 (July/August): 3–42.

Young, Iris Marion. 1990. *Justice and the Politics of Difference*. Princeton, NJ: Princeton University Press.

Zald, Mayer, and John McCarthy. 1987. "Resource Mobilization and Social Movements: A Partial Theory." In *Social Movements in an Organizational Society*, edited by M. Zald and J. McCarthy. New Brunswick: Transaction Publishers, 15–42.

Zaller, John. 1992. *The Nature and Origins of Mass Opinion*. Cambridge: Cambridge University Press.

Zinn, Maxine Baca, and Bonnie Thorton Dill, eds. 1994. *Women of Color in U.S. Society*. Philadelphia: Temple University Press.

Index